AF847828

This report contains the collective views of an international group of experts and does not necessarily represent the decisions or the stated policy of the United Nations Environment Programme, the International Labour Organisation, or the World Health Organization.

Environmental Health Criteria 88

544216

POLYCHLORINATED DIBENZO-*PARA*-DIOXINS AND DIBENZOFURANS

Published under the joint sponsorship of
the United Nations Environment Programme,
the International Labour Organisation,
and the World Health Organization

World Health Organization
Geneva, 1989

The **International Programme on Chemical Safety (IPCS)** is a joint venture of the United Nations Environment Programme, the International Labour Organisation, and the World Health Organization. The main objective of the IPCS is to carry out and disseminate evaluations of the effects of chemicals on human health and the quality of the environment. Supporting activities include the development of epidemiological, experimental laboratory, and risk-assessment methods that could produce internationally comparable results, and the development of manpower in the field of toxicology. Other activities carried out by the IPCS include the development of know-how for coping with chemical accidents, coordination of laboratory testing and epidemiological studies, and promotion of research on the mechanisms of the biological action of chemicals.

WHO Library Cataloguing in Publication Data

Polychlorinated dibenzo-*para*-dioxins and dibenzofurans.

(Environmental health criteria ; 88)

1. Dioxins 2. Benzofurans I.Series

ISBN 92 4 154288 8 (NLM Classification: QV 633)
ISSN 0250-863X

© World Health Organization 1989

Publications of the World Health Organization enjoy copyright protection in accordance with the provisions of Protocol 2 of the Universal Copyright Convention. For rights of reproduction or translation of WHO publications, in part or *in toto*, application should be made to the Office of Publications, World Health Organization, Geneva, Switzerland. The World Health Organization welcomes such applications.

The designations employed and the presentation of the material in this publication do not imply the expression of any opinion whatsoever on the part of the Secretariat of the World Health Organization concerning the legal status of any country, territory, city, or area or of its authorities, or concerning the delimitation of its frontiers or boundaries.

The mention of specific companies or of certain manufacturers' products does not imply that they are endorsed or recommended by the World Health Organization in preference to others of a similar nature that are not mentioned. Errors and omissions excepted, the names of proprietary products are distinguished by initial capital letters.

Printed in Finland

89/8268 — Vammala — 5000

CONTENTS

Page

Page

Page

Page

Page

WHO TASK GROUP ON CHLORINATED DIBENZO-*p*-DIOXINS AND DIBENZOFURANS

Members

Dr U.G. Ahlborg, Unit of Toxicology, National Institute of Environmental Medicine, Stockholm, Sweden
Dr J.S. Bellin, Office of Toxic Substances, US Environmental Protection Agency, Washington, DC, USA
Dr B. Birmingham, Ministry of the Environment, Hazardous Contaminants Section, Toronto, Ontario, Canada
Professor A.D. Dayan, Department of Health and Social Security, St Bartholomew's Hospital Medical College, London, United Kingdom (Chairman)
Dr A. di Domenica, Instituto Superiore di Sanita, Rome, Italy
Dr M. Greenberg, Department of Health and Social Security, Division of Toxicology and Environmental Protection, London, United Kingdom
Dr R.D. Kimbrough, United States Department of Health and Human Services, Center for Disease Control, Atlanta, Georgia, USA (Now at the US Environmental Protection Agency Washington, DC, USA)
Dr R. Koch, Department of Toxicology, Institute of Hygiene, Gera, DDR
Professor C. Rappe, Department of Chemistry, University of Umea, Umea, Sweden
Dr S. Safe, Texas A and M University, College Station, Texas, USA
Dr H. Spielmann, Max von Pettenkofer Institute, Bundesgesundheitsamt, Berlin (West)
Dr J. Vos, National Institute of Public Health and Environmental Hygiene, Bilthoven, Netherlands

Representatives

Dr A. Berlin, Health and Safety Directorate, Commission of the European Communities, Luxembourg
Mrs E. Cox, Department of the Environment, London, United Kingdom
Miss F.D. Pollitt, Department of the Environment, London, United Kingdom

Secretariat

Dr G.C. Becking, International Programme on Chemical Safety, World Health Organization, Research Triangle Park, North Carolina, USA (Secretary)

Secretariat (contd)

Dr H. Hakensson, Unit of Toxicology, National Institute of Environmental Medicine, Stockholm, Sweden (Temporary Adviser) (Rapporteur)
Dr E. Johnson, International Agency for Research on Cancer, World Health Organization, Lyons, France
Dr S. Tarkowski, Regional Office for Europe, World Health Organization, Copenhagen, Denmark

NOTE TO READERS OF THE CRITERIA DOCUMENTS

Every effort has been made to present information in the criteria documents as accurately as possible without unduly delaying their publication. In the interest of all users of the environmental health criteria documents, readers are kindly requested to communicate any errors that may have occurred to the Manager of the International Programme on Chemical Safety, World Health Organization, Geneva, Switzerland, in order that they may be included in corrigenda, which will appear in subsequent volumes.

* * *

A detailed data profile and a legal file can be obtained from the International Register of Potentially Toxic Chemicals, Palais des Nations, 1211 Geneva 10, Switzerland (Telephone No. 7988400 - 7985850).

ENVIRONMENTAL HEALTH CRITERIA FOR POLYCHLORINATED DIBENZO-PARA-DIOXINS AND DIBENZOFURANS

A WHO Task Group on Environmental Health Criteria for Polychlorinated Dibenzo-*para*-dioxins and Dibenzofurans met at the Monitoring and Assessment Research Centre, London, United Kingdom, from 9 to 13 February, 1987. Dr M. Berlin opened the meeting and welcomed the members on behalf of the host Institute and on behalf of the United Kingdom Department of Health and Social Security, who sponsored the meeting. Dr G.C. Becking addressed the meeting on behalf of the three cooperating organizations of the IPCS (UNEP, ILO, and WHO). The Task Group reviewed and revised the draft criteria document and made an evaluation of the risks for human health and for the environment from exposure to polychlorinated dibenzo-*p*-dioxins and dibenzofurans.

The drafts of this document were prepared by Dr U.G. Ahlborg, Dr H. Hakensson, and Dr B. Holmstedt, all of the National Institute of Environmental Medicine, Stockholm, Sweden, and by Professor C. Rappe of the University of Umea, Umea, Sweden.

The efforts of all who helped in the preparation and finalization of the document are gratefully acknowledged.

* * *

Partial financial support for the publication of this criteria document was kindly provided by the United States Department of Health and Human Services, through a contract from the National Institute of Environmental Health Sciences, Research Triangle Park, North Carolina, USA - a WHO Collaborating Centre for Environmental Health Effects. The United Kingdom Department of Health and Social Security generously supported the cost of printing.

ABBREVIATIONS

AHH	aryl hydrocarbon hydroxylase
ALA	aminolevulinic acid
BGG	bovine gammaglobulin
BHA	butylated hydroxyanisole
BP	benzo(a)-pyrene
CMI	cell-mediated immunity
DEN	diethylnitrosamine
diCDD	dichlorinated dibenzo-*p*-dioxin
diCDF	dichlorinated dibenzofuran
DMBA	dimethylbenzathraline
ECOD	7-ethoxycoumarin-*o*-deethylase
EGF	epidermal growth factor
EH	epoxide hydratase
EI	electron impact
EROD	7-ethoxyresurofin-*o*-deethylase
ETG	epidermal transglutaminase
fg	femtogram (10^{-15}g)
GC	gas chromatography
heptaCDD	heptachlorinated dibenzo-*p*-dioxin
heptaCDF	heptachlorinated dibenzofuran
hexaCDD	hexachlorinated dibenzo-*p*-dioxin
hexaCDF	hexachlorinated dibenzofuran
HMI	humoral-mediated immunity
HPLC	high pressure liquid chromatography
IARC	International Agency for Research on Cancer
ip	intraperitoneal
IR	infrared
LOEL	lowest-observed-effect level
MCPA	4-chloro-*o*-tolyloxyacetic acid
MFO	mixed-function oxidase
MS	mass spectrometry
MSW	municipal solid waste
ng	nanogram (10^{-9}g)
NMR	nuclear magnetic resonance
NOEL	no-observed-effect level
octaCDD	octachlorinated dibenzo-*p*-dioxin
octaCDF	octachlorinated dibenzofuran
PAH	polyaromatic hydrocarbons
PCB	polychlorinated biphenyl
PCDD	polychlorinated dibenzo-*p*-dioxin
PCDF	polychlorinated dibenzofuran
PCDPE	polychlorinated diphenylether
PCPY	polychlorinated pyrene
PCQ	polychlorinated quaterphenyl
pentaCDD	pentachlorinated dibenzo-*p*-dioxin
pentaCDF	pentachlorinated dibenzofuran

pg	picogram (10^{-12}g)
SC	subcutaneous
SCE	sister chromatid exchange
SD	standard deviation
SEM	standard error of the mean
SIM	selected ion monitoring
TCDD	2,3,7,8-tetrachlorinated dibenzo-*p*-dioxin
TCDF	2,3,7,8-tetrachlorinated dibenzofuran
TCP	trichlorophenol
tetraCDD	tetrachlorinated dibenzofuran
tetraCDF	tetrachlorinated dibenzofuran
TPA	12-*o*-tetradecanoylphorbol-13-acetate
triCDD	trichlorinated dibenzo-*p*-dioxin
triCDF	trichlorinated dibenzofuran
t_3	triiodothyronine
t_4	thyroxine
UDPGT	UDP-glucuronosyltransferase
UV	ultraviolet
2,4-D	2,4-dichlorophenoxyacetic acid
2,4,5-T	2,4,5-trichlorophenoxyacetic acid
3-MC	3-methylcholanthrene

1. SUMMARY AND RECOMMENDATIONS

1.1 Summary

1.1.1 Sources

Polychlorinated dibenzo-*p*-dioxins (PCDDs) and polychlorinated dibenzofurans (PCDFs) are two series of tricyclic aromatic compounds with similar chemical and physical properties; they are ubiquitous in the environment. They do not occur naturally, nor are they intentionally produced. There are 75 positional isomers of PCDDs and 135 isomers of PCDFs.

The most important sources of contamination with PCDDs and PCDFs include:

- contaminated commercial chemical products, such as chlorinated phenols and their derivatives, and PCBs;
- incineration of municipal, hazardous, and hospital wastes, and of sewage sludges;
- automobile operation;
- fossil fuel combustion;
- overheating and emissions from fires involving PCBs;
- disposal of industrial wastes resulting from processes such as the production of chlorophenols and their derivatives, chlorophenol wood treatment, use of PCB fluids in electrical equipment, and wastes from pulp and paper processing.

1.1.2 Ambient levels and routes of exposure

The limited data available indicate that ambient levels of these compounds are very low in air, soil, and sediment, i.e. fg/m^3 in air, ng/kg in soil and sediment. Levels of PCDDs and PCDFs up to 50 ng/kg have been found in aquatic organisms in the general environment. Data on contamination of drinking water and commercial food are very limited.

Exposure to these compounds in the general population probably occurs mainly through the food-chain.

Some workers engaged in the production, use, and destruction of materials containing PCDDs and PCDFs and their precursors may receive high exposure. For these persons, inhalation and dermal contact are the primary exposure routes of concern.

1.1.3 Toxicokinetics, biotransformation, and biological monitoring

The bioavailability of PCDDs and PCDFs depends on the matrix they are in and the route of exposure. Data on bioavailability through inhalation are not available for any species.

The quantity absorbed by humans after any route of exposure is not known.

Studies on rodents given single or repeated oral doses of 2,3,7,8-TCDD have shown that about half of the administered dose is absorbed from the gastrointestinal tract. The reported half-lives for elimination were between 12 and 94 days for rodents. The half-life of 2,3,7,8-TCDD in adipose tissue of the rhesus monkey is about 1 year.

Animal data on the toxicokinetics of PCDDs other than 2,3,7,8-TCDD are limited. The half-life for 2,3,7,8-TCDD has been reported to be in the range of 2 and 8 days for rats, mice, and monkeys and more than 20 days for guinea-pigs. Studies on rats have shown that 2,3,4,7,8-pentaCDF is more highly retained than is 2,3,7,8-TCDD.

Data on the retention of PCDDs and PCDFs in tissues of various species, exposed to synthetic mixtures or to environmental samples containing PCDDs and PCDFs, show a high variability in retention time between congeners with or without chlorine substitution in the 2,3,7, and 8 positions.

Limited human data indicate half-lives for some 2,3,7,8-substituted PCDDs and PCDFs in the range of 2-6 years.

The PCDDs and PCDFs are predominately stored in fat, but they are also excreted in milk and pass through the placenta. They also appear in the blood and vital organs at lower concentrations.

The tissue distribution in humans is not clear at present, although it has been suggested that the ratio between fatty tissue and liver is higher in humans than in rodents.

In human fat, background levels of TCDD up to 20 ng/kg have been found in the general population, with no known specific exposure, but higher levels have been reported in some cases without evidence of disease. None of these populations were randomly sampled. The more highly chlorinated PCDDs and PCDFs, particularly octaCDD, are also present in these samples. Average tissue levels of TCCD tend to increase with age.

1.1.4 Health effects

1.1.4.1 Animals

The toxic and biological effects resulting from exposure to 2,3,7,8-TCDD are dependent on a number of factors, which include the species, strain, age, and sex of the animals used. The toxic responses observed in several animal species include body weight loss, hepatotoxicity, porphyria, dermal toxicity, gastric lesions, thymus atrophy and immunotoxicity, teratogenicity, reproductive effects, and carcinogenicity. TCDD induces a wide spectrum of biological effects including enzyme induction and vitamin A depletion. Not all of these effects are observed in any single animal species. The most characteristic toxic effects observed in all laboratory animals are body weight loss, thymus atrophy, and immunotoxicity. Chloracne and related dermal lesions are the most frequently noted signs of 2,3,7,8-TCDD toxicosis in humans; dermal lesions are also observed in rhesus monkeys, hairless mice, and rabbits. In contrast, most rodents do not develop chloracne and related dermal toxic lesions after exposure to 2,3,7,8-TCDD. Many of the toxic lesions are noted primarily in epithelial tissues.

Reproductive effects have been reported in rhesus monkeys and rats. The lowest-observed-effect levels have been reported to be approximately 1-2 ng/kg body weight per day. In two cancer studies in rats, hepatocellular carcinomas were produced at approximate dose levels of 0.1 µg/kg body weight per day and 0.01 µg/kg body weight per day. Doses of 0.001 µg/kg body weight resulted in foci or areas of hepatocellular alteration. The incidence of certain hormone-dependent tumours was lower than in the control animals.

TCDD does not appear to have mutagenic properties, and is therefore not likely to be genotoxic. Thus, it is assumed to be carcinogenic through an indirect mechanism.

Several other PCDDs and PCDFs cause signs and symptoms similar to those of 2,3,7,8-TCDD, but there is a wide variation with regard to potency. There are 12 isomers that display higher toxicity, i.e., the tetra-, penta-, hexa-, and heptaCDDs and CDFs with four chlorine atoms in the symmetrical lateral positions 2,3,7, and 8. A mixture of two hexachlorodibenzo-p-dioxins (1,2,3,7,8,9- and 1,2,3,6,7,8-hexaCDD) has been demonstrated to possess carcinogenic properties in long-term animal studies, but at higher doses than those used in the study of TCDD. Dibenzo-p-dioxin and 2,7-diCDD failed to demonstrate carcinogenic properties. The relative toxic and biological potencies of PCDDs and PCDFs have been estimated using short-term studies in rats and mammalian cell cultures.

There are marked species differences in the susceptibility of animals to the biological and toxic effects elicited by 2,3,7,8-substituted PCDDs and PCDFs. For example, the oral LD_{50} values range from 0.6 µg/kg body weight in guinea-pigs, to 5051 µg/kg body weight in Golden Syrian hamsters for 2,3,7,8-TCDD. The tremendous variation in species and strain sensitivity to 2,3,7,8-TCDD and related compounds cannot be explained by the observed toxicokinetic differences. The toxicity and toxicokinetics of TCDD in monkeys most closely resemble the effects observed in humans. There is evidence in inbred mice that the cellular levels of the Ah receptor correlate, in part, with susceptibility to the biological and toxic effects of these compounds. The receptor has also been identified in other species including man. However, interspecies comparison of cellular Ah receptor levels do not explain fully the differences in sensitivity.

1.1.4.2 Humans

For occupational and accidental exposures to PCDDs and PCDFs, in spite of many clinical and follow-up studies, no clear-cut persistent systemic effects have been delineated except for chloracne. Other effects have been noted, but, apart from chloracne and perhaps minor functional disorders, none has been persistent.

In some epidemiological studies of people exposed to a mixture of dioxins, furans, and other chemicals, an increased incidence of cancer at different sites has been claimed, but a number of factors limits confidence in the findings.

In the Seveso accident, the only clear-cut adverse health effect recorded has been chloracne. Chloracne (193 cases) occurred in 1976 and 1977, and 20 of those individuals still had active chloracne in 1984. Many studies have been performed to find possible links between exposure to Agent Orange and health effects in civilians or military personnel in Viet Nam. However, the information available to date does not allow definite conclusions to be drawn with regard to effects on human reproduction or any other significant health effects.

In the Missouri incident, children who showed acute illness when the contamination occurred in 1971 are now reportedly in good health. Furthermore, epidemiological studies in Missouri on populations exposed to lower concentrations of dioxins over longer periods of time have so far not revealed any significant health effects. Although no clinical symptoms were observed, there were indications of an effect on the cell-mediated immune system.

The only documented intoxications with PCDFs in humans are the two instances of contamination of rice oil with PCDFs, PCBs, and PCQs, i.e., Yusho in Japan, 1968, and Yu-cheng in Taiwan, 1979. In total, several thousand people were acutely intoxicated. From the data it appears most likely that the causative agent was the PCDFs. The general symptomatology was similar to that seen in intoxications with TCDD, with the differences reflecting the intensity of exposure and the ages and sex of those exposed.

The average daily intake of 2,3,7,8-substituted PCDFs by Yusho patients was estimated to be 0.1-0.2 μg/kg body weight for a period of several months, while the lowest dose causing disease was estimated to be 0.05-0.1 μg/kg body weight per day over a period of 30 days.

1.1.5 Conclusion

PCDDs and PCDFs occur throughout the environment and we all probably carry a body burden of them. They have sometimes produced complex toxic effects following occupational and accidental exposure.

Based on the Yusho disease and experiments in sensitive species of monkeys, and making assumptions about the relative potencies of PCDDs and PCDFs, man and certain monkeys may have comparable sensitivity to these compounds. However, the uncertainties related to the real dose received by humans and the difficulties of assessing toxic effects other than chloracne in humans prevents a firm conclusion as to the relative resistance of humans to the toxic effects of these compounds. Exposure should be reduced to levels as low as reasonably practicable.

1.2 Recommendations

1. Analytical interlaboratory validation and "round-robin" studies using standardized quality assurance and quality control procedures are needed to improve analytical methodology.

Sampling strategy and analytical procedures and data interpretation should be optimized and standardized before undertaking surveys.

2. Further information is required about the origins and environmental distributon and fate of PCDDs and PCDFs.

Further monitoring data, including time trends and determinations of isomer patterns, are required for environmental levels of PCDDs and PCDFs, especially for food, ambient air, and sediments.

3. Data should be obtained about the effects of PCDDs and PCDFs on environmental biota.

4. More information is required on the bioavailability of PCDDs and PCDFs from different matrices in the environment and from the diet. Exposure from these sources should be correlated with agricultural and industrial practices.

5. Simpler and less expensive chemical and biological methods suitable for screening for the presence of PCDDs and PCDFs should be developed and validated.

6. Studies to determine the mechanisms of toxicity of PCDDs and PCDFs are needed to support an evaluation of the differ-

ences in effects between species and to support an extrapolation to man.

7. Further investigation of immunotoxicity is important, including cytotoxic T-lymphocyte function. Studies of the effects of perinatal exposure and of the duration of actions on the immune system are important.

8. Long-term toxicity studies should be carried out, including multigeneration reproductive studies in different species with three of the most widespread PCDDs and PCDFs, namely 2,3,4,7,8-pentaCDF, 1,2,3,7,8-pentaCDD, and octaCDD.

9. Because humans are exposed to complex mixtures of PCDDs and PCDFs, test systems, including human cell culture systems, should be developed further and validated for evaluating the toxic potency of these compounds and other mixtures. These systems can be used to study mechanisms of action, structure activity relationships, and interactive effects.

10. Investigations to examine the body burden and to correlate it with clinical effects and laboratory findings are indicated. Follow-up studies of previously exposed groups are important.

2. IDENTITY, PHYSICAL AND CHEMICAL PROPERTIES, ANALYTICAL METHODS

2.1 Identity

The polychlorinated dibenzo-para-dioxins (PCDDs) and polychlorinated dibenzofurans (PCDFs) are two series of almost planar tricyclic aromatic compounds with very similar chemical properties. The general formulae are given in Fig. 1.

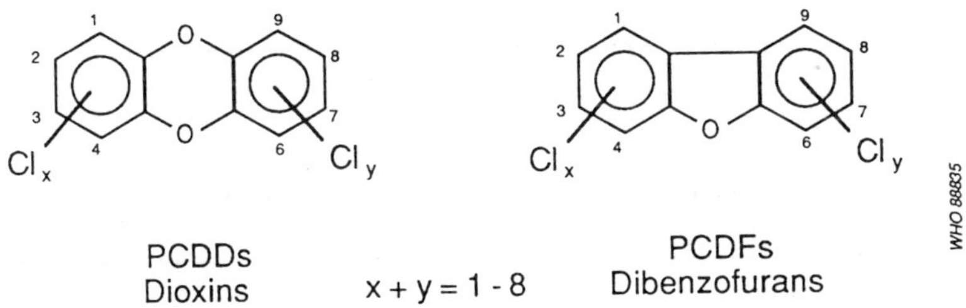

Fig. 1. Structural formulae of PCDDs and PCDFs.

The number of chlorine atoms can vary between 1 and 8. The term isomers refers to comparisons between compounds with the same empirical formulae. The term congeners refers to comparisons between compounds within the same series but with a different number of chlorine atoms. The number of positional isomers is quite large; in all there are 75 PCDDs and 135 PCDFs and the number of isomers for a certain number of chlorine atoms is given in Table 1.

The nomenclature used in this document is based on the system used by Chemical Abstracts. The Chemical Abstracts System Registry Numbers (CAS RN) for a few PCDDs and PCDFs that have been cited in the literature are provided in Table 2.

2.2 Physical and Chemical Properties

A large number of the individual PCDDs have been synthesized by various methods and characterized, mainly by gas chromatography-mass spectrometry (GC/MS) (Buser & Rappe, 1980, 1984; Taylor et al., 1985; Rappe et al., 1985a) but also by

Table 1. Number of PCDD and PCDF isomers

Number of chlorine atoms	Number of PCDD isomers	Number of PCDF isomers
1	2	4
2	10	16
3	14	28
4	22	38
5	14	28
6	10	16
7	2	4
8	1	1
	75	135

Table 2. CAS RN for some PCDDs and PCDFs

PCDD congener	CAS RN	PCDF congener	CAS RN
2,3,7,8-TetraCDD	1746-01-6	2,3,7,8-TetraCDF	51207-31-9
1,2,3,7,8-PentaCDD	40321-76-4	1,2,3,7,8-PentaCDF	57117-41-6
1,2,3,6,7,8-HexaCDD	57653-85-7	2,3,4,7,8-PentaCDF	57117-31-4
1,2,3,7,8,9-HexaCDD	19408-74-3	1,2,3,4,7,8-HexaCDF	70648-26-9
1,2,3,4,6,7,8-HeptaCDD	35822-46-9	1,2,3,6,7,8-HexaCDF	57117-44-9
1,2,3,4,7,8,9-HeptaCDD	58200-70-7	1,2,3,7,8,9-HexaCDF	72918-38-8
OctaCDD	3268-87-9	2,3,4,6,7,8-HexaCDF	60851-34-5

using nuclear magnetic resonance (NMR) or ultraviolet (UV), infrared (IR), (Pohland & Yang, 1972; Kende et al., 1974), or X-ray analyses (Boer et al., 1973; Slonecker et al., 1983).

Pyrolysis of chlorinated phenols yields small amounts of one or more PCDD isomers. Using this technique all the 22 tetraCDDs have been prepared (Nestrick et al., 1979; Buser & Rappe, 1980) as well as the 14 pentaCDDs (Buser & Rappe, 1984) and 10 hexaCDDs (Lamparski & Nestrick, 1981; Buser & Rappe, 1984).

Taylor et al. (1985) have synthesized, separated, and isolated all the 22 tetraCDD isomers. In Table 3 are listed some other isomers that have been synthesized and isolated.

Table 3. Synthetic method and melting point for some PCDDs

PCDD Isomer	Synthetic method[a]	Melting point °C	Reference
1-Chloro-	1	80-90	Pohland & Yang, 1972
2-Chloro-	1	88-89	Pohland & Yang, 1972
1,3-Dichloro-	1	113.5-114.5	Kende et al., 1974
2,3-Dichloro-	1	163-164	Pohland & Yang, 1972
2,7-Dichloro-	2	209-210	Pohland & Yang, 1972
2,8-Dichloro-	3	150.5-151	Pohland & Yang, 1972
1,2,4-Trichloro-	4	128-129	Pohland & Yang, 1972
2,3,7-Trichloro-	1	157-158	Kende et al., 1974
2,3,7,8-Tetrachloro-	2	305-306	Pohland & Yang, 1972
2,3,7,8-Tetrachloro-	5	305-307	Kende et al., 1974
1,2,3,4-Tetrachloro-	4	188-190	Pohland & Yang, 1972
1,3,7,8-Tetrachloro-	1	193.5-195	Kende et al., 1974
1,3,6,8-Tetrachloro-	2	219-219.5	Pohland & Yang, 1972
1,2,3,4,7-Pentachloro-	5	195-196	Kende et al., 1974
1,2,3,4,7,8-Hexachloro-	5	275	Pohland & Yang, 1972
1,2,4,6,7,9-Hexachloro-	2	238-240	Pohland & Yang, 1972
Octachloro	2	330	Pohland & Yang, 1972

[a] Synthetic methods as follows:

1 = Catechol + chlorobenzene
2 = Pyrolysis of chlorphenols
3 = Cyclization of chlorophenoxyphenol
4 = Catechol + chloronitrobenzene
5 = Chlorination of chlorodibenzodioxin

The most toxic and most extensively studied representative of the chlorinated dioxins (PCDDs) is 2,3,7,8-tetrachlorodibenzo-*para*-dioxin (2,3,7,8-tetraCDD) (Fig. 2). It is commercially available, as are more than 10 other PCDD congeners.

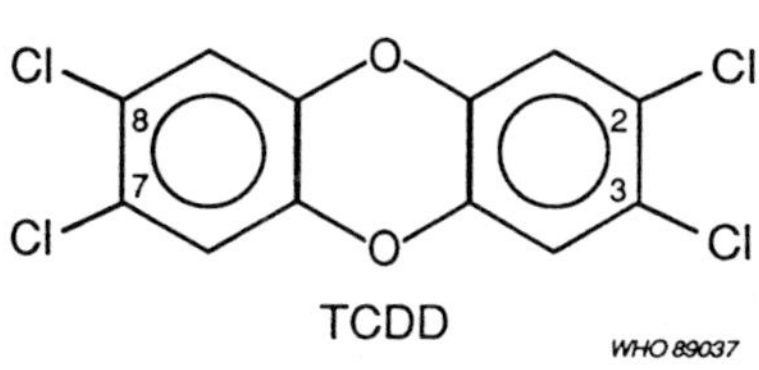

Fig. 2. Structural formula of TCDD.

The empirical formulae, molecular weights, and some physical properties of a few PCDDs are given in Table 4.

Table 4. Physical properties of some PCDDs

Compound	Molecular formulae	Molecular weight	Absorption maximum (chloroform) (nm)	Reference
2,3,7,8-TCDD	$C_{12}H_4Cl_4O_2$	321.9	310	Pohland & Yang (1972)
1,2,3,7,8-PentaCDD	$C_{12}H_3Cl_5O_2$	356.5	308	Gray et al. (1976)
1,2,3,6,7,8-HexaCDD	$C_{12}H_2Cl_6O_2$	390.9	316	Gray et al. (1975)
1,2,3,7,8,9-HexaCDD	$C_{12}H_2Cl_6O_2$	390.9	317	Gray et al. (1975)

Although tetraCDD is lipophilic, it is only slightly soluble in most solvents and very slightly soluble in water (Table 5).

Table 5. Solubility of 2,3,7,8-tetraCDD in various solvents[a]

Solvent	Solubility at 25 °C g/litre	g/kg
O-Dichlorobenzene	1.8	1.4
Chlorobenzene	0.8	0.72
Perchloroethylene	0.68	0.48
Chloroform	0.55	0.37
Benzene	0.47	0.57
Acetone	0.09	0.11
Dimethylsulfoxide[b]	< 0.1	< 0.1
Methanol	0.01	0.01
Water	2×10^{-7}	2×10^{-7}

[a] From: Crummett & Stehl (1973).
[b] DMSO caused detector fouling and a better value could not be obtained.

Marple et al. (1986a) have reanalysed the water solubility of 2,3,7,8-TCDD and found it to be considerably less (12.5-19.2 ng/litre). The log water-octanol partition coefficient (K_{ow}) has been determined as 6.64 by Marple et al. (1986b).

Friesen et al. (1985) have determined the water solubility for some PCDDs other than the 2,3,7,8-TCDD compound and these are given in Table 6.

Table 6. Water solubility of PCDDs[a]

Compound	Water solubility (g/litre) 20.0 °C	40.0 °C
1.3.6.8-TetraCDD	(3.2+0.2) x 10^{-7}	(3.9+0.4) x 10^{-7}
1.2.3.7-TetraCDD	(4.3±0.1) x 10^{-7}	(12.7±0.8) x 10^{-7}
1.2.3.4.7-PentaCDD	(1.2±0.1) x 10^{-7}	(4.6±0.1) x 10^{-7}
1.2.3.4.7.8-HexaCDD	(4.4±0.1) x 10^{-9}	(19.0±0.1) x 10^{-9}
1.2.3.4.6.7.8-HeptaCDD	(2.4±0.3) x 10^{-9}	(6.3±0.2) x 10^{-9}
OctaCDD	(0.4±0.1) x 10^{-9}	(2.0±0.2) x 10^{-9}

[a] From: Friesen et al. (1985).

Similarly Webster et al. (1985) have determined the log octanol-water partition coefficients for a number of PCDDs (Table 7).

2,3,7,8-TetraCDD is considered to be a stable compound, but due to its extreme toxicity its chemistry has not been fully evaluated. However, it undergoes substitution reactions (Baughman, 1974) as well as photochemical dechlorination (Crosby et al., 1971; Crosby & Wong, 1977; Gebefugi et al., 1977). Thermally it is very stable and rapid decomposition of 2,3,7,8-tetraCDD occurs only at temperatures above 750 °C (Stehl et al., 1973). The other PCDDs have been much less studied; however, octaCDD is completely destroyed by treatment with hot alkali (Albro & Corbett, 1977).

The first synthesis of 2,3,7,8-tetraCDD was reported by Sandermann et al. (1957), who used catalytic chlorination of the unchlorinated dioxin. It has also been prepared in good yields by the dimerization of 2,4,5-trichlorophenol salts (Buu-Hoi et al., 1971b; Langer et al., 1973).

In the PCDF series, Mazer et al. (1983) synthesized all the 38 positional tetraCDF isomers. The products were mixtures of isomers, and each of these isomers could be ident-

Table 7. Values for log K_{ow} for some PCDDs from linear and quadratic plots

Compound	log K_{ow} (linear) Waters Bondapak	log K_{ow} (linear) Waters Bondapak (Woodburn data)	log K_{ow} (quadratic) Waters Bondapak	log K_{ow} (quadratic) Waters Bondapak (Woodburn data)
Dibenzo-p-dioxin	4.26	4.01	4.34	4.17
1-MonoCDD	4.81	4.52	4.91	4.75
2-MonoCDD	5.33	5.00	5.45	5.29
2,7-DiCDD	6.27	5.86	6.39	6.17
1,2,4-TriCDD	7.36	6.86	7.45	7.11
1,2,3,7-TetraCDD	8.15	7.58	8.19	7.72
1,2,3,4-TetraCDD	8.63	8.02	8.64	8.07
1,3,6,8-TetraCDD	8.70	8.08	8.70	8.12
1,2,3,4,7-PentaCDD	9.48	8.80	9.40	8.64
1,2,3,4,7,8-HexaCDD	10.40	9.65	10.22	9.19
1,2,3,4,6,7,8-HeptaCDD	11.38	10.55	11.05	9.69
OctaCDD	12.26	11.35	11.76	10.07

[a] From: Webster et al. (1985).

ified. Later Bell & Gari, (1985) isolated and characterized all the 38 tetraCDFs, 28 pentaCDFs, and 16 hexaCDFs.

Kuroki et al. (1984) have synthesized 51 congeners of PCDFs by a structure specific method from chlorophenols and chloronitrobenzenes or chlorophenols and chlorodiphenyls iodonium salts. The structures were confirmed by MS and NMR.

Safe & Safe (1984) described the synthesis of 22 PCDF congeners resulting in quantities of 10-320 mg of purified product. They also reported NMR data on the compounds synthesized.

Sarna et al. (1984) and Burkhard & Kuehl, (1986) have documented the octanol/water partition coefficients for some PCDFs (Table 8). The disagreement for OCDF arises because of uncertainties in the K_{ow} values of reference compounds of high K_{ow}. The partitioning of organic chemicals between lipid and water is an important determinant of the bioconcentration potential of a toxicant and has sometimes been effectively used as an indicator of the preferred degradative in *in vivo* pathways.

Table 8. The logarithm of the octanol/water partition coefficients (K_{ow}) of some PCDFs using HPLC methods

PCDF	log K_{ow}	Reference
2,8-dichloro-	5.95 5.30[b]	Sarna et al. 1984[a] Burkhard & Kuehl, 1986[c]
2,3,7,8-tetrachloro-	5.82±0.02	Burkhard & Kuehl, 1986[c]
octachloro-	13.37 8.78	Sarna et al. 1984[a] Burkhard & Kuehl, 1986[c]

[a] Quadratic equation treatment: Biorad Biosil (10 μm) data.
[b] Quadratic equation treatment: unspecified "microbore" HPLC column.
[c] Sarna et al. (1984) data recalculated from experimental data.

2.3. Analytical Methods

2.3.1 General aspects

The earliest reported method used to detect 2,3,7,8-tetraCDD was a rabbit skin test (Adams et al., 1941). Test samples were applied to the inner surface of the ear and to the shaven belly of albino rabbits, and inflammatory responses were observed. Subsequently, Jones & Krizek (1962) developed a test based on the recovery and weight of the keratin formed on the rabbit ear after application of a sample. These biological methods were non-specific as to isomers and not sufficiently sensitive to detect low levels of contamination.

In the late 1960s and early 1970s, gas chromatographic methods were used for the quantification mainly of 2,3,7,8-tetraCDD in commercial 2,4,5-T formations. The detection level was normally in the range of μg/g. These analyses were not isomer-specific and the results could not be confirmed. Ryhage (1964) solved the problem of combining a gas chromatograph with a mass spectrometer. During the 1970s and 1980s, various types of mass spectrometer and gas chromatograph/mass spectrometer combinations were used in analytical work. Use of these more sophisticated instruments allowed for the development of isomer-specific and validated analyses for the tetraCDDs in the very late 1970s and for the other PCDDs and PCDFs in the early 1980s.

A number of spectroscopic methods are available for the laboratory identification of 2,3,7,8-tetraCDD, but their use is highly restricted, with the exception of mass spectroscopy (MS). Data on X-ray, infra-red (IR), ultra-violet (UV), nuclear magnetic resonance (NMR), electron spin resonance (ESR), and mass spectra were obtained by Pohland & Yang (1972), Baughman (1974), and Slonecker et al. (1983).

Because of the large number of isomers and congeners, and due to the extreme toxicity of some PCDD and PCDF isomers, highly sensitive and specific analytical techniques are required for the measurements. Detection limits for the analysis of environmental and human samples should be orders of magnitude lower than the usual detection levels required for pesticide analysis. A detection level of 1 pg or less might be required to measure 2,3,7,8-tetraCDD and the other toxic isomers in a 1-g environmental sample. Analyses at such low levels are complicated by the presence of a multitude of other interfering compounds and clean-up procedures are required.

The mono-, di-, and trichloro congeners are not usually included in these analyses. Such compounds are considered to be much less toxic than the higher chlorinated congeners and are also much more volatile and losses may occur during clean-up.

It should be mentioned that the level of sophistication needed in the analyses for PCDD and PCDFs will depend upon the objectives thereof. In cases where the objectives were primarily to screen samples to identify groups of PCDDs and/or PCDFs (in a qualitative or semiquantitative manner), routine assays and bioassays were adequate. In other instances, where the objective of the analysis was to quantify accurately specific PCDD and/or PCDF isomers in the samples, sophisticated analytical procedures were required. Clearly, both types of analyses can be useful, depending on the purpose for which the analytical results are to be used.

Many analytical methods have been developed in recent years for the analysis of trace amounts of PCDDs and PCDFs in environmental samples, especially for 2,3,7,8-tetraCDD. The most specific of these methods are based on MS. There are many requirements to be met by such an analytical method, including representative sampling and appropriate storage, efficient extraction, high selectivity in the clean-up, high specificity in the gas chromatography, high sensitivity in the detection, safe and reliable quantification, good reproducibility, useful confirmatory information.

Several review articles discussing methods of analyzing PCDDs and PCDFs have appeared (McKinney, 1978; Esposito et al., 1980; Rappe & Buser, 1980; Harless & Lewis, 1982; Karasek & Anuska, 1982; Tiernan, 1983; Crummett et al., 1985). Most of the older methods have been critically reviewed by a panel of experts assembled by the National Research Council of Canada (1981).

2.3.2 Sampling strategy and sampling methods

The quality and utility of analytical data depend on the validity of the sample and the adequacy of the sampling program. The purpose of sampling is to obtain specimens that represent the situation being studied. Sampling plans may require that systematic samples be obtained at specified times and places, or simple random sampling may be necessary. Generally, the sample should be an unbiased representation of the environmental situation.

All aspects of a sampling programme should be planned and documented in detail, and the expected relationship of the sampling protocol to the analytical result should be defined. A sampling programme should include reasons for choosing sampling sites, the number and type of samples, the timing of sample acquisition and the sampling equipment used. A detailed sampling procedure should include a description of the sampling situation, the sampling methodology, labelling of samples, field blank preparation, pretreatment procedures, and transportation and storage procedures.

The quality assurance programme should include means to demonstrate that containers or storage procedures do not alter the qualitative or quantitative composition of the sample. Special transportation and storage procedures (refrigeration or exclusion of light) should be described, if they are required.

Because environmental samples are typically heterogeneous, a sufficiently large number of samples (ten or more) must normally be analyzed to obtain meaningful data on chemical composition. The number of individual samples that should be analyzed will depend on the kind of information required by the investigation. If an average compositional value is required, a number of randomly selected individual samples may be obtained, combined, and blended to provide a homogeneous composite sample from which a sufficient number of subsamples could be analyzed. If composition profiles, time trends, or the variability of the sample population are of interest, many samples need to be collected and analyzed individually.

If field blanks are not available, efforts should be made to obtain blank samples that best simulate a sample that does not contain the specific chemical. In addition, measurements should be made to ascertain whether, and to what extent, any reagent or solvent used may contribute to or interfere with the analytical results (laboratory and solvent blanks).

The recovery tests are frequently used and necessary to evaluate the analytical methodology. Uncontaminated samples from control sites that have been spiked with the chemical of interest provide the best information because they simulate any matrix effect. When feasible, isotopically labelled

(^{13}C, ^{37}Cl) chemicals spiked into the sample provide the greatest accuracy since they are subjected to the same matrix effects. The ^{13}C- and ^{37}Cl-labelled compounds can be used to validate:

(a) sampling (sampling surrogate),
(b) analytical pretreatment (clean-up surrogate),
(c) quantification (internal standard).

Very few laboratories in the world have access to and experience in working with these complicated analyses.

In order to be able to compare data generated in different laboratories, the same quantitative standard compounds should be used. Interlaboratory calibrations or "round-robin" studies have been performed in very few cases.

2.3.3 Extraction procedures

In this step, the sample is homogenized or digested and extracted with a suitable solvent or solvent mixture to remove the bulk of the sample matrix and transfer the PCDD and PCDF residue into the solvent. Both the selection of the proper solvent and the method of extraction can be critical in obtaining a satisfactory recovery of PCDDs and PCDFs from the sample matrix.

Many different procedures for the extraction of PCDDs/PCDFs from various samples are described. In some cases this involves digestion or destruction of the matrix. Some of these methods have been evaluated in the report from the National Research Council of Canada (1982), while other methods are discussed by Tiernan (1983).

An interlaboratory "round-robin" study involving 13 laboratories was carried out to evaluate the reliability of data on 2,3,7,8-tetraCDD in fish samples. No significant differences were found from methods differing in the digestion or extraction procedures (Ryan et al., 1983b).

In a study described by Albro et al. (1985), eight different approaches were applied in eight laboratories to quantify four PCDDs (2,3,7,8-tetraCDD; 1,2,3,7,8-pentaCDD; 1,2,3,4,7,8-hexaCDD; and octaCDD) and three PCDFs (2,3,7,8-tetraCDF; 2,3,4,7,8-pentaCDF; and 1,2,3,7,8,9-hexaCDF) in spiked samples of an extract from human adipose tissue. Levels of fortification, unknown to the participating laboratories, were in the 5-50 ng/kg range, except for octaCDD (up to 500 ng/kg). The results indicated that most of the procedures tested gave a high degree of qualitative reliability. However, other methods were not so accurate, a large portion of the reported data consisting of false positives or false negatives.

Lustenhouwer et al. (1980) studied the extraction of PCDDs and PCDFs from a fly ash sample. A dramatic difference was found between different solvents.

2.3.4 Sample clean-up

In the sample clean-up, the PCDDs and PCDFs present in the sample should be separated from a multitude of other co-extracted and possibly interfering compounds. The clean-up methods, normally three steps or more, can vary for different sample matrices. Two different procedural trends can be recognized:

(a) all PCDD and PCDF isomers can be analyzed in one single fraction by the containment enrichment procedure (Norstrom et al., 1982; Stalling et al., 1983; Tiernan, 1983; Rappe, 1984),

(b) specific isomers are analyzed in different fractions mainly after normal-phase and reverse-phase high pressure liquid chromatography (HPLC) separation (Lamparski et al., 1979; Niemann et al., 1983; Tosine et al., 1983).

This latter method allows the identification of only a few PCDD isomers in each fraction, and is mainly used to monitor TCDD and a few other congeners. For a monitoring program of all PCDDs and PCDFs a more general method might be preferred.

The method described by Stalling et al. (1983) was originally designed for the analyses of fish samples. In a "round-robin" study of fish samples it gave good results (Ryan et al., 1983b). This method has now been used for the clean-up of other biological samples like bird muscle, seal fat, turtle fat, and human adipose tissue - blood, liver, kidney, and milk (Rappe et al., 1983c; Nygren et al., 1986; Rappe et al., 1986b).

2.3.5 Isomer identification

The purified extracts are used directly for the final analyses with the aid of a gas-chromatograph/mass spectrometer (GC/MS) equipped with a glass capillary or a fused-silica column. The column leads directly into the ion source of the mass spectrometer, which operates either in the electron impact (EI) or the negative ion-chemical ionization (NCI) mode. In view of the large variation in toxicological and biological effects of the PCDD and PCDF isomers, it is imperative that the isomers, particularly those having high toxicity, be identified. For an unambiguous isomer identification it is necessary to have access to all analytical standards within a specific group of isomers, e.g. all the 22 tetraCDDs and all the 38 tetraCDFs. All the 22 tetraCDDs have been prepared and, using a Silar 10c glass capillary column, the 2,3,7,8-tetraCDD can be separated from all the other 21 tetra isomers (Buser & Rappe, 1980). Recently all the 14 pentaCDDs and the 10 hexaCDDs have been prepared. Using the Silar 10c column all the 2,3,7,8- substituted isomers can be separated from all the other isomers (Buser & Rappe, 1984). The SP 2330 fused silica column can also be used for this separation (Rappe, 1984).

In the PCDF series, Mazer et al. (1983) have synthesized all the 38 positional tetraCDF isomers. The products were mixtures of isomers, and each of these isomers could be identified using both an SP 2330 and an SE 54 capillary column. Later, Bell & Gara (1985) isolated and characterized all tetra-, penta- and hexaCDFs. The SP 2330 column can separate most of these isomers (Rappe, 1984). The 1,2,3,7,8-pentaCDF co-elutes with the 1,2,3,4,8-isomer and the 1,2,3,4,7,8-hexaCDF with the 1,2,3,4,7,9-isomer, but they can be separated on less polar columns like OV-17 and DB-5.

A very limited number of investigations has been performed using these complete sets of synthetic standards.

2.3.6 Quantification

Mass selective detection (mass fragmentography) has been used to quantify trace amounts of PCDDs and PCDFs in the samples by selectively monitoring M, M + 2, and/or M + 4 ions (SIM). The quantification is based on peak area measurements and a comparison of these areas using either isotopically labelled internal standards (^{13}C or ^{37}Cl) or calibration curves of external standards. As a first approach, it has been generally assumed that with the MS quantification technique, all isomers of a particular congener of PCDD or PCDF (e.g. the tetrachloro- isomers) have the same response factors. However, an investigation of 13 well-defined tetraCDF isomers has shown a three-fold variation in response factors with the EI mode and up to a 20-fold variation with the negative ion-chemical ionization mode. For the higher chlorinated homologues (penta, hexa) the variation was found to be less (Rappe et al., 1983b).

Fung et al. (1985) have studied the mass spectra of 26 PCDF congeners. They found that the EI spectra are not particularly isomer specific, while positive ion chemical ionization spectra show a greater degree of isomer distinction.

2.3.7 Confirmation

Quality control and quality assurance programs help to assure that positive data reported actually refer to specific PCDDs and PCDFs (Kloepfer et al., 1983). To provide reliable data:

(a) isomer specificity must be demonstrated initially and verified daily,
(b) the retention time must equal (within 3 seconds) the retention time for the isotopically labelled congener,
(c) the signal to noise ratio must be 2.5:1 or higher,
(d) the chlorine cluster must be within $\pm$ 10% of the theoretical values, given in Table 9,
(e) correct fragments, e.g., M^{+}-COCl ions, must be with correct chlorine clusters.

For confirmation, mass spectroscopy is the best technique now available. The EI mass spectral properties of PCDFs and PCDD have been described (Buser, 1975). The molecular (M^{+}) and fragment ions of PCDDs and PCDFs show the typical, expected clustering due to the chlorine isotopes (Table 9). The typical fragmentation is $M^{-}COCl^{+}$, which is a useful fragment to study.

Buser & Rappe (1978) have shown that observation of low mass ions can be used for the identification of the substitution pattern of PCDDs, which can be defined as the number of chlorine atoms on each carbon ring of the dioxin molecular; the 2,3,7,8-isomer has a 2:2 pattern while 1,2,3,4-tetraCDD has a 4:0 pattern. However, these low mass ions may not be observed in spectra from environmental or biological samples.

In the negative ion-chemical ionization mode, the PCDFs have the base peak due to M^{-}, and the fragmentation produces the unusual M^{-}-34 ions (uptake of H and loss of Cl). Fragmentation of PCDDs in this mode is more conventional via loss of Cl yielding M^{-}-35 ions (Buser et al., 1985).

Using EI technique and a quadropole instrument, the detection limits are 1-10 pg for the tetrachloro compounds and up to 10-50 pg for the octachloro compounds using selected ion monitoring or multiple ion detection (SIM or MID). Full mass spectra require 0.1-1 ng of compound (Buser et al., 1985). High resolution instruments can improve the sensitivity by one order of magnitude.

The negative ion-chemical ionization mode, using methane gas as reagent, gas provides extremely good sensitivity for all PCDFs (tetra- to octachloro- compounds) and for the higher chlorinated PCDDs (penta- to octaCDD). The detection limits are in the 10-100 fg (10^{-15}g) range using SIR or MID, which is 1 to 2 orders of magnitude better than EI (Buser et al.,

Table 9. Isotopic abundance ratio ("cluster") of polychlorinated dioxins and dibenzofurans

Number of chlorine atoms	M	M + 2	M + 4	M + 6	M + 8	M + 10	M + 12	M + 14
1	100.0	33.7						
2	100.0	66.1	11.3					
3	100.0	98.4	32.7	3.8				
4	76.4	100.0	49.4	11.0	1.0			
5	61.2	100.0	65.5	21.6	3.6	0.3		
6	51.1	100.0	81.7	35.8	8.9	1.2	0.1	
7	43.8	100.0	97.9	53.4	17.6	3.5	0.4	
8	33.7	87.6	100.0	65.3	26.8	7.0	1.2	0.1

1985). However, the negative ion-chemical ionization mode has very poor sensitivity for 2,3,7,8- tetraCDD under these conditions.

Using low resolution MS instruments, a series of interfering compounds has been identified (Table 10). Some of this interference can be eliminated using high resolution MS instruments operating at 8000 - 10 000 daltons. However, compounds with the same empirical formulae cannot be separated by MS technique; they are normally eliminated during the clean-up or separated by the gas chromatography step.

2.3.8 Other analytical methods

Paasivirta et al. (1977) have shown that 2,3,7,8-tetraCDD can be detected down to the pg level using a glass capillary column and a ^{63}Ni electron-capture detector. Combined with efficient clean up procedures, this method has shown to be useful down to a level of 9 ppt (Niemann et al., 1983), although positive samples need confirmation by mass spectroscopy (MID, SIM).

Other techniques, such as enzyme induction and radioimmunoassay have been described and discussed by Firestone (1978) and McKinney (1978). McKinney et al. (1982) have used the radioimmunoassay method for determining 2,3,7,8-tetraCDD in human fat, and found the reliable sensitivity at 95% confidence interval to be 100 pg per sample.

An analytical method based on the keratonization response of epithelial cells in an *in vitro* system has been described by Gierthy & Crane (1985b). This method can be an assay for dioxin-like activity in environmental and biological samples. A positive response was found for 2,3,7,8-tetraCDD at a concentration of 10-11 mol/litre.

Table 10. List of molecular ions of polychlorinated compounds present in some human and environmental samples and possibly interfering in the mass spectral analysis of PCDFs and PCDDs[a]

Compounds	Molecular ions ($m/z, m^+, m^-$) (chlorination)									
	mono-	di-	tri-	tetra-	penta-	hexa-	hepta-	octa-	nona-	deca-
PCDDs				320	354	388	422	456	-	-
PCDFs				304	338	372	406	440	-	-
PCBs				290	324	358	392	426	460	494
PCNs				264	298	332	366	400	-	-
PCTs		298	332	366	400	434	468	502	536	570
PCDPEs[b]		238	272	306	340	374	408	442	476	510
PCPYs[c]	36	270	304	338	372	406				

[a] From: Buser et al. (1985).
[b] PCDPEs: Polychlorinated diphenylethers.
[c] PCPYs: Polychlorinated pyrenes.

3. SOURCES OF ENVIRONMENTAL POLLUTION

3.1 Production, Synthesis, and Use

PCDDs and PCDFs are not produced commercially. These compounds are in fact formed as trace amounts of undesired impurities in the manufacture of other chemicals such as chlorinated phenols and their derivatives, chlorinated diphenyl ethers, and polychlorinated biphenyls (PCBs). There is no known technical use for the PCDDs and PCDFs.

The amount of total PCDDs entering the Canadian environment/year has been estimated to be about 1500 kg, and 75% of this amount has been estimated to be due to octaCDD alone (National Research Council of Canada, 1981). There is no estimation of the amount of PCDFs entering the environment anywhere in the world.

Although the polychlorinated dioxins and dibenzofurans are not commercially produced, most of these compounds have been synthesized for research purposes in small quantities according to the reactions discussed in section 2.

3.2 Industrial Processes

In addition to the synthetic methods mentioned in section 2, 2,3,7,8-tetraCDD may be formed during the industrial preparation of 2,4,5-trichlorophenol from 1,2,4,5-tetrachlorobenzene. This substitution reaction takes place at about 180 °C, and when the solvent is methanol, the pressure rises to about 7 KPa. The formation of TCDD is an unwanted side reaction which takes place when the reaction mixture is heated to 230-260 °C (Milnes, 1971). This reaction is exothermic, so that even higher temperatures may be attained resulting in uncontrolled conditions.

In some factories ethylene glycol is used as a solvent in order to avoid the high pressure. As already pointed out by Milnes (1971), however, use of this solvent requires special precautions because of the occurrence of a base-promoted polymerization of ethylene glycol and decomposition reactions that produce ethylene oxide. These reactions are also exothermic; they may start spontaneously at temperatures above 180 °C and proceed rapidly and uncontrollably to result in the formation of relatively large amounts of TCDD.

After most of the solvent has been removed, the reaction mixture is acidified; the 2,4,5-trichlorophenol can be separated from 2,3,7,8-tetraCDD by one or two distillations, with the result that 2,3,7,8-tetraCDD is concentrated in the still-bottom residues. Up to 1 mg/g of 2,3,7,8 tetraCDD in such residues has been reported (Kimbrough et al., 1984). Improper disposal of such residues is discussed in sections 4.4.2 and 9.

Most of the 2,4,5-trichlorophenol produced is used for the preparation of herbicides such as 2,4,5-T (including various esters and salts, and the bactericide hexachlorophene).

PCDDs and PCDFs are both formed as by-products during the manufacture of chlorinated phenols (2,4-dichloro-, 2,4,6-trichloro-, 2,3,4,6-tetrachloro- and pentachlorophenol). The commercial chlorophenols are produced by two processes, i.e., by chlorination of the phenol using various catalysts and by the alkaline hydrolysis of an appropriate chlorobenzene. Apparently both reactions can lead to the formation of PCDDs as well as PCDFs, and the level of contamination is normally much higher here than in the production of 2,4,5-trichlorophenol (see section 3.3).

PCDDs and PCDFs are also formed during the preparation of chlorinated diphenyl ether herbicides (Yamagishi et al., 1981) and hexachlorobenzene (Villeneuve et al., 1974). A series of PCDFs are formed during the production of PCBs (see section 3.3).

Production equipment is often used for the production of several different chemicals. In the manufacture of chemicals on such equipment previously contaminated by PCDDs and PCDFs, both the products and waste generated can be contaminated. Thus, manufactured 2,4-dichlorophenoxyacetic esters (2,4-D), which otherwise should not be contaminated by 2,3,7,8-tetraCDD, did indeed contain this dioxin because the equipment used had been employed previously to produce 2,4,5-T and had not been cleaned properly (Federal Register, 1980).

It should be pointed out that the primary occurrence of TCDD in the environment is possibly related to the synthesis of 2,4,5-trichlorophenol, the use of products prepared from this compound (Table 11), and to incinerations reactions. The occurrence of the other PCDDs and PCDFs is related to the synthesis and use of a variety of other products (Table 12), some of which are quite common.

The other PCDDs and PCDFs are also formed in a variety of incineration reactions (see section 4.5).

3.3 Contamination of Commercial Products

3.3.1 Chlorophenoxyacetic acid herbicides

Depending on the temperature control and purification efficiency, the levels of 2,3,7,8-tetraCDD in commercial products may vary greatly. For example, the levels of 2,3,7,8-tetraCDD in drums of the herbicide Agent Orange placed in storage in the USA and in the Pacific before 1970 were between 0.02 and 47 μg/g. More than 450 samples were analyzed in this

Table 11. Some commercial products that may be contaminated with 2,3,7,8-tetraCDD, depending on the method of preparation

Common name	Chemical name
2,4,5-T[a]	2,4,5-Trichlorophenoxyacetic acid
2,4,5-T esters[a]	*n*-butyl-, butoxy ethyl-, and *iso*-octyl-esters of 2,4,5-trichlorophenoxyacetic acid
2,4,5-T salts[a]	dimethylamine salts of 2,4,5-trichlorophenoxyacetic acid
Fenoprop	esters of 2-(2,4,5-trichlorophenoxy)-propanoic acid
Erbon	ethyl ester of 2-(2,4,5-trichloro-phenoxy)-2,2-dichloropropanoic acid
2,4,5-Trichlorophenol	2,4,5-Trichlorophenol
Fenochlorphos	*O*,*O*-Dimethyl-*O*-2,4,5-trichlorophenyl phosphonothioate
Trichloronate	*O*-Ethyl-*O*-2,4,5-trichlorophenyl ethylphosphonothioate
Hexachlorophene/isobac 20	2,2'-Methylene-bis-(3,4,6-trichloro-phenol)

[a] There are numerous trade names for this product.

Table 12. Some commercial products which may be contaminated with PCDDs other than 2,3,7,8-tetraCDD, and with PCDFs, depending on the method of preparation

Common name	Chemical name
Bifenox	Methyl-5-2,4-dichlorophenoxy-2-nitrobenzoate
Chloranil	2,3,5,6-Tetrachloro-2,5-cyclohexadiene-1,4-dione.
2,4-D (esters and salts)	2,4-Dichlorophenoxyacetic acid and esters and salts
2,4-DB and salts	2,4-Dichlorophenoxybutyric acid and salts
Dicamba	3,6-Dichloro-2-methoxybenzoic acid
Dicamba, dimethylamine salt	3,6-Dichloro-2-methoxybenzoic acid, dimethylamine salt
Dicapthon	Phosphorothioic acid o-(2-chloro-4-nitrophenyl) o,o-dimethyl ester
Dichlofenthion	Phosphorothioic acid o-2,4-dichlorophenyl o,o-dialkyl ester
Disul sodium (sesone)	2,4-Dichlorophenoxyethyl sulfate, sodium salt
2,4-DP	2- 2,4-Dichlorophenoxy propionic acid
HCB	Hexachlorobenzene
Nitrofen	2,4-Dichlorophenyl-p-nitrophenyl ether
PCP and salts	Pentachlorophenol and salts
PCB	Polychlorinated biphenyls
2,4,6-TCP	2,4,6-Trichlorophenol and salts 2,3,4,6-Tetrachlorophenol and salts
CNP	1,3,5-Trichloro-2-(4-nitrophenoxy) benzene
NIP	2,4-Dichloro-1-(4-nitrophenoxy) benzene
X-52	2,4-Dichloro-1-(3-methoxy-4-nitrophenoxy) benzene

study, and the mean value was 1.98 µg/g (Young et al., 1983). Since Agent Orange was formulated as a 1:1 mixture of the butyl esters of 2,4,5-T and 2,4-D, the levels of 2,3,7,8-tetraCDD in individual 2,4,5-T preparations manufactured and used in the 1960s could have been as high as 100 µg/g.

In analyses using high-resolution GC-MS, Rappe et al. (1978a) have reported that in other samples of Agent Orange (as well as in European and the USA 2,4,5-T formulations from the 1950s and 1960s), 2,3,7,8-tetraCDD was the dominating compound of this group of contaminants. Only minor amounts of other PCDDs and PCDFs could be found, primarily lower chlorinated PCDDs, in samples of Agent Orange.

As a result of governmental regulations, efforts were made during the 1970s to minimize the formation of 2,3,7,8-tetraCDD during 2,4,5-T production, and now all producers claim that their products contain less than 0.1 µg 2,3,7,8-tetraCDD/g of product (Rappe et al., 1978a). At present, the chlorophenoxy herbicides are not the major source of PCDDs and PCDFs in the environment.

Sixteen samples of 2,4-D esters and amine salts from Canada were analyzed for the presence of PCDDs. Eight out of nine esters and four out of seven amine salts were found to be contaminated, with the esters showing significantly higher levels (210-1752 ng/g) than the salts (20-278 ng/g). The tetraCDD observed was the 1,3,6,8-isomer, as verified by a synthetically prepared authentic standard (Cochrane et al., 1981). In other studies, it has been found that no tetraCDD other than the 1,3,6,8-isomer elutes in this window. Hagenmaier et al. (1986) has reported that, unexpectedly, a German 2,4-D formulation contained 6.8 ng of 2,3,7,8-tetraCDD/g.

3.3.2 Hexachlorophene

The bactericide hexachlorophene is prepared from 2,4,5-trichlorophenol, also the key intermediate in the production of 2,4,5-T. Due to additional purification, the level of 2,3,7,8-tetraCDD in this product is usually < 0.03 mg/kg (Baughman, 1974). Ligon & May (1986) reported 0.0047 mg/kg of TCDD in one hexachlorophene sample. However, hexachlorophene also contains about 100 mg/kg of a hexachloroxanthene, the 1,2,4,6,8,9-substituted isomer (Göthe & Wachtmeister, 1972).

3.3.3 Chlorophenols

Chlorophenols have been used extensively since the 1950s as insecticides, fungicides, mold inhibitors, antiseptics, and disinfectants. In 1978 the annual world production was estimated to be approximately 200 000 tons. The most important use of 2,4,6-tri-, 2,3,4,6-tetra-, and pentachlorophenol, and their salts, is for wood preservation. Pentachlorophenol is also used as a fungicide for slime control in the manufacture of paper pulp and for a variety of other purposes such as in cutting oils and fluids, for tanning leather, and in paint, glues, and outdoor textiles. 2,4-Di- and 2,4,5-trichlorophenol are used for the production of 2,4-D and 2,4,5-T herbicides (phenoxy acids), and 2,4,5-trichlorophenol for the production of hexachlorophene.

Chlorophenols are produced industrially either by direct chlorination of phenol or by hydrolysis of chlorobenzenes, the actual process used depending on the isomer desired. Chlorination of phenol yields 2,4-di-, 2,4,6-tri-, 2,3,4,6-tetra-, or pentachlorophenol, while hydrolysis of chlorobenzenes is mainly used for the production of 2,4,5-tri- and pentachlorophenol (Nilsson et al., 1978). Chlorophenols may contain a variety of by-products and contaminants, such as other chlorophenols, polychlorinated phenoxyphenols, and neutral compounds like polychlorinated benzene and diphenyl ethers (PCDPEs), PCDDs, and PCDFs. Some of these contaminants may also occur in chlorophenol derivatives like phenoxy acids, other pesticides, and hexachlorophene. The possible presence of PCDDs and PCDFs in commercial products is of special significance because of their extraordinary persistence and toxicological properties (see sections 7-9). A scientific criteria document for chlorophenols and their impurities in the Canadian environment has been prepared by Jones (1981, 1984). Chlorophenols were estimated to be the major chemical sources of PCDDs and PCDFs in the Canadian environment (Sheffield, 1985).

Buser & Bosshardt (1976) reported on the results of a survey of the PCDD and PCDF contents of pentachlorophenol (PCP) and PCP-Na from commercial sources in Switzerland. From the results, a grouping of the samples into two series can be observed: a first series with generally low levels (hexaCDD <1 μg/g) and a second series with much higher levels (hexaCDD >1 μg/g) of PCDDs and PCDFs. Samples with high PCDD values had also high PCDF values. For most samples, the contents of the PCDF contaminants were in the order:

tetra- = penta- < hexa- < hepta- < octaCDD/CDF.

The ranges of the combined levels of PCDDs and PCDFs were 2-16 and 1-26 μg/g, respectively, for the first series of samples, and 120-500 and 85-570 μg/g, respectively, for the second series of samples. The levels of octaCDD and octaCDF were as high as 370 and 300 μg/g, respectively.

Some PCP-Na samples analyzed showed the unexpected presence of a tetraCDD (0.05-0.25 μg/g), which was later identified by Buser & Rappe (1978) as the unusual 1,2,3,4-substituted isomer. Table 13 collects a number of relevant analyses of these chlorophenol formulations. The levels of

Table 13. Levels of PCDDs and PCDFs in commercial chlorophenols (μg/g)[a]

	2,4,6-Trichlorophenol	2,3,4,6-Tetrachlorophenol	PCP Sample A	PCP Sample B
TetraCDDs	< 0.1	< 0.1	< 0.1	< 0.1
PentaCDDs	< 0.1	< 0.1	< 0.1	< 0.1
HexaCDDs	< 1	< 1	< 1	2.5
HeptaCDDs	< 1	10	0.5	175
OctaCDD	< 1	2	4.3	500
TetraCDFs	1.5	0.5	< 0.1	< 0.1
PentaCDFs	17.5	10	< 0.1	< 0.1
HexaCDFs	36	70	0.03	< 0.3
HeptaCDFs	4.8	70	0.5	19
OctaCDF	< 1	10	1.1	25

[a] From: Rappe et al. (1979).

PCDDs and PCDFs are higher than for the phenoxy-acetic acid herbicides.

It has also been reported that several positional isomers of PCDDs and PCDFs are present in the chlorophenols. However, isomer-specific methods have not been used in most of these investigations, and more research is necessary to identify all the isomers present for a risk evaluation of these products.

Miles et al. (1985) have analyzed PCP samples for hexaCDDs from five different manufacturers using an isomer-specific analytical method. The study included both free PCPs as well as the sodium salts. Total hexaCDDs in PCPs ranged from 0.66 to 38.5 mg/kg, while in the sodium salts levels of hexaCDDs between 1.55 and 16.3 mg/kg were found. The most abundant hexaCDD isomer found in the free PCPs was the 1,2,3,6,7,8 isomer; however, in the sodium salts the 1,2,3,6,7,9- and 1,2,3,6,8,9-hexaCDD pair was the most abundant.

Hagenmaier & Brunner (1987) has reported that 2,3,7,8-tetraCDD can be found in commercial pentachlorphenol formulation at levels of 0.21-0.56 ng/g, while Hagenmeyer & Brunner (1986) report that 1,2,3,7,8-pentaCDD was found in pentachlorophenol and Na-pentachlorophenates in concentrations of 0.9-18 ng/g.

3.3.4 Polychlorinated biphenyls (PCBs)

Vos et al. (1970) were able to identify PCDFs (tetra- and pentaCDFs) in samples of European PCBs (Phenoclor DP-6 and Clophen A 60) but not in a sample of Aroclor 1260. The toxic effects of these PCB products were found to parallel the levels of PCDFs present. Bowes et al. (1975) examined a series of Aroclors, as well as the samples of Aroclor 1260, Phenoclor DP-6, and Clophen A-60 previously analyzed by Vos et al. (1970). They used packed columns and very few standard compounds, and reported that the most abundant PCDFs had the same retention time as 2,3,7,8-tetraCDF and 2,3,4,7,8-pentaCDF. Using a complete set of PCDF standards and an isomer-specific analytical method, Rappe et al. (1985d) determined the levels of 2,3,7,8-substituted PCDFs in commercial PCB products (see Table 14).

3.3.5 Chlorodiphenyl ether herbicides

In 1981, Yamagishi et al. reported on the occurrence of PCDDs and PCDFs in the commercial diphenyl ether herbicides 1,3,5-trichloro-2-(4-nitrophenoxy) benzene (CNP), 2,4-dichloro-1-(4-nitrophenoxy)benzene (NIP), and 2,4-dichloro-1-(3-methoxy-4-nitrophenoxy)benzene (X-52). The total tetraCDD found was 14.0 mg/kg in CNP, 0.38 mg/kg in NIP, and 0.03 in X-52. Very few synthetic standards were used, but the major tetraCDDs were identified as the 1,3,6,8- and 1,3,7,9-isomers, the expected impurities in the starting material 2,4,6-trichlorophenol. No 2,3,7,8-tetraCDD could be detected in these samples. In all three herbicides, total tetraCDF was between 0.3 and 0.4 mg/kg.

3.3.6 Hexachlorobenzene

Hexachlorobenzene was used for the control of wheat bunt and fungi. Villeneuve et al. (1974), analyzing three commercial hexachlorobenzene preparations, identified octaCDD and hepta- and octaCDFs. The levels and identity of the heptaCDF isomers were not given. Great variation in levels of octaCDDs between the three samples (0.05-211.9 mg/kg) was noted, as well as in the level of octaCDF (0.35-58.3 mg/kg).

3.3.7 Rice oil

In 1968 more than 1500 people in southwest Japan were intoxicated by the consumption of a commercial rice oil accidentally contaminated by PCBs, PCDFs, and polychlorinated quarterphenyls (Masuda & Yoshimura, 1982; Masuda et al., 1985). In 1979 a similar episode occurred in central Taiwan, the number of people involved here approaching 2000 (Chen et al., 1980, 1981). Both these accidents have been referred to as Yusho episodes, but now the Taiwan episode has been renamed Yu-cheng (see section 5.4.4.4).

The total level of PCDFs in the Japanese rice oil was reported to be 5 μg/g (Nagayama et al., 1976) and 5.6 μg/g

Table 14. PCDFs in commercial PCBs (ng/g)[a]

PCB-type	TRI-	TETRA-		PENTA-			HEXA-					HEPTA-
	Total	2378	Total	12348 12378	23478	Total	123479 123478	123678	123789	234678	Total	Total
Pyralene	700	53	630	10	T	35	ND	ND	ND	ND	ND	ND
A1254	63	19	1400	690	490	4000	2500	2100	190	130	10 000	960
A1260	10	13	110	48	56	260	500	120	190	27	1500	1300
A30	500	35	573	14	28	160	50	59	ND	ND	220	T
A40	1300	180	2600	96	8	1700	79	68	ND	T	310	ND
A50	7400	3300	20 000	760	1100	8000	700	360	18	98	3100	75
A60	770	840	6900	1100	990	8100	1600	330	170	330	6800	2000
T64	47	23	360	97	122	840	520	390	58	41	2600	220
Clophen C	710	54	1200	34	30	270	ND	T	ND	ND	T	ND

[a] From: Rappe et al. (1985d).
T = traces.
ND = not detected.

(Buser et al., 1978d). For the rice oil from Taiwan, Chen et al. (1985) reported the PCDFs levels to be in the range 0.18-1.68 µg/g.

Buser et al. (1978) analyzed the Japanese rice oil using glass capillary columns. They found about 50-60 PCDF congeners and also reported that the 2,3,7,8-tetraCDF was the major isomer among the tetraCDFs. However, it was later shown that in this column system the 2,3,4,8-tetraCDF co-elutes with the 2,3,7,8-isomer, and in fact the 2,3,4,8-isomer was the main constituent in this peak (Chen & Hites, 1983; Masuda et al., 1985). The 2,3,7,8-substituted congeners were estimated to account for 10-15% of the total amount of PCDFs (Buser et al., 1978).

3.4 Sources of Heavy Environmental Pollution

3.4.1 Industrial accidents

Several industrial accidents occurring during the production of 2,4,5-trichlorophenol have been described in the literature. In most of these accidents the pollution of 2,3,7,8-tetraCDD has been to factories with circumscribed occupational exposure (section 9). However, on 10 July, 1976, a runaway reaction in a factory at Meda near Seveso in Northern Italy resulted in the escape of a chemical cloud of trichlorophenol/phenate containing 2,3,7,8-tetraCDD.

The cloud initially covered an area outside the factory 5 km long and 700 m wide. On the basis of the TCDD levels found in the contaminated soil samples, it has been estimated that 2-3 kg of TCDD was released in this accident. About 80% of this amount was deposited in an area of 15 ha, within a distance of about 500 m from the plant. The levels of soil contamination in three zones are given in Table 15 (Pocchiari, 1978).

3.4.2 Improper disposal of industrial waste

In 1973, three horse arenas in Missouri, USA, were found to be contaminated by high levels of 2,3,7,8-tetraCDD; the highest value reported was about 30 µg/g of soil (Kimbrough et al., 1977). This contamination resulted from the application, in 1971, of contaminated waste oil to control dust at these locations. The TCDD had originated at a hexachlorophene-producing factory in Verona, Missouri. Additional tri- and tetraCDDs were also found, but the major component was 1,2,4,6,8,9-hexachloroxanthene, a compound which apparently can serve as a marker for this type of contamination. The xanthene is a normal by-product of hexachlorophene production and has never been associated with the production of 2,4,5-tri-

Table 15. Distribution of TCDD contamination in the Seveso area on the basis of soil sample analyses[a]

Range ($\mu g/m^2$)	Number of soil samples		
	Zone A	Zone B	Surrounding monitored area
< 0.750	32	25	249
0.750 - 4.99	32	53	128
5.0 - 14.99	6	19	2
15.0 - 49.99	18	6	0
50.0 - 499.99	31	0	0
500.0 - 4999.99	18	0	0
> 5000	3	0	0

[a] From: Pocchiari (1978).
Zone A: high-level contamination, about 115 ha.
Zone B: low level contamination, about 255 ha.
Surrounding area: about 1400 ha.

chlorophenol or 2,4,5-T derivatives (Viswanathan & Kloepfer, 1986).

In 1982, numerous sites of potential 2,3,7,8-tetraCDD contamination were discovered in eastern Missouri. The contamination originated from the same waste oil from the factory in Verona. The streets of the entire town of Times Beach, Missouri, had been sprayed. More than 10 000 soil samples from Missouri were analyzed. In this state more than 40 hazardous waste sites containing 2,3,7,8-tetraCDD were identified. Most of these contaminated sites resulted from the disposal of waste from the same factory in Verona. The highest level reported in these soil samples was 9648 µg TCDD/g (Viswanathan & Kloepfer, 1986).

Another location of great concern is Love Canal, Niagara Falls, USA. Here, Smith et al. (1983) found high levels of 2,3,7,8-tetraCDD in storm sewer sediments taken from around the Love Canal waste disposal site. The highest value was 312 ng/g sediment.

3.4.3 Heavy use of chemicals

The Eglin Air Force Base in Northwest Florida, USA, has been used for the development and testing of aerial spraying equipment for military defoliation operations. During the period 1962-1970, a 3-km^2 test area was sprayed with 73 tons of 2,4,5-T. Analyses of archived samples of the formulations indicated that approximately 2.8 kg of 2,3,7,8-tetraCDD had been applied as a contaminant of the herbicide. However, one 37-ha test grid received 2.6 kg of this TCDD from 1962 to 1964. Levels of 10-1500 ng/kg were found in 22 soil samples (the top 15 cm) collected and analyzed 14 years after the last application of herbicide to this site (Young, 1983).

3.5 Other Sources of PCDDs and PCDFs in the Environment

3.5.1 Thermal degradation of technical products

The formation of 2,3,7,8-tetraCDD as a result of thermal reactions of 2,4,5-T and 2,4,5-T derivatives has been the subject of controversy. Heating 2,4,5-T salts at 400-450 °C for 30 minutes or longer yielded approximately 1 g of 2,3,7,8-tetraCDD per kg of 2,4,5-T salt, while no TCDD was identified from the same treatment of 2,4,5-T acid or esters (Langer et al., 1973; Baughman, 1974). Using a more sensitive analytical method, Ahling et al. (1977) reported that 0.2-3 mg of 2,3,7,8-tetraCDD was formed per kg of 2,4,5-T esters during combustion at 500-850 °C. Two reports (Stehl & Lamparski, 1977; Andersson et al., 1978) have shown that 2,3,7,8-tetraCDD could not be found after burning samples of spiked or sprayed vegetation at 600 °C. The combustion gases, soot, particles, and ashes were analyzed and the detection limit was 4 mg of TCDD/kg 2,4,5-T burned.

Rappe (1978b) have studied the burning of material impregnated with various salts of chlorophenols. Very carefully purified 2,4,6-tri- and pentachlorophenate were studied, in addition to a commercial formulation of 2,3,4,6-tetrachlorophenate. The analytical method used in this study was not isomer specific, but the following conclusions can be drawn concerning the formation of PCDDs by thermal reactions:

(a) the expected dimerization products and the products formed in the "Smiles rearrangement" are the major PCDDs;
(b) no other thermal isomerization of the PCDDs formed can be observed;
(c) no formation of higher chlorinated PCDDs can be observed;
(d) octaCDD and other higher chlorinated PCDDs yield lower chlorinated dioxins in a nonspecific dechlorination reaction;
(e) a series of PCDFs was also observed.

It has been found that PCBs can be converted to PCDFs under pyrolytic conditions. The pyrolysis of commercial PCBs in sealed quartz ampoules in the presence of air yielded about 30 major, and more than 30 minor, PCDFs. The optimal yield of PCDFs was about 10%, calculated on the amount of PCB decomposed. Thus, uncontrolled burning of PCBs can be an important environmental source of hazardous PCDFs. Therefore, it was recommended (Buser et al., 1978a, 1978d) that all destruction of PCB-contaminated waste using incinerators must be carefully controlled. In the temperature range 300-400 °C, the conversion yield seems to be in the part-per-million range (Morita et al., 1978).

Buser & Rappe (1979) studied the pyrolysis of 15 individual synthetic PCB congeners and showed that the formation of PCDFs can follow several competing reaction pathways. In another study where a series of chlorobenzenes were pyrolyzed in the same way, Buser (1979) found that significant amounts (> 1%) of PCDDs and PCDFs were formed. A complex mixture of isomers of PCDDs and PCDFs was found, suggesting several reaction routes. Using the same technique as above, Lindahl et al. (1980) studied the thermal decomposition of polychlorinated diphenyl ethers. Both PCDDs and PCDFs were formed, involving several pathways. The temperature range was 500-600 °C and the yields varied from 0.1 to 4.5%.

Bergman et al. (1984) studied the thermal degradation of two polychlorinated alkanes containing 59% and 70% chlorine, respectively, and also a commercial chlorinated paraffin containing 70% chlorine. Their studies indicated the presence of at least mono- and diCDFs.

Ahling et al. (1978) reported that chlorinated benzenes can be found in the pyrolysis of PVC.

Direct evidence for the conversion of PVC to PCDDs and PCDFs has recently been reported by Marklund et al. (1986). They found that laboratory pyrolysis of PVC resulted in the formation of PCDDs and PCDFs, mainly hexa- and heptaCDDs, and tetra- to heptaCDFs. In some cases, the pattern of isomers seemed to be similar to those found in municipal and hazardous waste incinerators, e.g. the pentaCDFs (Rappe et al., 1987).

The data discussed in this section are summarized in Table 16.

3.5.2 Incineration of municipal waste

For some time, emissions from municipal incinerators, heating facilities, and thermal power plants have been the subject of concern. Whereas previously the emission of dust, smoke, toxic metals, and noxious gases were of prime concern, the presence of potentially hazardous organic compounds from these emissions has been recognized only recently. Lahaniatis et al. (1977) reported the presence of chlorinated organic compounds (chlorinated aliphatics, benzenes, PCBs, and pesticides) in fly ash from a municipal incinerator.

Table 16. Formation of PCDDs and PCDFs by thermal processes

Precursor	Conditions	Products
2,4,5-T salt	Pyrolysis	2,3,7,8-tetraCDD
2,4,5-T (vegetation)	Pyrolysis	No TCDD
	Burning	No TCDD
Cl-phenate	Burning	PCDDs[a] + PCDFs
PCBs	Pyrolysis	PCDFs[b]
PCBz[c]	Pyrolysis	PCDFs + PCDDs[d]
Cl-Diphenyl ethers	Pyrolysis	PCDFs + PCDDs
Cl-Alkanes (Paraffins)	Pyrolysis	PCDFs
PVC	Pyrolysis	PCDDs + PCDFs

a = PCDDs formed by dimerization and a non-specific dechlorination.
b = other products: hexa- and pentaCBs.
c = polychlorinated benzenes.
d = other products: PCBs, polychlorinated naphthalenes.

Olie et al. (1977) reported the occurrence of PCDDs and PCDFs in fly ash from three municipal incinerators in the Netherlands. Their results indicated the presence of up to 17 PCDD peaks, but isomer identification and quantification was not possible due to the lack of synthetic standards. Buser & Bosshardt (1978) studied fly ash from a municipal incinerator and an industrial heating facility, both in Switzerland. In the former, the level of PCDDs was 0.2 µg/g and of PCDFs 0.1 µg/g. In the industrial incinerator, the levels were 0.6 µg/g and 0.3 µg/g, respectively.

During the period 1978-1982 a series of papers, reports, and reviews were published confirming the original findings of Olie et al. (1977) and Buser & Bosshardt (1978) regarding fly ash. Less data have been published on the levels of PCDDs and PCDFs in other incineration by-products, e.g., particulates and flue gas condensate, and in total flue gas, which are the true emissions (Marklund et al., 1986).

A risk evaluation should be based on the emission levels of PCDD and PCDF isomers found in isomer-specific analyses using validated sampling and clean-up methods. However, in many studies non-validated sampling and analytical methods are used and the results are given in terms of total levels of tetra-, penta-, hexa-, hepta-, and octaCDDs and CDFs. The value of such studies is limited, particularly in this situation where the number of isomers is quite large. More than 30 PCDDs and 60 PCDFs have been found in fly ash samples (Buser et al., 1978b, 1978c).

In March 1986, a working group of experts convened by the World Health Organization Regional Office for Europe reviewed the available data on emissions of PCDDs and PCDFs from municipal solid-waste (MSW) incinerators. It was found that the origin of these compounds was not completely understood, but they appear to result from complex thermal reactions occurring during periods of poor combustion. Because of their high thermal stability, the PCDDs and PCDFs can be destroyed only after adequate residence times at temperatures above 800 °C (WHO/EURO, 1987).

Available data on total emissions of PCDDs and PCDFs from tests on MSW incinerators range between a few and several thousand ng/Nm^3 dry gas at 10% carbon dioxide (CO_2). The working group prepared a table giving a range of estimated isomer specific emissions for those isomers of major concern with respect to MSW incinerators operating under various conditions (Table 17).

The emissions tabulated in column 1 are those which the working group considered to be achievable in the most modern, highly controlled, and carefully operated plants in use at the present time. Such results do not represent what is considered to be achievable by the use of acid gas cleaning equipment; use of such equipment should result in much lower values (probably at least one order of magnitude). The results given in column 1 are not representative of emissions that might be expected from such plants during start-up or during occasional abnormal conditions. Emission levels listed in column 2 were considered by the working group to be indicative of the higher limit of emissions from modern MSW incinerators. These plants might experience such emissions during start-up or during occasional upset conditions. Consequently, the majority of the available concentration data falls between columns 1 and 2. Some of the data reviewed has shown that the figures in column 2 should not be considered an absolute maximum. However, most existing plants, if carefully operated, will have PCDD and PCDF emissions in the range between columns 1 and 2.

The highest values for MSW incinerators (column 3) were obtained by multiplying the values in column 2 by a factor of 5. Column 3 includes emission data that were reported to the working group from all tests and under all circumstances. Generally, these emission levels are associated with irregular or unstable operating conditions, high moisture content of the MSW, low combustion or afterburner temperatures, less than adequate technologies, etc.

The working group was aware of both lower and higher emission levels than those included in Table 17. However, it was felt that the values included in Table 17 were likely to be representative of emissions from current facilities (WHO/EURO, 1987).

Table 17. Estimated range of emissions from municipal solid waste (MSW) and municipal sewage sludge (MSS) incinerators[a]

Congeners	Emissions from MSW combustion			Emissions from MSS combustion
	1 Achievable with modern plants with no acid gas cleaning	2 Maximum from average operation	3 High emissions	4 Most likely highest emissions
	(ng/Nm^3, dry, at 10% CO_2)			
2, 3, 7, 8-TetraCDD	0.1	1.5	7.5	0.1
1, 2, 3, 7, 8-PentaCDD	0.3	14	70	0.3
1, 2, 3, 4, 7, 8-HexaCDD	0.2	31	155	0.2
1, 2, 3, 6, 7, 8-HexaCDD	0.6	56	280	0.6
1, 2, 3, 7, 8, 9-HexaCDD	0.4	20	100	0.4
2, 3, 7, 8-TetraCDF	0.9	10	50	0.9
1, 2, 3, 7, 8-/1, 2, 3, 4, 8-PentaCDF	2.3	52	260	2.3
2, 3, 4, 7, 8-PentaCDF	2.0	40	200	2.0
1, 2, 3, 4, 7, 8/1, 2, 3, 4, 7, 9-HexaCDF	1.1	48	240	1.1
1, 2, 3, 6, 7, 8-HexaCDF	1.3	40	200	1.3
1, 2, 3, 7, 8, 9-HexaCDF	0.06	52	260	0.06
2, 3, 4, 6, 7, 8-HexaCDF	2.0	36	180	2.0

[a] From: WHO/EURO (1987).

Of special importance is the observation that the emission of 1,2,3,7,8-pentaCDD normally exceeds the emission of 2,3,7,8-tetraCDD by a factor of three to ten.

3.5.3 Incineration of sewage sludge

Sludge from municipal waste water treatment plants may be incinerated after being dewatered. The WHO working group (see 3.5.2) reviewed the available data from municipal sewage sludge (MSS) incinerators, and found that PCDD and PCDF emissions from this type of plant were generally lower than emissions from MSW incinerators (see Table 17, column 4) (WHO, 1986).

3.5.4 Incineration of hospital waste

Doyle et al. (1985) claimed that the incomplete combustion of certain hospital waste containing halogenated organics could produce high levels of PCDDs and PCDFs. They found the mean values of total PCDDs to be 69 ng/m^3 and total PCDFs to be 156 ng/m^3. No isomer-specific data seems to be available. Hagenmaier et al. (1986) reported the analyses of stack gas from 10 hospital waste incineration plants. The mean value of 2,3,7,8-tetraCCD emitted was 0.28 ng/m^3, the mean of all TCDDs being 20 ng/m^3. The mean value for total PCDDs was 118 ng/m^3 and for total PCDFs 434 ng/m^3.

3.5.5 Incineration of hazardous waste

Analyses from a test burn of pentachlorophenol waste have been reported by Rappe et al. (1983c). PCP is a well known precursor to octaCDD (section 2). Samples of baghouse ash and bottom ash were analyzed. In the baghouse ash the total level of octaCDD was only 0.2 µg/g. The major constituents were lower chlorinated PCDDs such as hepta-, hexa-, penta , and tetraCDDs. The isomeric distribution was reported to be very similar to a "normal" fly ash. In both cases 2,3,7,8-tetraCDD was a very minor constituent. The level of PCDD in the bottom ash was 0.31 µg/g. The baghouse ash was also reported to contain PCDFs at a total level of 2.5 µg/g. For the tetra- and penta chlorinated compounds, equal amounts of PCDDs and PCDFs were reported.

Oberg & Bergstrém (1986) reported on test data from a Swedish hazardous waste incinerator equipped with a rotary kiln, an afterburner, and a dry scrubbing unit. Combustion tests were performed with PCB (Aroclor 1242) as a fluid, and as a contaminant in solid waste (Aroclor 1016 in capacitors). The results of these tests indicated no correlation between the amount of PCB incinerated and the amount of PCDDs and PCDFs found in the emissions.

3.5.6 Metal industry and metal treatment industry

It has been reported by Marklund et al. (1986) that industrial high-temperature processes like copper smelters and electric arc furnaces in steel mills have been identified as sources of environmental contamination by PCDDs and PCDFs. The results are reported in "TCDD equivalents" according to US EPA (1987). The emission from the copper smelter contained 11 ng of TCDD equivalents/Nm^3 dry gas and 10% CO_2, while the dust from the steel mill contained 0.8 ng TCDD equivalents/g dust. Marklund et al. (1986) also considered the emissions from industrial incinerators to be of the same magnitude, or even higher, than the emissions from MSW incinerators.

Southerland et al. (1987) analyzed emissions from various incinerators within Tier 4 of the USA. The highest levels were found in a secondary copper smelter, which contained 170 ng of 2,3,7,8-tetraCDD/Nm^3 and 3% oxygen. This was by far the highest level found within the US EPA National Dioxin Strategy.

3.5.7 Wire reclamation

Hryhorczuk et al. (1981) studied a wire reclamation incinerator in the USA. Using a non-isomer-specific analytical method, they determined total levels of tetraCDDs and tetraCDFs. Two samples were analyzed, one from the furnace and one from the stack. The furnace sample contained 58 ng/kg of total TCDDs and 730 ng/kg of total TCDFs, whereas the stack sample contained 410 ng/kg of total TCDDs and 11 600 ng/kg of total TCDFs.

3.5.8 Traffic

Marklund et al. (1987) reported a study where automobile exhaust emissions were analyzed for PCDDs and PCDFs. Two groups of test cars were utilized: (1) cars equipped with a catalytic converter using unleaded gasoline with no halogenated scavengers; (2) cars with no catalytic converter using leaded gasoline (0.15 g/litre) and a dichloroethane scavenger (0.1 g/litre). Before the test runs, the motor oil was changed in all cars. No PCDDs and PCDFs could be identifed in the cars using the unleaded gasoline, while the average emission from the cars running on leaded gasoline was found to be 30-540 pg/kg of TCDD equivalents. It was assumed that the chlorinated scavenger (dichloroethane) was the precursor of the PCDDs and PCDFs formed. It was estimated that the total amount of PCDDs and PCDFs from cars in Sweden using leaded gasoline with halogenated scavengers is in the range of 10-100 g TCDD equivalents/year.

3.5.9 Fires and accidents in PCB-filled electrical equipment

In February 1981 a fire in the State Office Building in Binghamton, New York, USA, caused a transformer to rupture, releasing soot throughout the building. The dielectric fluid in the transformer consisted of a mixture of PCB (65%) and chlorinated benzenes (35%). The soot was found to be highly contaminated with PCDFs (total PCDFs > 2000 µg/g). The most toxic isomers (2,3,7,8-tetraCDF; 1,2,3,7,8- and 2,3,4,7,8-pentaCDF; and 1,2,3,4,7,8- and 1,2,3,6,7,8-hexaCDF) were found to be the major constituents within each group of congeners. Levels reported were 12 mg/g of 2,3,7,8-tetra CDF, 670 mg/g of total penta-CDFs, and 965 mg/g of total hexa-CDFs, 46 mg/g of total hepta-CDFs, and 460 mg/g of octa-CDFs (Rappe, 1984; Rappe et al., 1985b). In addition, a series of PCDDs were identified, including the highly toxic 2,3,7,8-tetraCDD, and 1,2,3,7,8-pentaCDD (Rappe et al., 1983a; Buser & Rappe, 1984). It is assumed that the chlorinated benzenes were the dioxin precursors.

Between 1981 and 1985, a series of transformer accidents (7 in all) similar to the one in Binghamton were reported in the USA and Canada (Rappe et al., 1986a). In January 1985, an explosion followed by a fire ruptured a transformer in the basement of a residential complex in Rheims, France. The transformer was filled with PCB (60%) and trichlorobenzene (40%). Total levels of PCDFs were as high as 2570 $\mu g/m^2$ before clean-up. Only traces of hepta- and octaCDD were found (Rappe et al., 1985a).

In Europe, between 1981 and 1985, 19 accidents involving indoor capacitor fires and explosions were reported from Scandinavian countries (Rappe et al., 1986a). All capacitors were mineral oil filled, and contamination of the sites averaged 1-5 µg total $PCDFs/m^2$.

3.5.10 Pulp and paper industry

Large amounts of chlorine or chlorine compounds are used in the pulp and paper industry for the bleaching of the pulp. Three black liquor boilers from the craft paper process were included in the US EPA study of combustion sources. No 2,3,7,8-tetraCDD was found in these emissions, but low levels of other PCDDs and PCDFs were found in one of the three incinerators and a yearly emission of 0.25 g was calculated (Southerland et al., 1987).

Rappe et al. (1987) recently identified both 2,3,7,8-tetraCDD (170 ng/kg) and 2,3,7,8-tetraCDF (890 ng/kg) in a sample taken in a sedimentation lagoon at a Swedish paper mill. A series of other PCDDs and PCDFs was also identified but at lower levels. The isomeric pattern in this sample differed markedly from other sediment samples, indicating pulping processes to be a source of environmental pollution by 2,3,7,8-tetraCDD and 2,3,7,8-tetraCDF (Rappe et al., 1987).

3.5.11 Incineration of coal, peat, and wood

The emissions of PCDDs and PCDFs from coal-fired power plants (Kimble & Gross 1980), wood stoves (Clement et al., 1985), and peat burning (Marklund et al., 1986) seem to be very low when calculated per m^3. However, the very high flow rates and the large number of units could make a significant total contribution. The occurrence of pentaCDDs and all PCDFs was not discussed in this report.

3.5.12 Inorganic chlorine precursors

It is well known that certain organochlorine compounds are efficient precursors to PCDDs and PCDFs during pyrolysis. However, it was proposed by scientists from Dow Chemical Company that PCDDs, and especially 2,3,7,8-tetraCDD, are ubiquitous and formed as trace level by-products of any normal combustion (Bumb et al., 1980). Consequently, dioxins should have been present in the environment since the advent of fire. This suggests that inorganic chloride can serve as a useful precursor to the formation of PCDDs and PCDFs. A recent survey of PCDD levels, in particular from residential wood combustion units, has been quoted in support of the above. The survey showed PCDD levels in the ng/kg range (see also section 3.5.11). However, this hypothesis has been criticized. One of the main arguments against such a hypothesis is that 2,3,7,8-tetraCDD does not appear to be formed in coal-fired power plants (Kimble & Gross, 1980; Junk & Richard, 1981). Another argument is that the Dow studies lack data on levels of dioxin precursors in the material being burned, including the air in the flames (Rappe, 1984).

The analyses of historical samples gives additional support to the theory that organochlorine compounds are more important as precursors than inorganic chloride. When Czuczwa & Hites (1985) analyzed sediment core samples from Lake Huron, N. America, the first indication of PCDDs and PCDFs was found in sediments from 1940. There was also a good correlation between the trend in the levels of PCDDs and PCDFs in these sediments and the trend in the production of chlorinated aromatic compounds (section 5.4).

Schecter et al. (1986a) were unable to detect PCDDs and PCDFs in human liver and lung tissue from two female Eskimos frozen over one hundred years ago (see also section 4.4.4).

3.5.13 Photochemical processes

Sundström et al. (1979) studied the formation of 2,3,7,8-tetraCDD in six re-forestation areas that were sprayed with 2,4,5-T esters. Leaf samples from the areas were analyzed for 2,4,5-T esters and TCDD. TCDD was found in one leaf sample only, at levels lower than expected from the level of dioxin contamination of the herbicide formulations used.

The photochemical formation of PCDDs and PCDFs has also been studied in laboratory experiments.

The photochemical dimerization of chlorophenols to PCDDs was studied by Crosby & Wong (1976). The only PCDD formed in this study was the octaCDD. Other PCDDs can be formed by photochemical cyclization of chlorinated o-phenoxyphenols, also called pre-dioxins (Nilsson et al., 1974). These pre-dioxins are very common impurities (1-5%) in commercial chlorophenols (Nilsson et al., 1978), but the cyclization is only a minor reaction pathway; the main reaction being the dechlorination of the pre-dioxin.

Akermark (1978) studied the formation of 2,3,7,8-tetraCDD from the appropriate pre-dioxins. He could identify the product, but claimed the reaction to be very inefficient.

Another photochemical process of potential environmental importance is dechlorination of the higher chlorinated PCDDs and PCDFs, e.g., octaCDD and octaCDF. The products formed by photolysis of octaCDD in organic solvent have now been identified (Buser & Rappe, 1978). By comparison with authentic standards, it was found that the main tetrachloro isomer was the 1,4,6,9-tetraCDD; the major pentachloro compound was expected to be the 1,2,4,6,9-isomer, and the main hexa- and heptachloro compounds were the 1,2,4,6,7,9- (or 1,2,4,6,8,9-) and the 1,2,3,4,6,7,9-isomers, respectively. The reaction scheme deduced from this data indicates that the chlorine atoms are removed preferentially from the lateral positions on the carbon rings. Consequently, the most toxic PCDD isomers, such as 2,3,7,8-tetraCDD, are not likely to be formed from the photolysis of the higher PCDDs in solution.

Crosby et al. (1973) studied the photolysis of a series of PCBs dispersed in water. For two isomers, the 2,5-dichloro- and 2,2',5,5'-tetrachlorobiphenyls, small amounts (0.2%) of 2-mono-CDF could be found among the products (for photochemical transformations, see section 4.2.1).

3.6 Comparison of Isomeric Pattern and Congener Profiles From Various Sources

There is a pronounced difference between technical products and incineration emissions in both isomeric patterns and congener profiles of PCDDs and PCDFs. In technical products the number of isomers present is limited, whereas in incineration emissions most isomers seem to be present. Rappe (1987) has pointed out the large similarity qualitatively in isomeric patterns between different incineration sources.

4. ENVIRONMENTAL TRANSPORT, DISTRIBUTION, AND TRANSFORMATIONS

4.1 Environmental Transport

4.1.1 Air

The PCDDs and PCDFs are believed to be transported in the atmosphere. The transport of these compounds from stacks and other stationary point sources, as well as from waste disposal sites and other area sources, can be predicted from dispersion modelling (SAI, 1980). In the case of the accidental release of a toxic cloud containing 2,3,7,8-tetraCDD at Seveso, Italy, Cavallaro et al. (1982) determined the transport pattern and the ground deposition. They determined that the deposition of 2,3,7-8-tetraCDD from air to soil should follow an exponential decay pattern in the Gaussian-distribution along the cross-section of the downwind direction. Thibodeaux (1983) studied the air transport of 2,3,7,8-tetraCDD at a herbicide production facility in Jacksonville, Arkansas, USA.

The dispersion modelling has limitations. If possible, the modelling calculations should be combined with true air measurements.

4.1.2 Water

The solubility of 2,3,7,8-tetraCDD in water has been extensively studied (see section 2), but much less data are available for the other PCDDs and PCDFs. However, data from microbiological experiments indicate that 2,3,7,8-tetraCDD is highly adsorbed to sediments and biota. Matsumura et al. (1983) suggested that more than 90% of the 2,3,7,8-tetraCDD in an aquatic medium could be present in the adsorbed state. Rappe et al. (1985c) studied a suspension of soot/dust in the wash water from a PCB fire. The suspension contained 100 ng/ml of various PCDFs, but when the soot was settled the water contained no detectable levels of PCDFs (detection level: 0.1 ng/ml of each isomer). Most of the PCDDs and PCDFs, if present in waterways, should be in the sediments or attached to suspended particles.

Thibodeaux (1983) has calculated the amount of 2,3,7,8-tetraCDD transported by a creek within the contaminated herbicide factory in Jacksonville, Arkansas, USA. The value was 0.89 g/year as an average rate, and a maximum of 2.1 g/year.

4.1.3 Soil and sediments

The mobility of 2,3,7,8-tetraCDD and of a dichlorodioxin in soils has been studied by Helling et al. (1973). Both were found to be immobile in all soils and, therefore, would not be leached out by rainfall or irrigation, though lateral transport during surface erosion of the soil could occur.

The US Air Force conducted studies in an area of north west Florida that had been heavily sprayed with the herbicide Agent Orange between 1962 and 1964 (Young et al., 1975). This herbicide mixture was contaminated with TCDD (section 3.2). A 7.8-ha test grid received a total of 40 metric tons of 2,4,5-T between 1962 and 1964. When 15-cm soil core samples were taken in 1974, they showed TCDD concentrations ranging from 10 to 710 ng/kg. This study illustrates that significant levels of TCDD residues remained 10 years after the last herbicide application. Similar TCDD concentrations were obtained from areas that had been sprayed between 1962 and 1969 (Bartelson et al., 1975).

In another study Young (1983) measured the concentration of 2,3,7,8-tetraCDD in a soil profile. The samples were collected in 1974 and the data suggested that most of the 2,3,7,8-tetraCDD would be found in the top 15 cm of the soil profile (Table 18).

Table 18. Concentration of 2,3,7,8-tetraCDD in a soil profile[a,b]

Depth (cm)	2,3,7,8-tetraCDD (ng/kg)
0 - 2.5	150
2.5 - 5.0	160
5.0 - 10	700
10 - 15	44
15 - 90	ND[c]

[a] From: Young (1983).
[b] The area received 1,069 kg/ha of 2,4,5-T Agent Orange during 1962-1964. The soil samples were collected and analyzed in 1974.
[c] None detected (minimum detection limit: 10 ng/kg).

The probable media and modes of transport of PCDDs from soils are the following: (1) to air via contaminated airborne dust particles; (2) to surface water via eroded soil transported by water; (3) to groundwater via leaching; (4) to air via volatilization. Movement of particulate matter containing adsorbed PCDDs and PCDFs has been considered to be a much more important transport mechanism than leaching and volatilization because of the low water solubility and volatility of these compounds (Josephson, 1983). However, the monitoring of Seveso soil one year after the accident showed that the highest 2,3,7,8-tetraCDD levels were not present in the topmost soil layer (0.5 cm), but very often in the second (0.5-1.0 cm) or third (1.0-1.5 cm) layers. This disappearance of at least a part of the 2,3,7,8-tetraCDD from the topmost soil layer was speculated to be due to volatilization or vertical movement through the soil (DiDomenico et al., 1980). Therefore, it appears that volatilization from soil and leaching to groundwater can be responsible for the transport of PCDDs and PCDFs from soils under certain conditions, namely, heavy rainfall on sandy soils. Studies by Young (1983) indicate that the half-life for 2,3,7,8-tetraCDD in soil is 10-12 years.

Thibodeaux (1983) has calculated the vaporization of 2,3,7,8-tetraCDD from a herbicide plant in Jacksonville, Arkansas, USA. The vaporization can take place from soil surfaces, from landfill cells, and from the surface of a pond. In Table 19 a summary of yearly emission rates from these sources is presented.

Table 19. Surface source areas and emission rates of 2,3,7,8-tetraCDD[a]

Source	Area (m^2)	Emission rate (g/year)
Blow-out area, volatilization	753	120-1200
Blow-out area, entrainment	753	28-37
Rocky Branch Creek, dissolved		0.89-2.1
Reasor-Hill dump	1129	0.1-1.0
Rocky Branch Creek, sediment		0.094-0.22
Cooling water pond	15050	0.015-0.016
Total		150-1240

[a] From: Thibodeaux (1983).

It was found that vaporization from the soil surface in the highly contaminated blow out area was the major contributing source of emissions from this plant.

Freeman et al. (1986) have developed a model to describe the vaporization and diffusion through a column of soil of low volatility organic chemicals like PCDDs and PCDFs. This model has been used to make predictions on the transport of 2,3,7,8-tetraCDD at a site in Times Beach, Missouri, USA. The model predicted that the 1983 levels in this soil would be only 10% of the original loading. The model also predicted that 57% of the initial amount of 2,3,7,8-tetraCDD was vaporized through the soil column to the surface in the first year after the spraying and that most transport of the vapour occurred during the summer months. The same results were also obtained in studies reported by Facchetti et al. (1986) and Palausky et al. (1986).

4.2 Environmental Transformation

4.2.1 Abiotic transformation

Like other PCDDs and PCDFs, 2,3,7,8-tetraCDD is chemically quite stable, and is not likely to be degraded at a significant rate by hydrolytic reactions under environmental conditions. Under these conditions, TCDD seems also to be rather stable to photochemical degradation (Crosby et al., 1971). The half-life of TCDD of about 10-12 years, as found by Young et al. (1983) for soil, is in agreement with this observation.

However, three reports on rapid photochemical degradation of 2,3,7,8-tetraCDD under experimental conditions make the situation more complicated. In a methanol solution, TCDD is fairly easily degraded by photolysis in the laboratory (Crosby et al., 1971). Other studies using 2,4,5-T ester formulations with known amounts of TCDD and exposed to natural sunlight on leaves, soil, or glass plates showed that most of the TCDD was lost during a single day (Crosby & Wong, 1977). In these two studies, a "hydrogen donor", such as methanol or 2,4,5-T ester, enhanced the photochemical dechlorination (Akermark, 1978); they do not therefore truly reflect environmental conditions, where the 2,4,5-T ester would be rapidly hydrolyzed on the surface of the leaves. At Seveso the TCDD was released together with salts of 2,4,5-trichlorophenol, ethylene glycol, and inorganic constituents (Rappe, 1978b). Like water, none of these is a potent hydrogen donor.

According to Bertoni et al. (1978), the addition of a solution of ethyl oleate in xylene enhances the breakdown of TCDD in soil by UV light. Similarly, a cationic surfactant, 1-hexadecylpyridinium chloride, was also reported to enhance photodecomposition (Botre et al., 1978).

Another experiment, which might be a good model for the degradation of TCDD bound to dust particles in the air, has shown that TCDD adsorbed on silica gel undergoes rapid photochemical degradation (Gebefugi et al., 1977).

In order to explain the longer half-life of 2,3,7,8-tetraCDD in a model laboratory ecosystem than in an outdoor pond, Matsumura et al. (1983) speculated that photolysis was the most likely cause. In the outdoor environment, algae-mediated photosensitization of 2,3,7,8-tetra-CDD may have caused some photodecomposition of this compound.

An increase in chlorine substitution is expected to decrease the rate of photodegradation. For example, Crosby et al. (1971) showed that although complete decompostion of 2,3,7,8-tetraCDD in methanol occurred in 24 h under UV irradiation, > 80% octaCDD in methanol remained unreacted during the same period under similar irradiation conditions.

Although the degree of photolysis may be related to the extent of chlorination, different chlorine substitution patterns also play a critical part. In higher chlorinated PCDDs, there appears to be preferential loss of chlorine from the 2,3,7, and 8 positions (Buser & Rappe, 1978). Thus, PCDDs with chlorine substitutions in positions 2,3,7, and 8 are likely to be photochemically degraded faster than compounds not having these positions substituted. For example, the photolysis half-life of 1,2,3,7,8-pentaCDD has been estimated to be 7.8 h in n-hexadecane solution under sunlamp irradiation (Nestrick et al., 1980). Similarly, the photolytic half-lives of 1,2,3,7,8-pentaCDD, 1,2,3,6,7,9-, and 1,2,4,6,7,9-hexaCDD in hexane solutions under sunlight irradiation have been determined to be 5.4, 17, and 47 hours, respectively (Dobles & Grant, 1979). Nestrick et al. (1980) reported a half-life value of 6.8 h for 1,2,3,6,7,8-hexaCDD in n-hexadecane under sunlamp irradiation. The primary intermediates of the photodegradation of higher chlorinated PCDDs are probably lower chlorinated dioxins (Buser & Rappe, 1978), but the pathways of degradation are not known with certainty (National Research Council of Canada, 1981).

From these discussions of the photolysis of PCDDs in the presence of organic hydrogen-donating substrates, it is difficult to predict the photolytic fate of these compounds in natural aquatic media, where hydrogen donors may or may not be available. The situation is complicated further by the fact that a predominant amount of PCDDs in surface water may be adsorbed or suspended on particles and sediments, rather than in solution. Moreover, since the penetration of UV light into natural water may be very limited, photolytic degradation of PCDDs in water is not likely to be of environmental importance.

Hutzinger et al. (1973) have studied the photochemical degradation of 2,8-diCDF and octaCDF. They found that a reductive dechlorination takes place, especially in methanolic solution. The reaction was much slower when a thin film was exposed to sunlight.

Thermally, 2,3,7,8-tetraCDD is quite stable, rapid decomposition occurring only at temperatures above 750 °C (Stehl et al., 1973).

4.2.2 Biotransformation and biodegradation

The 2,3,7,8-tetraCDD isomer is very resistant to biodegradation. Only 5 of about 100 microbial strains with the ability to degrade persistent pesticides were able to degrade 2,3,7,8-tetraCDD (Matsumura & Benezet, 1973). Ward & Matsumura (1978) studied the biodegradation of ^{14}C-labelled 2,3,7,8-tetraCDD in lake waters and sediments from Wisconsin, USA, and observed a half-life of 2,3,7,8-tetraCDD in lake waters containing sediment of 550-590 days. In lake water alone, about 70% of the 2,3,7,8-tetraCDD remained after 589 days. Using an outdoor pond as a model aquatic ecosystem, and dosing it with ^{14}C-labelled 2,3,7,8-tetraCDD, Matsumura et al. (1983) estimated the half-life of 2,3,7,8-tetraCDD to be approximately 1 year. Although biodegradation may have been responsible for part of the degradation, it is almost impossible to estimate the biodegradation half-life of 2,3,7,8-tetraCDD in aquatic systems from this experiment.

Philippi et al. (1982) detected a polar metabolite of 2,3,7,8-tetraCDD in several microbiological cultures after long-term incubation. They reported chromatographic and MS data that supported the conclusion that the metabolite was 1-hydroxy-2,3,7,8-tetraCDD, although a synthetic standard compound was not available.

Tulp & Hutzinger (1978) reported that in rats, dibenzo-*p*-dioxin, 1-monoCDD, 2-monoCDD, 2,3-diCDD, 2,7-diCDD, 1,2,4-triCDD, and 1,2,3,4-tetraCDD are metabolized to mono- and dihydroxy derivatives. In the case of dibenzo-*p*-dioxin and both of the two monochloro isomers, sulfur-containing metabolites were also excreted. Primary hydroxylation exclusively took place at the 2, 3, 7, or 8 positions in the molecule. In these studies, no metabolites resulting from fission of the C-O bonds (*ortho*, *ortho*'-dihydroxychlorodiphenyl ethers, chlorocatechols), or hydroxylated derivatives thereof, were detected. No metabolites were found from octaCDD.

4.3 Bioaccumulation

The bioaccumulation of 2,3,7,8-tetraCDD has been investigated in several studies, using several aquatic species and different model ecosystems. In the experiments in which ^{14}C-TCDD was introduced into the model ecosystem in the form of residues on sand, particularly high values were found in the mosquito (*Aedes egypti*) larvae, the level exceeding that found in water by more than 9000 times. Under similar conditions, the level in brine shrimp (*Artemia salina*) was 1570 times higher than that found in water (Matsumura & Benezet, 1973). In the second study (Isensee & Jones, 1975; Isensee, 1978), ^{14}C-TCDD was absorbed, at a broad range of levels, into soil and placed at the bottom of an aquarium. Five species of organisms were added (though not simultaneously) 1-30 days after flooding, and exposed for 3-32 days. The correlation between the TCDD level in the water and in the organisms of each species was highly significant (correlation coefficient of 0.94 or higher).

Bioaccumulation factors for 2,3,7,8-tetraCDD are given in Table 20 (US EPA, 1985).

4.4 Levels in Biota

4.4.1 Vegetation

When ^{14}C-labelled 2,3,7,8-tetraCDD was added to soil, both oats and soya beans accumulated small quantities of TCDD, at all stages of growth. TCDD was also detected in control plants housed with the experimental plants after treatment (Isensee & Jones, 1971). A maximum of 0.15% of the TCDD present in the soil was translocated to the aerial portion of the oats and the soya beans, but neither the grain nor the beans harvested at maturity showed any detectable level of ^{14}C-labelled TCDD. When TCDD was applied to the central leaflet of 3-week-old soya bean plants and 12-day-old oat plants, very little TCDD was lost from the soya bean leaves in 21 days, but there was a gradual loss (38% in 21 days) from the oat leaves.

Analyses of vegetation from Seveso, Italy, after the industrial accident, gave values of up to 50 mg TCDD/kg (Firestone, 1978). In the following years, when there was no direct contact of the newly grown vegetation with the aerosol cloud, the levels of dioxin in plants decreased by several orders of magnitude (Wipf & Schmid, 1983). In 1977 (one year after the accident in Seveso), no traces of TCDD were found in the flesh of apples, pears, and peaches, or in corn cobs or kernels, grown near the factory (the detection limit for the analyses was 1 ng/kg). At the same time about 100 ng TCDD/kg was detected in the fruit peels. This strongly suggests that the contamination was due to dust and not from plant uptake. The TCDD level in the soil was found to be in the order of 10 ng/g, which corresponds to about 1000 $\mu g/m^2$ (Wipf et al., 1982).

Facchetti et al. (1986) studied plants grown in soil spiked with 2,3,7,8-tetraCDD in the range 1-752 ng TCDD/kg. At the end of cultivation, root samples were collected, carefully washed, and analyzed. The levels of TCDD in the roots were found to be higher than the levels found in the soil in which the plants were grown. On the parts above ground, Facchetti et al. (1986) could not find any significant increase in the levels of TCDD. However, the TCDD concentration

Table 20. Measured bioaccumulation factor for 2,3,7,8-TCDD in freshwater aquatic organisms[a]

Species	Tissue	Duration (days)	Bioconcentration factor	Reference
Alga (*Oedogonium cardiacum*)		33	3094[b]	Isensee (1978)
Alga (*Oedogonium cardiacum*)		32	2075[c]	Isensee (1978) Yockim et al. (1978)
Snail (*Physa* sp.)	whole body	33	5471[b]	Isensee (1978)
Snail (*Physa* sp.)	whole body	32	3095[c] 3731	Isensee (1978) Yockim et al. (1978)
Cladoceran (*Daphnia magna*)	whole body	32	3895[b]	Isensee (1978)
Cladoceran (*Daphnia magna*)	whole body	30	7070[c] 7125	Isensee (1978) Yockim et al. (1978)
Catfish (*Italurus punctatus*)	whole body	28	4875	Yockim et al. (1978)
Mosquitofish (*Gambusia affinis*)	whole body	14	4850[c] 4875	Isensee (1978) Yockim et al. (1978)

[a] From: US EPA (1985).
[b] Arithmetic mean of several values reported.
[c] Tissue concentrations at equilibrium.

was found to vary with the location, being higher if the plants were grown in the vicinity of other pots containing contaminated soil. The conclusion was drawn that evaporation is the predominant process for the contamination of the aerial parts of plants. However, studies by Sacchi et al. (1986) indicated that maize and bean plants grown in soil contaminated by ^{3}H-2,3,7,8-tetraCDD accumulated radioactivity in the aerial parts progressively with time and with soil contamination (Sacci et al., 1986). It was suggested that the distribution of the TCDD into the leaves occurred via the transpiration stream.

Very few analyses of sprayed vegetation have been reported. A rough estimate of 20-1000 ng/kg for 2,3,7,8-tetraCDD contamination can be made on the basis of the level of 2,4,5-T found in newly sprayed vegetation and the level of 2,3,7,8-tetraCDD in the spray formulation used. Higher values could be obtained for Agent Orange. Sundström et al. (1979) reported data in agreement with this estimate. However, the analytical technique used in their study was not isomer specific. Vegetation was sprayed with 2,4,5-T ester contaminated by only 0.06 µg 2,3,7,8 tetraCDD/g. A sample of leaves collected 42-45 days after the spraying was found to have 170 ng TCDD/kg, somewhat lower than the expected value 600 ng TCDD/kg, indicating a slow photochemical breakdown.

4.4.2 Aquatic organisms

Fish and shellfish taken from areas in South Viet Nam that were heavily exposed to Agent Orange during military defoliation operations in the 1960s have been reported to contain 18-810 ng TCDD/kg (Baughman & Meselson, 1973). The analytical technique of direct-inlet high resolution MS used in this study is not considered isomer specific and did not include any GC separation at all.

In two streams associated with the US Air Force test area in north-west Florida (section 4.1.3), which had been heavily sprayed with Agent Orange between 1962 and 1964, the silt contained, 10 years later, 10 and 35 ng TCDD/kg where eroded soil entered the water. Concentrations of 12 ng TCDD/kg were found in two species of fish from this stream, the sailfin shiner (*Notropis hypselopterus*) and the mosquito fish (*Gambusia affinis*). The spotted sunfish (*Lepomis punctatus*) contained 4 ng TCDD/kg in skin and muscle, 18 ng/kg in the gonads, and 85 ng/kg in the gut (Young et al., 1976).

The levels of TCDD in fish from the Atlantic or from ponds in the USA in areas sprayed with 2,4,5-T were below the detection levels (1-2 ng/kg) (Baughman, 1974; Shadoff et al., 1977).

Mitchum et al. (1980) reported levels of 400 ng 2,3,7,8-tetraCDD/kg in fish samples collected in Bayou Meto/Arkansas River, USA, a waterway associated with industrial plants for the production of 2,4,5-T (Thibodeux, 1983) (see Table 21).

Table 21. Levels of TCDDs in fish and shellfish[a]

Sample number	Tissue type[b]	Concentration of 2,3,7,8-TCDD (ng/kg)[c]
1	Fish (edible flesh)	480
2	Catfish	40
3	Buffalo fish	ND(13)
4	Fish (predator)	230
5	Fish (bottom feeder)	77
6	Catfish	50
7	Buffalo fish	ND(7)
8	Catfish	ND(7)

[a] From: Mitchum et al. (1980).
[b] All samples were obtained from the Arkansas River, USA, or a tributary, the Bayou Meto.
[c] These are averages of samples that had detectable levels of TCDD.
ND = none detected; the number in parenthesis is the measured detection limited for that sample.

Levels ranging from 4-695 ng TCDD/kg were found in the edible portion of channel catfish, carp, yellow perch, small-mouth bass, and suckers from Saginaw Bay, Michigan, USA, near facilities used for the production of 2,4,5-T herbicides. The highest concentrations were detected in bottom-feeding catfish and carp, while the lowest concentrations were detected in bass, perch, and suckers (see Table 22) (Harless et al., 1982).

Rappe et al. (1981) identified a series of tetra- to octaCDFs in fat samples of a snapping turtle from the Hudson River and of gray seal from the Baltic Sea. The total levels of PCDFs in these samples were 3 ng/g and 40 ng/kg, respectively. In both samples the major PCDFs consisted of the most toxic isomers (2,3,7,8-tetra-; 2,3,4,7,8-penta-; and 1,2,3,4,7,8- and 1,2,3,6,7,8-hexaCDFs).

Norstrom et al. (1982) have analyzed pooled samples of herring gull eggs collected in 1982 from various parts of the Great Lakes, N. America. In all samples, 2,3,7,8-tetraCDD was found in levels ranging from 9 to 90 ng/kg. The identity of the 2,3,7,8-isomer was confirmed by retention times on three capillary columns. In another study Stalling et al. (1983) were not able to detect measurable levels of tetraCDDs and

Table 22. Analytical results for 2,3,7,8-tetraCDD residues in fish from Saginaw Bay Region, Michigan, USA[a]

Species	Number of samples[b]	Number of positive samples	TCDD detected (ng/kg)[c] low	high	mean
Channel catfish	8	8	28	695	157 (13)
Carp	14	10	20	153	55 (7)
Yellow perch	6	3	10	20	13 (5)
Smallmouth bass	2	2	7	8	8 (6)
Sucker	4	3	4	21	10 (4)
Lake trout	2	0	0	0	0 (5)

[a] From: Harless et al. 1982).
[b] Mean % recovery for 2.5-10 ng $^{37}Cl_4$-TCDD added to 5 or 10 g of tissue prior to sample preparation was between 78 and 100%.
[c] Corrected for losses in efficiency of sample preparation for particular species. The numbers in parenthesis indicate the limit of detection for TCDD.

other PCDDs in fish samples from Lake Superior, N. America (the detection level was 2-5 pg/g). The difference could be explained by the migration of the herring gulls during the winter. On the other hand, a series of PCDFs could be identified in the Lake Superior fish samples, indicating more widespread background levels for the PCDFs than for the PCDDs. Stalling et al. (1983) found the total levels of PCDFs in fish samples from Lakes Michigan, Huron, and Ontario, N. America, to be 12-290 ng/kg. The toxic 2,3,7,8-substituted PCDDs and PCDFs were present in all samples, the highest levels being found in samples from Lake Huron, Lake Ontario, and the Tittabawasee River, which flows into Saginaw Bay. The residue pattern found in the fish and locally high levels suggest a strong influence by local point source discharges (Stalling et al., 1983). The data of O'Keefe et al. (1983) are also in agreement with this theory.

Norstrom et al. (1986) have studied the long-term trends of 2,3,7,8-substituted PCDDs and PCDFs in herring gull eggs in the Great Lakes. The levels of 2,3,7,8-tetraCDD were found to decline exponentially in Lake Ontario, with a half-life of

3-4 years, from a high of 2000-5000 ng/kg in the early 1970s to a level of 80-100 ng/kg in 1984/1985. The levels of TCDD in Lake Michigan were 249 ng/kg in 1971, 70 ng/kg in 1972, and 10-20 ng/kg in 1984/1985. These levels have not changed significantly since 1979. This suggests that an equilibrium between input and removal mechanisms has been established in this water system for most PCDDs and PCDFs. The same trend is reported for various fish species in Lake Ontario (Ontario, 1986).

Ryan et al. (1983a) analyzed a series of commercial and sport fish from the Great Lakes and from the Pacific coast of Canada for 2,3,7,8-tetraCDD (Table 23). The highest levels were found in Lake Huron and Lake Ontario. In a preliminary study they also reported finding levels of 2,3,7,8-tetraCDFs and other unidentified tetraCDFs of 3-200 ng/kg of fish.

Table 23. Levels of 2,3,7,8-tetraCDD and PCB in Great Lakes Canadian sport fish (1980) and smelt (1979)[a]

Species	Origin	TCDD (ng/kg)	PCB (μg/g)
Lake trout[b]	Lake Ontario	58	7.28
	Lake Huron	37	5.03
Rainbow trout[b]	Lake Ontario	33	1.77
Coho salmon	Lake Ontario	28[c]	7.39
	Pacific Coast	ND[d] (4)	0.03
Smelt	Lake Ontario	11	
		16	
		11	
	Lake Erie	ND[d] (2)	

[a] From: Ryan et al. (1983a).
[b] Whole fish.
[c] Also contained 36 ng hexaCDD/kg (three isomers) and 93 ng octaCDD/kg.
[d] ND = not detected at bracketed detection limit.

The Baltic Sea is an area of interest because this region is without any known point sources of dioxins. Rappe et al. (1987) reported on the analyses of two samples of homing salmon and two samples of pooled herring; one herring sample from the Baltic Sea (Karlskrona) and the other from the northern part of the Gulf of Bothnia (Lulea) (Table 24). As

Table 24. Levels of PCDDs and PCDFs in fish samples from the Baltic Sea (pg/g)[a,b]

	Salmon Ume River 1985	Salmon Ume River 1985	Herring Karlskrona 1983	Herring Lulea 1983
2,3,7,8-TetraCDF	29	12	5.5	3.0
2,3,7,8-TetraCDD	1.9	1.3	< 0.3	< 0.6
1,2,3,7,8-/1,2,3,4,8-PentaCDF	6.9	3.3	1.4	0.9
2,3,4,7,8-PentaCDF	49.0	23.0	6.8	8.8
1,2,3,7,8-PentaCDD	8.8	4.3	1.1	4.7
1,2,3,4,7,8-/1,2,3,4,7,9-HexaCDF	1.1	0.7	0.4	0.3
1,2,3,6,7,8-HexaCDF	1.3	0.8	0.4	0.3
1,2,3,7,8,9-HexaCDF	ND	ND	0.4	0.2
2,3,4,6,7,8-HexaCDF	1.1	0.6	0.4	0.2
1,2,3,4,7,8-HexaCDD	ND	0.4	0.2	ND
1,2,3,6,7,8-HexaCDD	4.6	2.3	ND	8.1
1,2,3,7,8,9-HexaCDD	ND	ND	ND	ND
Total HeptaCDFs	ND	2.7	0.8	ND
Total HeptaCDDs	ND	ND	ND	ND
OctaCDF	ND	1.0	ND	ND
OctaCDD	ND	ND	ND	ND

[a] From: Rappe et al. (1987).
[b] ND indicates a level < 0.1 pg/g.

expected, the levels in the salmon muscle were much higher than the levels found in the herrings, but, unexpectedly, the levels in the herring sample from the Gulf of Bothnia (Lulea) were somewhat higher than levels found in the sample from the Baltic Sea (Karlskrona).

An interesting observation is that in the majority of the aquatic samples only the 2,3,7,8-substituted PCDD and PCDF congeners were found. However, crustaceans seemed to be an exception from this general trend. Norström et al. (1988) reported that crab hepatopancreas from the Canadian Pacific Coast contain other congeners, e.g. 1,2,4,7,8-pentaCDD and 1,2,3,6,7,9-/1,2,3,6,8,9-hexaCDD. Rappe et al. (1987) collected and analyzed crab hepatopancreas from three different locations along the west coast of Sweden. The crab samples from the locations Grebbestad and Idefjord should represent background levels, while Väröfjord has a potential point source of dioxins from a pulp mill using chlorine for bleaching. The results are given in Table 25.

Low background levels of series PCDDs and PCDFs were found in all samples. In addition, the sample from the Väröfjord also contained much higher levels of some congeners, es-

Table 25. Levels of PCDDs and PCDFs in samples of crab hepatopancreas from the west coast of Sweden[a]

	Crab Idefjorden (pg/g)	Hepatopancreas Grebbestad (pg/g)	Väröfjord (pg/g)
2,3,7,8-tetraCDF	31	47	590
Total tetraCDFs	90	114	800
2,3,7,8-tetraCDD	17	17	170
Total tetraCDDs	17	17	170
1,2,3,7,8-pentaCDF[b]	6	7.6	45
2,3,4,7,8-pentaCDF	44	50	130
Total pentaCDFs	130	150	490
1,2,3,7,8-pentaCDD	13	11	28
Total pentaCDDs	86	76	270
1,2,3,4,7,8-hexaCDF[c]	12	16	50
1,2,3,6,7,8-hexaCDF	3	5	10
1,2,3,7,8,9-hexaCDF	3	3	11
2,3,4,6,7,8-hexaCDF	16	18	63
Total hexaCDFs	70	88	280
1,2,3,4,7,8-hexaCDD	8	5	14
1,2,3,6,7,8-hexaCDD	26	18	71
1,2,3,7,8,9-hexaCDD	3	4	7
Total hexaCDDs	154	170	465
Total heptaCDFs	23	28	90
Total heptaCDDs	32	30	85
octaCDF	< 1	< 1	< 2
octaCDD	< 1	< 1	< 2

[a] From: Rappe et al. (1987).
[b] Not separated from 1,2,3,4,8-pentaCDF.
[c] Not separated from 1,2,3,4,7,9-hexaCDF.

pecially 2,3,7,8-tetraCDF and 2,3,7,8-tetraCDD. This is another indication that pulp bleaching could be a potential source of 2,3,7,8-tetraCDD and 2,3,7,8-tetraCDF (see section 3.5.10).

4.4.3 Terrestrial animals

In a heavily sprayed test area in north-west Florida (Young et al., 1976), a total of 106 adult and 67 fetuses of beach mice (Peromysous polionotus) were collected in 1973 and 1974 and examined (method not specified). Livers from the beach mice contained from 540-1300 ng TCDD/kg and the pelts 130-140 ng/kg. The visceral mass of race runners (Cnemidophorus sexlineatus) which were caught in that area contained 360 ng TCDD/kg and the trunk of the reptiles contained 370 ng/kg.

At the time of the accident in Seveso, Italy, more than 81 000 animals were inhabiting the contaminated zones. Most were rabbits (25 000), poultry, and other small animals (55 500), with 349 cattle, 233 pigs, 49 horses, 21 sheep, and 49 goats also in the zones. Many of these animals died and others were killed. A large number of these animals were analyzed for 2,3,7,8-tetraCDD by a method with a detection level of 250 ng/kg (Pocchiari et al., 1983). The results are summarized in Tables 26 and 27.

Table 26. TCDD content of the livers of farm animals from Seveso contaminated zones and surrounding areas (1976-1979)[a]

Animal	Number of samples	TCDD-containing samples	TCDD maximum level (ng/g)
Rabbits[b]	698	433	633
Poultry	83	35	24
Cattle	43	21	94
Horses	12	2	88
Pigs	13	0	-
Goats	25	17	1
Cats	1	0	-

[a] From: Pocchiari et al. (1983).
[b] Figures include rabbits kept in the special test plots on contaminated ground for experimental purposes.

Harless et al. (1983) reported a study in which 2,4,5-T containing less than 0.1 mg of 2,3,7,8-tetraCDD/kg was applied at a rate of 3.4 kg/ha to approximately 3 ha of an enclosed plot (4.5 ha). Twelve deer were placed in the enclosure prior to the application of 2,4,5-T. One deer died two days later of unknown causes. The remaining deer were sacrificed prior

Table 27. CDD analyses of wildlife from Seveso contaminated zones and surrounding areas (1976-1979)[a]

Animal	Tested organs and number of samples	Number of TCD-containing samples	Maximum level of TCDD (ng/g)
Rabbits	6 (liver)	4	13
Field mice	14 (whole body)	14	49
Rats	1 (pool-4 livers)		28
Earthworms	2 (pool)		12
Frogs	1 (liver)		0.2
Snakes	1 (liver)		3

[a] From: Pocchiari et al. (1983).

to, and at specific intervals during, the course of the 30-day study. The analytical results are summarized in Table 28.

Table 28. Analytical results for 2,3,7,8-tetraCDD residues[a]

Sections of eleven deers in study	No. of deer samples analyzed	No. of positive samples	Concentration range of TCDD detected (ng/kg)[b]	Limit of detection range (ng/kg)[b]
Muscle	11	3	12 - 27	0.5 - 5
Adipose tissue	10	8	3 - 12	1 - 3
Liver	11	4	2 - 5	0.4 - 4
Bone marrow	5	0	ND	1 - 3

[a] From: Harless et al. (1983).
[b] Results corrected for efficiency of sample preparation.
ND = not detected.

In another study (Hryhorczuk et al., 1981), samples from a horse grazing close to a wire reclamation incinerator were analyzed and found to contain unspecified tetraCDFs (165 ng/kg in the fat, 57 ng/kg in the liver) and unspecified tetraCDDs (45 ng/kg in the fat and less than 6 ng/kg in the liver) (compare section 3.5.7).

In order to identify PCDD and PCDF levels in the general terrestrial background, Nygren et al. (1986) analyzed bovine samples - fat, liver, and milk - and identified the same 2,3,7,8-substituted PCDDs and PCDFs as were found in the aquatic samples. However, the levels were lower and normally close to the detection limit.

4.4.4 Human data

Occupational exposure to 2,3,7,8-tetraCDD can occur during the production of 2,4,5-trichlorophenol and the subsequent production and use of 2,4,5-T acid and esters. The first commercial production of 2,4,5-T in the United States was in 1944, and the use of 2,4,5-T herbicides increased in the 1940s and 1950s. However, the problem of dioxin contamination in 2,4,5-T was not recognized until 1957 (Kimmig & Schulz, 1957a, b).

During the normal production of 2,4,5-T, the heaviest exposure to TCDD is during purification steps. The residues are far more contaminated than the purified products. Only limited information is available on the levels of TCDD contamination of products prepared prior to the 1970s, and absolutely no information is available on the dioxin levels in the corresponding residues. Consequently it is a difficult task to estimate the levels of occupational and general population exposures during the period prior to 1970.

4.4.4.1 Adipose tissue

Gross et al. (1984) reported a study in which 30 coded samples of adipose tissue from Viet Nam veterans were analyzed for TCDD. The TCDD levels found for two of the three heavily exposed men were 99 pg/g and 63 pg/g, which is higher than for the other Viet Nam veterans or for the controls (all well below 15 pg/g). Only one single isomer of tetraCDDs was found, and it was assumed that this was the 2,3,7,8-isomer. The data in this study has also been discussed by Young et al. (1983). These authors concluded that the levels do not correlate well with known exposure data or with health status.

Rappe et al. (1984) reported the presence of 2,3,7,8-substituted PCDDs and PCDFs in samples of human adipose tissue from Northern Sweden. A series of reports presented during the period 1984-1986 confirms these observations and it has been clearly shown that there is a background of 2,3,7,8-substituted PCDDs and PCDFs in the general population in the industrialized part of the world. Most of these reports are lacking data on how the sampled people were selected and possible exposure to PCDDs and PCDFs. Consequently, these studies might not be representative. A series of earlier studies failed to detect these background levels due to insufficiently low detection levels. The Swedish study included 31 people, of which 18 were exposed to phenoxy esters and 13 were nonexposed. The group included 17 cancer patients and 14 non-cancer patients. The different groups were matched against each other. No difference in the levels, isomer patterns, or ranges could be found between these subgroups (Nygren et al., 1986). The mean values for these 31 people are given in Table 29.

Schecter et al. (1986a) reported the mean levels of PCDDs and PCDFs in 46 samples of adipose tissue collected in Canada and in 8 samples from the USA (see Table 29). The Canadian samples were taken from people who had died in 1976 from car accidents, drownings, trauma, and suicide. The samples included all ages and both sexes and came from all over the country. The USA samples, (1983-1984), were taken from biopsies from New York State residents during the course of normal medical procedures, and also from autopsies. Table 29 also includes the PCDD and PCDF levels in adipose tissue samples from Viet Nam (Schecter et al., 1986b) and from cancer patients in Japan (Ono et al., 1986).

It is interesting to note the similarity between isomers present, levels of isomers, isomeric patterns, and congener profiles in samples collected from the general population in industrialized countries on three continents. The profile of the PCDD isomers shows increasing levels with an increasing number of chlorine atoms; the level of OCDD is 230-900 pg/g. On the other hand, the profile of PCDFs shows a maximum for 2,3,4,7,8-penta- or 1,2,3,6,7,8-hexaCDF. The difference in levels found between samples from South and North Viet Nam may be explained by spraying during the war in the 1960s and by the difference in industrial activities between the two parts of the country.

Four samples of adipose tissue taken from German workers exposed to TCDD in the early 1950s have also been analyzed (Rappe et al., 1987). In spite of the fact that these workers were exposed more than 30 years before collecting the samples, enhanced levels of 2,3,7,8-tetraCDD could be identified, but the levels of the other PCDDs and PCDFs seem to be in the normal range (Table 29, last column).

Patterson et al. (1986) studied the levels of 2,3,7,8-tetraCDD in the adipose tissue of 39 exposed people and 57 controls in Missouri, USA. The exposed group had subgroups of recreational, residential, and occupational exposure. All persons in both the exposed and control groups had detectable levels of 2,3,7,8-tetraCDD in their adipose tissue. Nineteen of the 39 exposed people had measurements higher than the highest level in the control group and six of the exposed people had levels greater than 100 ng/kg, which was five times higher than the highest control (Table 30).

Table 29. Levels of PCDDs and PCDFs in human adipose tissue (ng/kg wet weight)

Isomer	Sweden n=31[a]	USA/NY[f] n=8[b]	Canada[f] n=46[b]	Japan[f] n=13[c]	N Viet Nam[f] n=9[d]	S Viet Nam[f] n=15[d]	FRG n=4[e]
2,3,7,8-tetraCDD	3	7.2	6.4 (25)	9 (12)	< 2	28 (12)	150
1,2,3,7,8-pentaCDD	10	11.1	10 (46)	15 (13)	< 2	15 (14)	19.2
1,2,3,6,7,8-hexaCDD	15	96	81 (46)	70 (12)	11 (6)	100 (15)	77
1,2,3,7,8,9-hexaCDD	4	NA	NA	12 (10)	NA	NA	9.4
1,2,3,4,6,7,8-heptaCDD	97	164	135 (46)	77 (12)	28 (6)	178 (15)	56
octaCDD	414	707	830 (46)	230 (12)	104 (8)	1256 (15)	267
2,3,7,8-tetraCDF	3.9	NA	NA	9 (13)	NA	NA	0.9
2,3,4,7,8-pentaCDF	54	14.3	15 (46)	25 (13)	13 (7)	21 (15)	44
1,2,3,4,7,8-hexaCDF	6	NA	NA	15 (11)	NA	NA	10.0
1,2,3,6,7,8-hexaCDF	5	31.3	16 (34)	14 (11)	13 (7)	58 (15)	6.7
2,3,4,6,7,8-hexaCDF	2	NA	NA	8 (3)	NA	NA	3.8
1,2,3,4,6,7,8-heptaCDF	11	16.5	30 (44)	NA	7 (3)	29 (15)	19.5
octaCDF	4	NA	NA	NA	NA	NA	1

n = number of tissue samples.
NA = not analyzed.
a Nygren et al. (1986).
b Schecter et al. (1986a).
c Ono et al. (1986).
d Schecter et al. (1986b).
e Refers to occupationally exposed workers. Rappe et al. (1987).
f Mean values of positives. Number of positives within brackets. Levels below the detection level (< 1.0 ng/kg) not included.

Table 30. Comparison of Levels of 2,3,7,8-Tetrachlorodibenzo-*p*-dioxin (ng/kg) in Adipose Tissue of Exposed and Control Groups[a]

Variable	Controls	Exposed			
		Total	Recreational	Residential	Occupational
Number of subjects	57	39	8	16	15
Arithmetic mean	7.4	79.7	90.8	21.1	136.2
Median	6.4	17.0	23.5	14.5	24.7
Range	1.4-20.2	2.8-750	5.0-577	2.8-59.1	3.5-750
Geometric mean	6.4	21.8	24.8	15.3	29.8
Mean age, years (SD)	52.6 (15.7)	44.3 (13.7)	42.1 (14.7)	39.7 (14.9)	50.3 (9.8)
% Men	35.1	61.5	37.5	43.8	93.3

[a] From: Patterson et al. (1986).

Ryan et al. (1986) analyzed autopsy tissue samples that were collected from three subjects who died in New York State, USA, from natural causes. The tissue types were: fat (both abdominal and subcutaneous), adrenal, bone marrow, liver, muscle, spleen, kidney, and lungs. As far as could be ascertained, no subjects had known abnormal exposure to PCDDs or PCDFs, yet these chemicals were found in all tissues analyzed. The highest concentrations of all PCDDs and PCDFs were found in adipose tissue. In individual tissues of the three subjects, the levels of individual congeners detected were within a narrow range, with much higher levels of the higher chlorinated PCDDs and PCDFs (e.g. hepta- and octa-CDD). In adipose tissue, the level of 2,3,7,8-tetraCDD was 3.7-8.4 ng/kg and that of 2,3,4,7,8-pentaCDF 5.2-13 ng/kg, while octaCDD ranged between 430 and 700 ng/kg. No major differences were seen between abdominal and subcutaneous fat samples or between these two types and perirenal fat when the lower lipid content of the latter was considered. Smaller concentrations of PCDDs and PCDFs were measured (on a wet weight basis) in decreasing order: adrenal, bone marrow, liver, muscle, spleen, kidney, and lungs.

The high levels found in exposed Viet Nam veterans and German workers indicate a very slow excretion rate or metabolism of TCDD in humans. This indicates a dramatic difference between man and rodents; in the latter the half-life of TCDD is reported to be in the range of a few weeks.

4.4.4.2 Blood plasma

Analysis of blood plasma has been used to evaluate occupational exposure to PCDDs and PCDFs, which can occur during the production or use of 2,4,6-tri-, 2,3,4,6-tetra-, and pentachlorophenol. Rappe et al. (1983) investigated such exposure through the analysis of blood plasma of exposed workers and unexposed controls. Good correlations were found between the plasma levels and:

(a) the nature of exposure - dermal contact with liquids resulted in higher levels than inhalation of contaminated dust;
(b) the duration of exposure - higher levels for longer exposure times.

The isomers present in the formulations used could also be found in the blood plasma.

Kochman et al. (1986) studied a group of people exposed to PCBs and PCDFs after a transformer fire in Rheims, France in 1985. Low levels (1-25 pg/g) of 2,3,7,8-substituted penta-, hexa-, hepta-, and octaCDFs were found in the blood plasma of these people, and there was a slight variation in the T-lymphocytes cells.

Kahn et al. (1986) measured the levels of PCDDs and PCDFs in the blood plasma from 10 heavily exposed Viet Nam veterans and their 17 controls. The levels of TCDD was much higher in the exposed men than in their controls.

5. ENVIRONMENTAL LEVELS AND HUMAN EXPOSURE

5.1 Air

Owing to sampling and analytical problems, very few data are available on the levels of 2,3,7,8-TCDD and other PCDDs and PCDFs in normal urban air.

Rappe & Kjeller (1987) reported the levels of PCDDs and PCDFs in total air samples collected in Hamburg, FRG, and samples of air particulates collected in Sweden (Table 31). Sample 1 was collected on the outskirts of Hamburg (representing an urban area), sample 2 in a traffic tunnel, sample 3 downwind from a MSW incinerator, and sample 4 in the vicinity of a dumpsite and metal refinery. PCDDs and PCDFs were found in all samples. Lower levels of PCDDs and PCDFs were found in air particulates than in total air samples (Table 31). Sample 5 was taken when "clean air" was blowing into a street in Gothenburg, Sweden, and sample 6 was taken in the same street during an inversion situation. Samples 7 and 8 were taken at a rural research station outside Gothenburg when the air was blowing from the sea (sample 7) or from Gothenburg (sample 8). The isomeric pattern found in these samples were very similar (Rappe & Kjeller, 1987).

Airborne dust was monitored in 1977 in the Seveso area to evaluate the possibility that 2,3,7,8-tetraCDD-contaminated particles might have drifted outside the contaminated areas. A high-volume sampling technique was used. When pooled particulate samples were analyzed, levels of 0.17-0.50 pg TCDD/m^3 were reported (Wipf et al., 1982).

The atmospheric concentrations of 2,3,7,8-tetraCDD near two hazardous waste sites have been monitored. In one study, US EPA (1982) failed to detect (detection limit: 1-20 pg/m^3) any 2,3,7,8-TCDD in the atmosphere at the Love Canal (New York, USA) area. In another study of a waste disposal site (near Jacksonville, Arkansas, USA), Thibodeaux (1983) reported an average concentration of 1100 pg of 2,3,7,8-TCDD/g in two air particulate samples collected near the disposal site.

Rappe et al. (1985c) analyzed indoor air samples for PCDFs resulting from fires and explosions in PCB-filled electrical equipment, and in an industrial situation (locomotive shop) (Table 32).

O'Keefe et al. (1985) analyzed air samples collected in an office building in Binghamton, New York, USA, after a transformer accident in the basement in February 1981. The samples were collected after a primary clean-up and the values are given in Table 33.

Table 31. Levels of PCDDs and PCDFs in samples of total air and air particulates[a]

Total air samples	1 pg/m^3	2 pg/m^3	3 pg/m^3	4 pg/m^3	Air particulates 5 fg/m^3	6 fg/m^3	7 fg/m^3	8 fg/m^3
2,3,7,8-tetraCDF[b]	0.04	0.72	0.38	0.18	30	240	5	62
Total tetraCDFs	0.36	6.2	4.9	3.3	320	2000	54	490
2,3,7,8-tetraCDD	0.02	0.06	0.02	0.08	3	9	< 1	5
Total tetraCDDs	0.10	0.22	0.21	1.5	150	350	9	130
1,2,3,7,8-pentaCDF[c]	0.04	0.36	0.42	1.0	39	190	7	58
2,3,4,7,8-pentaCDF	0.04	Int[e]	0.43	1.2	51	240	6	69
Total pentaCDFs	0.51	4.1	5.0	10	470	2500	85	610
1,2,3,7,8-pentaCDD	< 0.02	0.28	0.22	0.6	17	66	5	35
Total pentaCDDs	0.07	1.3	2.4	5.0	200	840	31	280
1,2,3,4,7,8-hexaCDF[d]	0.03	0.13	0.27	1.1	23	100	8	38
1,2,3,6,7,8-hexaCDF	0.03	0.15	0.24	1.4	20	78	8	33
1,2,3,7,8,9-hexaCDF	< 0.01	< 0.05	< 0.02	0.33	4	17	3	14
2,3,4,6,7,8-hexaCDF	< 0.01	< 0.05	0.12	0.80	10	84	7	32
Total hexaCDFs	0.18	1.1	2.2	9.5	180	800	70	310
1,2,3,4,7,8-hexaCDD	< 0.08	< 0.17	0.19	1.0	3	19	< 1	7
1,2,3,6,7,8-hexaCDD	0.23	0.66	0.71	2.2	11	46	4	14
1,2,3,7,8,9-hexaCDD	< 0.08	< 0.17	0.36	5.2	6	92	5	32
Total hexaCDDs	0.74	2.7	5.3	24.	100	520	32	190
Total heptaCDFs	0.10	1.2	2.0	5.	200	1100	120	500
Total heptaCDDs	0.60	3.4	5.3	15.	380	2900	140	1000
OctaCDF	< 0.11	< 1.0	0.78	7.0	150	480	100	440
OctaCDD	0.37	6.4	7.4	40.0	290	1900	64	540

[a] From: Rappe & Kjeller (1987).
[b] Not separated from 2,3,4,8-tetraCDF.
[c] Not separated from 1,2,3,4,8-pentaCDF.
[d] Not separated from 1,2,3,4,7,9-hexaCDF.
[e] Int = Interferences.

5.2 Water and Leachate

Shadoff et al. (1977) failed to identify 2,3,7,8-tetraCDD in water from areas in the USA where 2,4,5-T herbicides had been used.

In the 2,4,5-T plant in Jacksonville, Arkansas, USA, Thibodeaux (1983) could not detect any 2,3,7,8-tetraCDD in the creek water (no limit of detection levels given).

Table 32. Analyses of PCDFs in air samples (pg/m3)[a]

Sample	total tetra-CDF	2,3,7,8-tetraCDF	penta-CDF	hexa-CDF	hepta-CDF	octa-CDF
Surahammar (during cleaning)	< 20	< 2	< 10	< 10	< 10	< 10
Surahammar (after cleaning)	< 10	< 2.5	< 10	< 10	< 10	< 10
Railway locomotive (during cleaning operations)	500	50	50	30	20	20

[a] From: Rappe et al. (1985c).

Since August 1976, a number of tests have been periodically conducted in Seveso on streams running through the affected area, as far south as the River Lambro, with consistently negative results. During the same period sediment samples were taken from Torrents, Certesa, and Seveso. Positive results of the order of 1 pg/g were obtained within the first few kilometers downstream from their confluence, but further downstream results were negative. The intensive rainfalls after the accident caused the Seveso to repeatedly overflow its embankments at the point of entry into Milan, thus depositing silt on adjacent areas. Tests conducted to determine TCDD in these silts yielded negative findings for the first four floods while the fifth flood yielded positive findings (pg/g). Since August 1976, the monthly determinations conducted on pipeline and ground waters have consistently yielded negative results, even when the analytical detection threshold was as low as 1 pg/litre (parts per quadrillion) (Pocchiari, 1983).

During 1983 and 1984, the Dow Chemical Company conducted a study to determine the 2,3,7,8-tetraCDD contamination at its plant in Midland, Michigan, USA. It was estimated that 0.6 g of 2,3,7,8-tetraCDD was being emitted per year in 2.5×10^7 m^3 of wastewater effluent (Lamparski et al., 1986).

The Ontario Ministry of Environment has included PCDDs and PCDFs in its Drinking Water Surveillance Program for the St Clair/Detroit River area (Ontario, 1986). No 2,3,7,8-tetraCDD has been found in any sample of raw or treated

Table 33. Concentrations of PCDFs in air samples collected on various floors of a Binghamton, New York (USA) office after primary cleanup

	Analytical results (pg/m^3)			
Floor/sample type[a]	2,3,7,8-tetraCDF	Total tetraCDFs	Penta-CDFs	Hexa-CDFs
3	16	151	43	
5	11	126	30	2.0
5 (NE)	20	195	60	8.7
7	11	121	36	
9 volatiles	14	140	42	
9 particulates	1.8	4.8	4.7	
9 (SE) volatiles	13	146	31	3.7
9 (SE) particulates	0.8	3.9	3.2	
11	23	76	16	
11 (SE + NW)	16	133	19	
14	11	92	21	
14 (NE)	14	185	13	
16	16	118	21	
17 volatiles	12	79	24	
17 particulates	0.8	3.9	ND[b]	
17 volatiles	9	59	6.6	
17 particulates	0.9	ND[b]	2.9	

[a] Abbreviations in parentheses designate sampling location on the floor, e.g., SE = south-east corner. Unless otherwise specified samples were collected in the north-west corner and analyzed as combined particulates and volatiles.

[b] ND = not detected.

water. Unspecified congeners of PCDDs and PCDFs have been found mainly in raw water, octaCDD being the most frequent congener found. The highest value reported was 1.1 pg octaCDD/litre raw water in Amherstburg. The octaCDD level in the treated water was below the detection level of 0.01 pg/litre.

Götz (1986) reported on levels of PCDDs and PCDFs in the oily leachate from a sanitary landfill in Georgswerder, Hamburg, FRG (Table 34).

5.3 Soil and Sediment

The levels of 2,3,7,8-tetraCDD in point sources after improper disposal of industrial waste are discussed in section 3.4.2.

Table 34. Levels (ng/g) of the 2,3,7,8-substituted PCDDs and PCDFs in leachate from a sanitary landfill[a]

Isomer	Concentration	Isomer	Concentration
2,3,7,8-tetraCDD	60	2,3,7,8-tetraCDF	9
1,2,3,7,8-pentaCDD	28	1,2,3,7,8-pentaCDF[b]	322
1,2,3,4,7,8-hexaCDD	476	2,3,4,7,8-pentaCDF	261
1,2,3,6,7,8-hexaCDD	1440	1,2,3,4,7,8-hexaCDF	748
1,2,3,7,8,9-hexaCDD	310	1,2,3,6,7,8-hexaCDF	336
		1,2,3,7,8,9-hexaCDF	558
		2,3,4,6,7,8-hexaCDF	114

[a] From: Götz (1986).
[b] Overlapping isomer: 1,2,3,4,8-pentaCDF.

Analytical results of the 1976-1977 survey of Zones B and R in Seveso were discussed by Pocchiari (1983). TCDD levels in Zones B and R were, in general, considerably lower than those in Zone A. In fact, most TCDD levels were lower than 50 μg/m^2 in Zone B and 5 μg/m^2 in Zone R. In 1980, a large part of Zone R was remonitored to evaluate the persistence of TCDD in the soil. This zone had been ploughed and worked since 1978. A comparison, as well as a statistical evaluation, of the relevant data indicated a significant decrease (40%) in the geometric mean level of TCDD in the soil of Zone R.

In 1980 and 1981, soil samples from ten sites in Zone R and five sites outside Zone R were analyzed using a high resolution GS-MS system to establish whether other isomers of 2,3,7,8-tetraCDD were also present. A significant percentage decrease in tetraCDDs could be accounted for by two isomers (1,3,6,8-tetraCDD and 1,3,7,9-tetraCDD) present in the majority of the samples tested. These two isomers were not related to the chemical accident at the factory.

Wipf & Schmid (1983) reported the presence of PCDDs other than 2,3,7,8-tetraCDD in the soil from Zone R (Table 35). They suggest that a municipal incinerator and the burning of wood shavings treated with chlorinated phenols could be the source of the other PCDDs.

Nestrick et al. (1986) reported the levels of 2,3,7,8-tetraCDD in soil samples collected from industrialized areas of US cities. They observed a widespread occurrence of 2,3,7,8-tetraCDD in urban soils, with levels of 1-10 ng/kg, and suggested that local combustion sources, including MSW and industrial incinerators, were the probable origin.

Table 35. PCDD contamination in soil from Zone R in Seveso (1981) (values in ng/kg)[a]

Sample	2,3,7,8[b] tetraCDD	TCDD[c]	Penta-CDDs	Hexa-CDDs	Hepta-CDDs	Octa-CDD	Total PCDDs
S1	0.8	0.3	0.4	6.0	1.4	1.7	10.6
S2	3.4	1.0	0.7	9.5	2.1	2.2	18.9
S3	4.0	1.9	1.2	8.2	8.6	27.0	50.9
S4	2.3	0.8	0.6	10.2	2.1	2.0	18.0
S5	< 0.1	< 0.3	0.5	9.5	1.9	1.4	13.7
S6	6.3	1.5	1.1	10.4	2.6	1.3	24.8
S7	1.7	1.0	0.8	12.4	1.9	1.8	19.6
S8	2.2	0.4	0.8	8.8	1.8	0.8	14.8
S9	1.0	2.8	2.3	21.2	9.6	13.5	50.4

[a] From: Wipf & Schmid (1983).
[b] Probably related to the accident.
[c] Total levels of isomers other than 2,3,7,8-tetraCDD, probably not related to accident.

McLaughlin & Pearson (1984) measured soil concentrations of PCDDs and PCDFs in the vicinity of a municipal refuse incinerator in Ontario, Canada. Urban and rural control locations were also sampled. All soil samples (14) had detectable quantities of at least one of the five PCDD congener classes (tetraCDD to octaCCD) tested for, whereas eight samples contained detectable levels of one or more of the five PCDF congener groups (tetraCDF to octaCDF). The levels ranged from non-detectable (0.003 - 0.008 ng/g) to 3.5 ng/g (octaCDD); only one site had a measurable quantity (0.007 ng/g) of tetraCDD in the soil. The most abundant PCDD or PCDF congener was octaCDD, which had similar levels whether samples were taken close to or remote from the incinerator. Similarly, no concentration gradients, relative to distance from the incinerator, were apparent for any of the other PCDDs or PCDFs.

Soil samples near a chemical waste incinerator in Scotland have also been analyzed for PCDDs and PCDFs, together with samples from control locations (Edulgee et al., 1986). Detectable levels of all PCDFs or PCDFs that were examined were found in each of the soil samples (13). Levels found ranged from 1.2 ng/kg (2,3,7,8-tetraCDD) to 1900 ng/kg (total hexaCDF). No consistent pattern was observed to differentiate levels found in control samples from levels in soil near the incinerator.

These studies from widely separate areas of the world support the suggestion that diffuse combustion sources are the major source of PCDDs and PCDFs in the soil.

Rappe & Kjeller (1987) analyzed soil samples from various parts of Europe (Table 36). They represent rural areas (samples 1, 2, and 3) as well as more industrialized areas (samples 4 and 5). PCDDs and PCDFs could be identified in all samples. The 2,3,7,8-tetraCDD concentration was below the detection level in the soil samples from the non-industrialized areas. Trapped sediments from the archipelago of Stockholm, Sweden, were also analyzed. The samples were collected in the inner (sample 6), middle (sample 7), and outer archipelago (sample 8). Levels decreased with increasing distance from the city of Stockholm. The isomeric patterns for tetra- and pentaCDF isomers are very similar to those found for samples of total air and air particulates (section 6.1). A sediment sample from the mouth of River Viskan, Sweden, was also analyzed (sample 9). A slight difference in congener profile was found between this sample and the sediments from the archipelago of Stockholm.

Czuczwa & Hites (1985) found PCDDs and PCDFs in sediment samples from several locations in Saginaw River and Bay, and southern Lake Huron, levels ranging from 100 ng/g in urban areas to 100 ng/kg at remote sites. Although no isomers were identified, the analytical profiles in the sediments followed closely those found in combustion samples, suggesting that combustion is the major source of PCDDs and PCDFs found in the sediments. Analyses of sediment cores showed a dramatic increase in the PCDD and PCDF concentrations at a depth corresponding to approximately the year 1940, and levels remained high up to the present. There is no good correlation between the trend in these levels and the trend for coal burning in the United States. However, the levels in the sediments correlate with the production and use of chlorinated aromatic compounds within this area of the Great Lakes.

5.4 Food

5.4.1 Meat and bovine milk

The levels of PCDDs and PCDFs in fish and other seafood are discussed in section 4.4.2.

The US Environmental Protection Agency (US EPA) initiated a 2,3,7,8-tetraCDD monitoring programme of beef fat samples taken from cattle that had grazed on rangelands known to have been treated with 2,4,5-T. The analytical collaborators in this programme were Dow Chemical Co. (USA), Wright State University, and Harvard University. All the laboratories used mass spectroscopic techniques for quantification. Two different

Table 36. Levels (pg/g) of PCDDs and PCDFs in samples of sediments and soil[a]

	Soil samples					Sediments			
	1	2	3	4	5	6	7	8	9
2,3,7,8-tetraCDF[b]	2.9	1.6	1.1	34	38	30	17	14	1.6
Total tetraCDFs	9.3	7.7	11	320	370	290	150	120	24
2,3,7,8-tetraCDD	< 2.0	< 2.1	< 0.2	2.4	0.8	2.4	2.0	< 2.0	0.2
Total tetraCDDs	-	-	3.2	55.5	11.2	69	21	23	6.4
1,2,3,7,8-pentaCDF[c]	2.5	1.6	0.5	17	31	16	8.6	8.5	1.3
2,3,4,7,8-pentaCDF	0.8	1.0	0.6	23	65	20	14	16	1.7
Total pentaCDFs	14	13	6.7	200	450	260	140	130	30
1,2,3,7,8-pentaCDD	< 2.0	< 2.0	< 0.1	18	34	7.6	5.2	5.5	0.9
Total pentaCDDs	-	-	4.6	220	270	230	99	86	13
1,2,3,4,7,8-hexaCDF[d]	3.8	2.2	0.9	30	45	16	10	8.8	1.9
1,2,3,6,7,8-hexaCDF	1.8	1.5	0.4	11	25	12	7.1	5.9	1.2
1,2,3,7,8,9-hexaCDF	1.0	0.9	4.3	110	1100	5	< 1	< 1	2.0
2,3,4,6,7,8-hexaCDF	1.9	1.0	0.7	26	57	16	31	23	1.6
Total hexaCDFs	16	12	11	270	1900	250	220	92	44
1,2,3,4,7,8-hexaCDD	< 2	< 2	< 0.1	13	28	1.6	0.8	1.0	1.6
1,2,3,6,7,8-hexaCDD	< 2	< 2	< 0.1	19	64	48	2.0	2.0	10
1,2,3,7,8,9-hexaCDD	< 2	< 2	< 0.1	6.2	19	2.5	0.9	1.0	4.3
Total hexaCDDs	-	-	4.7	200	330	49	16	19	64
Total heptaCDFs	22	14	18	260	4500	1300	1500	190	300
Total heptaCDDs	< 10	< 10	17	370	1600	5700	1200	880	190
OctaCDF	-	-	5.7	68	71	39	< 20	< 20	330
OctaCDD	-	-	14	140	180	3100	510	260	900

a From: Rappe & Kjeller (1987).
b Not separated from 2,3,4,8-tetraCDF, except in the case of sample 9.
c Not separated from 1,2,3,4,8-pentaCDF.
d Not separated from 1,2,3,4,7,9-hexaCDF.

extraction techniques were used. All three laboratories analyzed control samples taken from cattle that had grazed on non-treated areas. Some of these control samples were spiked with known amounts of TCDD. All the controls were prepared by the US EPA (Firestone, 1978). Good agreement was found between the amounts of TCDD spiked into the control beef fat samples and the reported levels found, even down to TCDD levels of 10 ng/kg. The average reported TCDD level was 10 ng/kg; the amount actually added by the EPA was 9 ng/kg. Of a total of 34 analyses of controls to which no TCDD was added, in only one case was there a false positive report of TCDD (O'Keefe et al., 1977). Of 52 samples of beef fat from 2,4,5-T-treated rangeland, 19 (37%) were reported by one or more laboratories to have TCDD. The average range of levels reported was 5-66 ng/kg, and the overall average was 7 ng/kg. If one considers only the 40 beef fat samples from areas receiving at least 1.1 kg of 2,4,5-T/ha, all 19 positive samples (48%) belong to this group, and the average reported TCDD level would be 9 ng/kg. The results indicated a consistent trend, relating the average reported TCDD level in beef fat to the intensity of the 2,4,5-T application to rangeland (O'Keffe et al., 1978; McKinney, 1978).

None of the three collaborating laboratories used the most selective and sensitive analytical method now known (capillary glass column gas chromatography - high resolution mass fragmentography).

Kocher et al. (1978) also analyzed specimens of fat taken from steers that had grazed on rangeland previously treated with 2,4,5-T herbicides. The limit of detection of TCDD (2.5 times peak to peak noise) was found to be in the 30-60 pg range (3-6 pg/g in beef fat using 10 gram samples). None of the sixteen samples analyzed in two of three studies revealed TCDD. In the third study, the animals were confined to a fenced pasture sprayed in its entirety with 2,4,5-T herbicides. The samples from three of the seven animals gave a positive response at the extremely low level of 3 to 4 ng TCDD/kg, which is at the detection limit; the highest reported value (without interfering components) was 13 pg/g. The level of 2,3,7,8-tetraCDD in the 2,4,5-T used was, however, unknown.

Beck et al. (1986) analyzed seven randomly collected samples of cow's milk from different areas of the Federal Republic of Germany and one sample from the German Democratic Republic. The cow's milk was taken from road transport tankers. In all samples, 2,3,7,8-substituted PCDDs and PCDFs were found at low levels of pg/g on a fat weight basis. Detection limits were in the range 0.1-0.3 ng/kg. The levels of PCDDs and PCDFs found in the milk samples were lower than those measured by Rappe et al. (1987b) in cow's milk from

Switzerland (Table 38). In addition, there was no evidence of high levels of the higher chlorinated congeners (e.g. hepta- and octa-) (see Table 37). Levels were much lower than those in human milk samples (see section 5.4.2).

Rappe et al. (1987b) analyzed PCDDs and PCDFs in six samples of bovine milk from various locations in Switzerland. In all samples, 2,3,7,8-substituted PCDDs and PCDFs were found at levels of pg/kg in whole milk (Table 38). However, the levels were lower in commercial milk samples than in samples collected directly from cows grazing in the vicinity of incinerators.

When Ryan et al. (1985) analyzed PCDDs and PCDFs in chicken and pork samples in Canada, the incidence of positives for hexa-, hepta-, and octaCDD in selected samples of chicken fat was 50, 62, and 46%, with averages of 27, 52, and 90 ng/kg, respectively. Similar levels of hexa and heptaCDFs were also found in some of these samples, but tetra- and pentaCDDs and tetra-, penta , and octaCDFs were not detected. A comparison between the tissue analyses and those of the wood (treated with pentachlorophenol) used to house the animals showed a marked similarity (see Table 38), indicating that pentachlorophenol was the probable source of contamination of the food samples.

Firestone et al. (1986) reported the analyses of various food items collected in the period beginning in 1979. Low levels (< 300 ng/kg) of 1,2,3,4,6,7,8- and 1,2,3,4,6,7,9-heptaCDD were found in some samples of chicken, bacon, pork chops, and beef liver. HexaCDD was not found in any of the foods. Several beef livers had high levels of OCDD residues, the highest reported value being 3830 ng/kg. No PCDDs (at a detection limit of 10-40 ng/kg) were found in ground beef.

5.4.2 Human milk

Rappe et al. (1984) reported low levels of 2,3,7,8-substituted PCDDs and PCDFs in five samples of human milk from the Federal Republic of Germany (FRG) (Table 39).

Table 39 also indicates the results of analyses of four samples of human milk from the Umea region of northern Sweden (Rappe, 1985), 92 samples from Rheinland-Westfalia in the FRG (Furst et al., 1987), 30 other samples from the FR (Beck et al., 1987), and five samples from the Netherlands or Yugoslavia (Rappe et al., 1987).

Van der Berg et al. (1986) also reported the levels of PCDDs and PCDFs in human milk samples from the Netherlands, but these levels were reported on milk basis, not on fat basis, and are therefore not included in Table 39.

A comparison between the isomers, levels, isomeric pattern, and congener profiles found in human milk (Table 39) and

Table 37. PCDD and PCDF levels in samples of cow's milk (ng/kg on a fat weight basis)[a]

	SAMPLE							
	1	2	3	4	5	6	7	8
2,3,7,8-tetraCDF	< 0.1	0.29	0.28	1.1	1.0	1.4	1.4	0.27
2,3,7,8-tetraCDD	0.33	< 0.2	< 0.2	< 0.2	ND	< 0.2	ND	ND
1,2,3,7,8-pentaCDF	ND	0.4	ND	0.26	0.24	ND	0.39	< 0.2
2,3,4,7,8-pentaCDF	1.3	0.91	1.1	1.6	1.5	1.3	2.9	0.8
1,2,3,7,8-pentaCDD	1.0	0.72	ND	0.81	0.6	0.78	1.2	< 0.5
1,2,3,4,7,8-hexaCDF	0.93	0.67	0.70	0.85	< 0.3	0.84	1.9	0.57
1,2,3,6,7,8-hexaCDF	0.73	0.58	0.57	0.85	< 0.3	0.73	2.1	0.41
2,3,4,6,7,8-hexaCDF	0.65	0.48	0.53	0.68	ND	0.64	1.8	0.37
1,2,3,4,7,8-hexaCDD	0.33	0.34	< 0.3	< 0.3	< 0.3	0.36	0.33	< 0.3
1,2,3,6,7,8-hexaCDD	1.3	1.2	1.0	0.82	0.32	1.7	1.9	0.80
1,2,3,7,8,9-hexaCDD	< 0.3	0.34	0.36	0.39	ND	0.55	0.48	< 0.3
1,2,3,4,6,7,8-heptaCDF[b]	< 0.5	< 0.5	< 0.5	< 0.5	< 0.5	< 0.5	< 0.5	< 0.5
1,2,3,4,6,7,8-heptaCDD[b]	< 2	< 2	< 2	< 2	< 2	< 2	< 2	< 2
octaCDD[b]	<10	<10	<10	<10	<10	<10	<10	<10
octaCDF[b]	< 1	< 1	< 1	< 1	< 1	< 1	< 1	< 1

[a] From: Beck et al. (1987).
[b] Not significantly higher than blanks.
ND = not detectable.

Table 38. PCDF and PCDD content of bovine milk from Switzerland. Results in ng/kg (ppt), whole milk basis[a]

Compound	Commercial			Incinerators		
	1	2	3	4	5	6
2,3,7,8-tetraCDF	< 0.028	< 0.035	< 0.021	< 0.022	< 0.032	< 0.028
1,2,3,7,8-pentaCDF	< 0.020	< 0.022	< 0.021	< 0.020	< 0.036	< 0.032
2,3,4,7,8-pentaCDF	0.084	0.066	0.069	0.43	0.22	0.23
1,2,3,4,7,8-hexaCDF	< 0.020	< 0.026	< 0.017	0.13	0.06	0.084
1,2,3,6,7,8-hexaCDF	0.028	< 0.018	< 0.021	0.19	0.095	0.059
2,3,4,6,7,8-hexaCDF	< 0.020	< 0.018	ND (< 0.02)	0.28	0.12	0.049
1,2,3,4,6,7,8-heptaCDF	< 0.12	ND (< 0.13)	ND (< 0.08)	0.49	0.28	< 0.18
octaCDF	< 0.20	ND (< 0.13)	ND (< 0.09)	ND (< 0.16)	ND (< 0.21)	< 0.52
2,3,7,8-tetraCDD	ND (< 0.012)	ND (< 0.013)	ND (< 0.013)	0.049	0.038	0.021
1,2,3,7,8-pentaCDD	ND (< 0.04)	ND (< 0.08)	ND (< 0.06)	0.25	< 0.086	ND (< 0.1)
1,2,3,4,7,8-hexaCDD	< 0.068	ND (< 0.1)	ND (< 0.06)	0.23	0.14	< 0.14
1,2,3,6,7,8-hexaCDD	< 0.068	ND (< 0.1)	ND (< 0.06)	0.29	0.16	< 0.21
1,2,3,7,8,9-hexaCDD	< 0.068	ND (< 0.1)	ND (< 0.06)	0.17	< 0.080	< 0.11
1,2,3,4,6,7,8-heptaCDD	< 0.064	< 0.066	< 0.064	0.26	< 0.095	0.42
octaCDD	< 0.16	< 0.26	< 0.12	0.28	< 0.16	0.59

[a] From: Rappe et al. (1987b).
ND = not detectable.

Table 39. Levels of PCDDs and PCDFs found in human milk (ng/kg of fat weight)

	Sweden n=4[a]	FRG n=5[b]	FRG n=92[c]	FRG n=30[d]	Netherlands n=3[e]	Yugoslavia n=2[e]
2,3,7,8-tetraCDD	0.6	1.9	< 5	3.4	9.7	< 1.0
1,2,3,7,8-pentaCDD	6.5	12.9	10.7	15	44	5.5
1,2,3,4,7,8-hexaCDD	2.5	4.6	8.1	12	25	3.5
1,2,3,6,7,8-hexaCDD	19	17.3	32.7	59	251	15
1,2,3,7,8,9-hexaCDD	6.3	1.6	6.4	11	23	ND
1,2,3,4,6,7,8-heptaCDD	59.5	72.8	49.9	61	130	106
octaCDD	302	434	181	530	744	106
2,3,7,8-tetraCDF	4.2	5.4	2.6	2.5	2.8	< 1.0
1,2,3,7,8-pentaCDF	< 1	< 1	1.8	< 1	ND	ND
2,3,4,7,8-pentaCDF	21.3	36.4	22.9	20	79	25
1,2,3,4,7,8-hexaCDF	4.7	11.4	8.2	8.5	8.9	3.7
1,2,3,6,7,8-hexaCDF	3.4	10.2	6.6	7.8	10.3	3.6
2,3,4,6,7,8-hexaCDF	1.4	4.3	3.3	3.0	6.4	1.3
1,2,3,4,6,7,8-heptaCDF	7.4	9.2	6.4	8.5	39	ND
octaCDF	3.2	2.4	22.8	< 3	ND	ND

ND = not detected; NA = not analyzed; n = number of samples.

[a] Rappe (1985).
[b] Rappe et al. (1984).
[c] Furst et al. (1987).
[d] Beck et al. (1987).
[e] Rappe et al. (1987) (pooled samples).

in adipose tissue (Tables 29 and 30) shows a remarkable degree of similarity.

5.4.3 Rice

Rice from fields in Arkansas, Louisiana, and Texas, USA, treated at a maximum rate to give 2.52 kg 2,4,5-T/ha, were analyzed for possible 2,3,7,8-tetraCDD residues. A specification of 1 µg 2,3,7,8-tetraCDD/g 2,4,5-T was given in the report, but no analytical data were given for the herbicide. No 2,3,7,8-TCDD was detected in the rice (detection limit = 2-7 mg/kg) and no 2,3,7,8-TCDD residues (detection limit = 2-10 mg/kg) were found in 30 samples of rice purchased in retail stores throughout the USA (Jensen et al., 1983).

5.5 Yusho and Yu-cheng Episodes

In 1968, more than 1500 people in south-west Japan were intoxicated through consuming commercial rice oil accidentally contaminated by PCBs, PCDFs, and polychlorinated quarterphenyls (Masuda & Yoshimura, 1982; Masuda et al., 1985). In 1979, a similar episode occurred in central Taiwan, the number of persons involved here approaching 2000 (Chen et al., 1980; Chen et al., 1985). In the past, both accidents were referred to as Yusho episodes, but now the Taiwan episode has been renamed Yu-cheng.

The Japanese rice oil contained more than 40 PCDF isomers (tri- to hexaCDFs) (Buser et al., 1978d), whereas the number of isomers in the Taiwanese oil seems to have been less (Chen & Hites, 1983). The toxic 2,3,7,8-substituted PCDFs were middle or minor constituents, about 10-15% of the total amount of PCDFs (Buser et al., 1978d; Masuda et al., 1985; Chen & Hites, 1983). The mean total consumption of PCDFs of the Yusho and Yu-cheng patients has been estimated to be 3.3-3.8 mg/person (Hayabuchi et al., 1979; Chen et al., 1985), or a daily intake of total PCDFs of 0.9 µg/kg body weight (Hayabuchi et al., 1979). The average intake of 2,3,7,8-substituted PCDFs was 90-135 ng/kg body weight per day. The smallest amount of total PCDFs causing chloracne has been estimated to be 0.16 µg/kg body weight per day (Hayabuchi et al., 1979) or 20-30 ng/kg per day of the 2,3,7,8-substituted congeners.

Analysis of liver samples taken from the Yusho patients about 18 months after the exposure showed a dramatic decrease in the number of PCDF isomers. Apparently most of the PCDF isomers were metabolized or excreted during the period between exposure and sampling (Rappe et al., 1979). A comparison between the PCDF isomers found in the Yusho oil and the liver samples revealed an interesting relationship. Most of the isomers retained had lateral positions (2, 3, 7, and 8) substituted with chlorine; these isomers have the highest toxicity (Rappe et al., 1979).

Kunita et al. (1984) studied the blood levels of PCDFs in people involved in the Japanese and Taiwanese episodes. They used a non-isomer-specific analytical method, and reported higher blood levels in persons with severe dermal symptoms than in persons with light symptoms. The levels 2 years after exposure were lower than 0.5 year after exposure; for the six persons studied the levels of total PCDFs decreased on average by 57% ± 12% (Kunita et al., 1984).

The rate of excretion of these toxic PCDF isomers is very low. Rappe & Nygren (1984) could detect 2,3,4,7,8-pentaCDF in blood plasma from Yusho patients when the samples were collected 11 years after exposure. However, higher levels were found in blood from Yu-cheng patients one year after exposure; these analyses also showed a 15-20% reduction in levels in one year (Rappe, 1984).

6. KINETICS AND METABOLISM OF 2,3,7,8-TETRACHLORO-DIBENZO P-DIOXIN (TCDD) AND OTHER PCDDs

6.1 Uptake, Distribution, and Excretion

Most of the available toxicokinetic data arise from studies of gastrointestinal exposure and oral or intraperitoneal administration. There has been one dermal study on rats, but no studies on exposure via the respiratory tract. Data on the gastrointestinal absorption, distribution, and elimination of TCDD in various species are summarized in Tables 40 and 41. Principle organ depots in all species studied are the liver and adipose tissue. In addition skin and muscle have been found to be organ depots in monkeys, and skin in guinea-pigs. In all species studied clearance of TCDD from the body follows apparent first-order kinetics.

6.1.1 Studies on rats

Male Sprague Dawley rats were dosed by gavage with ^{14}C TCDD in acetone: corn oil (1:9), at a concentration of 50 µg/kg body weight (Piper et al., 1973). Rats lost weight and their physical condition was generally poor, although no deaths occurred. Approximately 30% of the administered dose of radioactivity was eliminated in the faeces during the first 48 h, this being most probably unabsorbed TCDD. The total faecal TCDD content was equivalent to 53.2% of the dose over a 21-day period. During this time 13.2% was eliminated in the urine and 3.2% in the air. From these results the half-time for the clearance of TCDD was calculated as 17.4 ($\pm$ 5.6) days. In another study, groups of two to three rats were killed at different time intervals after administration of the same dose of ^{14}C-TCDD. The liver contained 3.2, 4.5, and 1.3% of the administered dose per gram of tissue 3, 7, and 21 days, respectively, after dosing. The concentrations in adipose tissue at the same time intervals were 2.6, 3.2, and 0.4% of the dose per gram of tissue. Other tissues showed lower concentrations.

In a study by Allen et al. (1975), male Sprague Dawley rats were given ^{14}C-TCDD in a single dose of 50 µg/kg body weight by stomach tube. Groups of five rats were sacrificed 1, 3, 5, 7, 14, and 21 days after dosing. The dose given resulted in marked liver hypertrophy, thymic regression, weight loss, and death in 50% of the animals within 25 days. Twenty-five percent of the dose was eliminated within the first 3 days through the faeces. During the next 18 days, 1 to 2% of the dose was found in the faeces daily. The total amount in

Table 40. Gastrointestinal absorption of TCDD

Species/Strain	Vehicle	Dose (μg/kg body weight)	% Absorption (mean ± SD)	Reference
Rats				
Sprague Dawley	acetone:corn oil (1:9)	50[a]	70	Piper et al. (1973)
Sprague Dawley	corn oil	50[a]	> 75	Allen et al. (1975)
Sprague Dawley	diet	7 or 20; for 42 days	50-60	Fries & Marrow (1975)
Sprague Dawley	acetone:corn oil (1:24)	1[a]	84±11	Rose et al. (1976)
Sprague Dawley	acetone:corn oil (1:24)	0.1 or 1.0; 5 days/week for 7 weeks	86±12	Rose et al. (1976)
Mice				
ICR/Ha Swiss	ethanol:Tween 80:saline (1:10:89)	135[a]	27-28	Koshakji et al. (1984)
Hamsters				
Golden Syrian	olive oil	650[a]	73.5±22.8	Olson et al. (1980a)

[a] Single dose.

Table 41. Elimination of TCDD in different species

Species/Strain	Route/Vehicle	Dose[a] (µg/kg body weight)	Duration of study (days)	Half-life for elimination (days)	Eliminated radioactivity (% of administered dose)		Reference
					Faeces	Urine	
Rats							
Sprague Dawley	oral/acetone: corn oil (1:9)	50	21	17.4 ± 5.6	53.2	13.2	Piper et al. (1973)
Sprague Dawley	oral/corn oil	50	21	21.3 ± 2.9	53.3	4.5	Allen et al. (1975)
Sprague Dawley	oral/acetone: corn oil (1:24)	1	22	31 ± 6	NR	ND	Rose et al. (1976)
Sprague Dawley	oral/acetone: corn oil (1:24)	1[b]	49	23.7	NR	3.1 ± 0.2 (m) 12.5 ± 5.1 (f)	Rose et al. (1976)
Sprague Dawley	ip/corn oil	400	7	NR	4.96 ± 0.3	0.51 ± 0.05	van Miller et al. (1976)
Mice							
C57BL/6	ip/olive oil	10	30	11	59.3	20.5	Gasiewicz et al. (1983b)
DBA/2	ip/olive oil	10	30	24.4	39.8	16.8	Gasiewicz et al. (1983b)
B6D2F$_1$	ip/olive oil	10	30	12.6	56.3	20.5	Gasiewicz et al. (1983b)
ICR/Ha Swiss	oral/ethanol: tween 80: saline (1:10:89)	135	11	20	78	4	Koshakji et al. (1984)
C57BL/6 Ah^b/Ah^d	ip/emulphor: ethanol:H_2O (1:1:18)	0.5	42	9.6	61.8	19.9	Birnbaum (1986)
C57BL/6 Ah^d/Ah^d	ip/emulphor: ethanol:H_2O (1:1:18)	0.5	42	9.6	55.9	26.8	Birnbaum (1986)
DBA/2 Ah^b/Ah^d	ip/emulphor: ethanol:H_2O (1:1:18)	0.5	42	10.8	71.5	13.6	Birnbaum (1986)

Table 41 (contd).

Species/Strain	Route/Vehicle	Dose[a] (μg/kg body weight)	Duration of study (days)	Half life for elimination (days)	Eliminated radioactivity (% of administered dose)		Reference
					Faeces	Urine	
Mice (contd)							
DBA/2 Ah^d/Ah^d	ip/emulphor: ethanol:H_2O (1:1:18)	0.5	42	10.8	76.1	11.1	Birnbaum (1986)
Guinea-pigs							
Hartley	ip/olive oil	2	23		33	2	Gasiewicz & Neal (1979)
NR	oral/NR	NR	22	22-43	ND	ND	Nolan et al. (1979)
Hartley	ip/olive oil	0.56	45	93.7 ± 15.5	26.2 ±3.6	3.1 ±1.2	Olson (1986)
Hamsters							
Golden Syrian	oral/olive oil	650	35	15.0 ±2.5	NR	NR	Olson et al. (1980a)
Golden Syrian	ip/olive oil	650	35	12.0 ±2.0	50.0±2.7	34.6±5.4	Olson et al. (1980a)
Monkeys							
Rhesus (adult)	ip/corn oil	400	7	NR	3.75	1.06	van Miller et al. (1976)
Rhesus (infant)	ip/corn oil	400	7	NR	1.26	2	van Miller et al. (1976)

[a] Single dose, unless otherwise stated.
[b] 5 days/week for 7 weeks.
ND = not detectable, NR = not reported, m = males, f = females, ip = intraperitoneal.

the faeces during the 21 days following administration was about 52%.

The authors concluded that the faecal content during the first 3 days represented mainly unabsorbed TCDD and that apparently more than 75% of the administered dose had been absorbed from the gastrointestinal tract. The radioactivity excreted daily through the urine ranged between 0.1 and 0.2% of the administered dose during the initial 12 days. Thereafter, the daily urinary radioactivity excretion increased from 0.25% of the administered dose to 0.43% by day 21. The total amount of ^{14}C excreted through the urine over a 21-day period was about 4.5% of the dose. On the basis of the daily faecal and urinary excretion, the authors calculated a half-time of 21.3 ($\pm$ 2.9) days. In the rats killed on days 1, 3, 5, 7, 14, and 21 after administration, the total liver content was 56 ($\pm$ 5), 54 ($\pm$ 14), 54 ($\pm$ 6), 54 ($\pm$ 8), 45 ($\pm$ 5), and 24 ($\pm$ 4)% of the administered dose, respectively. At all intervals, the levels found in the liver exceeded those found in other organs. On days 5, 7, and 14 about 90% of the total radioactivity in the liver was present in the microsomal fraction.

Fries & Marrow (1975) fed Sprague Dawley male and female rats a diet containing 7 or 20 µg ^{14}C-TCDD/kg diet for 42 days. Thereafter all rats received the control diet for another 30 days. Two animals of each sex and TCDD dietary level were sacrificed at 14-day intervals. This treatment resulted in decreased food consumption, decreased weight gain, and increased relative liver weight among both males and females. The concentration of TCDD-derived radioactivity in the liver, which was the principal tissue depot of both males and females, was directly proportional to the dietary intake of ^{14}C-TCDD. At the end of the 42-day feeding period, the ^{14}C levels in male livers indicated TCDD contents of 5.8 and 15.9 µg/kg of tissue for the lower and higher feed concentrations, respectively. The concentrations in the liver of female rats were similar. Analysis of the liver of rats killed 14 and 30 days after discontinuing TCDD exposure indicated a gradual decrease in TCDD liver concentration in both sexes. The steady-state body burden for TCDD was estimated to be 10-11 times the daily intake in both sexes. The whole-body and liver half-lives were calculated to be 12 and 11 days in males and 15 and 13 days, respectively, in females.

Rose et al. (1976) estimated the absorption of a single non-toxic dose of 1 µg ^{14}C-TCDD/kg body weight in male and female Sprague Dawley rats to be 84 $\pm$ 11% of the administered dose. The elimination of TCDD was followed for 22 days after administration and the faecal excretion accounted for most if not all of the elimination of TCDD and/or its metabolites. No radioactivity was detectable in urine and expired air. Twenty-two days after dosing, mean values of 1.26% and 1.25% of the dose/g liver and adipose tissue, respectively, were found. Much lower ^{14}C-activities were found in the thymus, kidney, and spleen, namely 0.09, 0.06, and 0.02% of the dose/g, respectively. The whole-body half-life was estimated to be 31 days. Rose et al. (1976) also followed the fate of 5 daily doses per week of 0.01, 0.1, and 1.0 µg ^{14}C-TCDD/kg body weight given for 1, 3, and 7 weeks to male and female Sprague Dawley rats (Table 42).

Table 42. Tissue distribution of TCDD-derived radioactivity in rats given oral doses of ^{14}C-TCDD[a]

	Tissue content of ^{14}C (µg equivalents of TCDD/kg tissue)[b]		
Tissue	1 week	3 weeks	7 weeks
	Exposure level: 1.0 µg/kg body weight per day		
liver	49.5±3.6	110.2±37.1	204.0±52.2
adipose tissue	10.0±3.0	23.5±7.5	61.4±36.7
thymus	0.9±0.2	7.3±4.5	6.9±2.5
kidney	0.9±0.2	1.9±0.9	5.5±5.1
spleen	0.4±0.1	1.6±0.8	1.9±1.1
	Exposure level: 0.1 µg/kg body weight per day		
liver	3.9±1.1	11.8±2.2	19.8±3.1
adipose tissue	0.9±0.6	2.7±0.8	4.5±0.7
thymus	ND	1.0±0.6	0.6±0.2
spleen	ND	0.6±0.4	0.3±0.1
kidney	ND	ND	ND
	Exposure level: 0.01 µg/kg body weight per day		
liver	ND	0.8±0.1	1.6±0.5
adipose tissue	ND	0.3 (2)[c]	0.3±0.1 (4)[c]
thymus	ND	0.6±0.1	ND
spleen	ND	0.6±0.3	ND
kidney	ND	ND	ND

[a] From: Rose et al. (1976).
[b] The mean ± standard deviation of 3 male and 3 female rats.
[c] Indicates the number of animals with detectable levels of ^{14}C-activity.
ND = not detected.

According to Kociba et al. (1976), a dose level of 0.01 µg/kg per day, 5 days/week for 13 weeks, produced no overt toxic effects, whereas 0.1 or 1.0 µg/kg per day produced adverse effects, including some deaths in the high dose group. In the study by Rose et al. (1976), the dose level of 0.01 µg/kg per day resulted in no detectable ^{14}C, except in liver, fat, and excreta. Thus no kinetic calculations on a truly non-toxic dose could be performed. Pooling the results for all rats receiving 0.1 or 1.0 µg/kg per day, the absorbed dose corresponded to 86 ± 12% of the administered dose, with an individual variation of 66 to 93%. The overall rate constant for elimination corresponded to a half-time of 23.7 days, with an individual variation of 16-37 days. The radioactivity was eliminated primarily in the faeces, but the percentage of the dose excreted in the urine compared to that eliminated in the faeces tended to increase with time. At the dose level of 1.0 µg/kg per day, males excreted in the urine 3.1 (± 0.2)% and females 12.5 (± 5.1)% of the cumulative dose over 7 weeks of exposure. The one female rat that died during the 7th week excreted 17.8% of the cumulative dose in the urine. Exhaled air was not examined in these studies. After 7 weeks of exposure, the average body burdens were 47.7 (± 8.8) and 37.1 (± 7.5)%, respectively, of the administered dose for the rats given 0.1 and 1.0 µg TCDD/kg per day. The main tissue depots of ^{14}C were the liver and adipose tissue. Radioactivity was also detected in thymus, kidney, and spleen at levels between 1 and 2% of that in liver. Direct chemical determination of liver samples confirmed the TCDD-concentrations calculated by radioactivity measurements. TCDD and/or its metabolites approached a steady-state body burden calculated to be 21.3 D_0 for rats given a daily dose (D_0, µg/kg body weight) on 5 consecutive days per week for an infinite number of weeks, within 13 weeks over the dose range 0.01 to 1.0 µg/kg per day. It was thought unlikely that the dietary intake of extremely low levels of TCDD would result in the accumulation of toxic amounts in the rat.

The excretion and distribution of a toxic dose of 400 µg ^{3}H-TCDD/kg body weight was followed in male Sprague Dawley rats (Van Miller et al., 1976). Within 7 days, about 5.0% of the dose had been excreted in faeces and 0.5% in urine. The principal tissue depots for radioactivity were liver, muscle, and skin, which contained 43.0, 4.6, and 4.4% of the administered dose, respectively.

Kociba et al. (1976) gave Sprague Dawley rats TCDD in daily doses of 0.01, 0.1, and 1 µg/kg body weight 5 days per week for 13 weeks by gavage. The liver contained TCDD at a level of 324 (± 53) µg/kg wet weight in males and 284 (± 21) µg/kg wet weight in females given repeated TCDD doses of 1 µg/kg body weight per day. For the dose level of

0.1 µg/kg body weight per day, the liver TCDD levels were 36 (± 4) and 35 (± 4) µg/kg wet weight for males and females, respectively. A dose of 0.01 µg/kg body weight per day resulted in TCDD liver levels of 2.6 (± 0.6) µg/kg wet weight in males and 3.7 (± 0.4) µg/kg wet weight in females.

After feeding diets with TCDD levels corresponding to daily dietary intakes of 0.001, 0.01, or 0.1 µg/kg body weight for 2 years, the average concentrations of TCDD found in the liver of female Sprague Dawley rats were 0.54, 5.1, and 24.0 µg/kg wet weight, respectively (Kociba et al., 1978). The corresponding levels in adipose tissue were 0.54, 1.7, and 8.1 µg/kg wet weight. A comparison of liver TCDD levels found in rats given comparable daily doses of TCDD for 13 weeks (Kociba et al., 1976) or 2 years (Kociba et al., 1978) indicates that with prolonged exposure the liver TCDD content reaches a plateau. This finding agrees well with the prediction obtained by mathematical analysis of the data resulting from experiments involving exposure of a few weeks (Rose et al., 1976).

The proportion of a single oral dose of ^{3}H-TCDD found in the liver of female Sprague Dawley rats was dependent both on the dose level and on the vehicle used (Poiger & Schlatter, 1980). Maximal retention occurred within 48 h after dosing. Increasing retention was observed up to a dose of 280 ng TCDD/rat. Hepatic retention 24 h after dosing was higher (36.7% of the dose) if TCDD was given in 50% ethanol than if it was given as an aqueous suspension of soil (37%, w/w), where it was 16-24.1% of the dose, or activated carbon (25%, w/w), where it was < 0.07% of the dose (see section 7.4).

Biliary excretion of radioactivity originating from ^{3}H-labelled TCDD occurred at a more or less constant rate of 0.5 to 1% of the administered dose per day for 12 days following the administration of 100 µg TCDD/kg body weight in a female Sprague Dawley rat (Poiger & Buser, 1983). No severe toxic effects were observed within that time period.

McConnell et al. (1984) dosed female Sprague Dawley rats orally with either pure TCDD in corn oil or amounts of contaminated soil giving similar doses of TCDD. In general TCDD in soil was as potent an inducer of aryl hydrocarbon hydroxylase (AHH) as pure TCDD in corn oil. The hepatic concentration of TCDD was 40.8 µg/kg in the corn oil group, receiving 5 µg TCDD/kg body weight, and 20.3 µg/kg in the soil group, receiving 5.5 µg TCDD/kg body weight (see section 7.4).

Poiger & Schlatter (1980) studied the dermal absorption of ^{3}H-TCDD in hairless rats of the Naked ex Back-Cross and Holzman strain (200-250 g). Using the amount of TCDD-derived radioactivity found in the liver as an indicator of its absorption, they reported that the permeation of TCDD across the epidermis was highly dependent on the formulation used. The highest radioactivity in the liver, 14.8% of the administered dose, was detected when TCDD was applied as a methanolic solution. The hepatic recovery of the administered dose observed when TCDD was applied in polyethylene glycol 1500 with and without 15% water was 14.1 and 1.4%, respectively. Dermal application of TCDD in vaseline or adsorbed onto soil or activated carbon decreased the percentage of the dose recovered in the liver to 1.4, 1.7-2.2, and < 0.05%, respectively.

In studies by van den Berg et al. (1983), fly ash and crude or purified toluene extracts of PCDD- and PCDF-containing fly ash from a municipal incinerator were mixed with ordinary laboratory diet for rats. Small portions (2 g) of these diets were fed to male Wistar rats (300 g) every 24 h for 19 days, at which time the animals were sacrified. Tetra-, penta-, and hexa-chlorinated PCDDs and PCDFs in the liver and adipose tissues of these rats were determined. Rats fed the fly ash containing diet stored PCDDs and PCDFs in their livers at concentrations that were at least 3 to 5 times lower than in the case of rats fed comparable amounts of fly ash extracts (for the pentaCDD, hexaCDF, and hexaCDD isomers, the concentrations were approximately 10-20 times lower). Generally PCDFs showed a higher retention in rat liver than did the corresponding PCDDs. In the adipose tissue of rats fed with fly ash extracts, retention was higher for penta- and hexaCDDs than for the corresponding PCDFs.

In further fly ash studies, male Wistar rats (275 g) were fed for up to 99 days a diet that included 2.5% HCl-pretreated fly ash (containing PCDDs and PCDFs) from a municipal incinerator (van den Berg et al., 1986a). A control group received standard diet. All congeners retained in the liver of the rats had a 2,3,7,8-chlorine substitution pattern. With the exception of 2,3,4,7,8-pentaCDF and 2,3,4,6,7,8-hexaCDF, liver retention for each congener was below 10% of the group dose. The retention percentages of the various congeners in the liver were almost equal at the time-points studied (34, 59, and 99 days), thus indicating a long half-life of these congeners in rat liver.

Male Wistar rats fed 22.7 (± 1) μg or 120.7 (± 2.8) μg octaCDD over a two-week period were found to retain about 1-2% of the given dose in the liver (Williams et al., 1972). The heart, kidneys, spleen, lung, skeletal muscle, testes, and urine contained no detectable levels of octaCDD, but minor amounts were found in the adipose tissue of the high-dose group. Faeces contained 61% and 37%, respectively, of the low and high dose given. The presence of a large quantity of octaCDD in the faeces compared to that in the bile 24-72 h after a single oral dose of 58 μg octaCDD to bile-cannulated male Wistar rats (400 g) indicated that the dioxin present in the faeces was mainly unabsorbed octaCDD (Williams et al., 1972).

After 21 daily doses of 100 µg octaCDD containing 12.6 pg ^{35}S-thio-heptaCDD to male Sprague Dawley rats, the radioactivity was mainly recovered in the faeces and urine, the percentages of the ingested radioactive dose being 93 (± 6) and 5.2 (± 0.8)% respectively (Norback et al., 1975). The high faecal excretion suggests poor absorption. Of the radioactive body burden, 50% was contained in the liver. The microsomal fraction contained 96.3 (± 8.2)% of the hepatic radioactivity.

6.1.2 Studies on mice

In studies by Vinopal & Casida (1973), male white mice (20 g) were given tritium-labelled TCDD intraperitoneally in a single dose of 130 µg/kg body weight. Three days after TCDD administration to one mouse, 13% of the administered tritium was recovered in the faeces and 0.3% in the urine, while 32% was found in the liver and 0.3% in the kidneys. In another study, groups of two to six mice were killed at various time intervals after similar treatment with the same dose of ^{3}H-TCDD. One and 4 days after dosing, the liver contained about 15% of the dose, on the 8th day, 26%, on the 11th day, 22%, and on the 15th and 20th days, about 10%. The highest amount of ^{3}H-activity was found in the microsomal fraction of the liver. Somewhat lower activity was detected in the mitochondrial fraction and the nuclei. The supernatant fraction was practically devoid of any radioactivity. On day 8 when the highest levels were observed, the whole liver homogenate contained 26.7 (± 4.8)% of the administered dose, the microsomes 12.6 (± 3.8)%, the nuclei 7.8 (± 1.2)%, the mitochondria 6.2 (± 1.3)%, and the supernatant fraction 0.1 (± 0.0)% of the administered dose.

Coccia et al. (1981) described the effect of adding different substances to food on the persistence of TCDD in the liver of male C57Bl/6 mice. In one of the experiments, the test diet was given immediately after the administration of a single oral dose of 7.6 µg ^{3}H-TCDD/kg body weight. The hepatic radioactivity 14 days after dosing was 17.3, 6.3, 13.1, and 14.5% of the administered dose in animals fed standard chow containing 5% vegetable charcoal, 0.5% cholic acid, and 4% cholestyramine, respectively. When feeding of the test diet started 3 days after dosing, the hepatic retention of ^{3}H-TCDD was decreased to a similar extent.

Faecal and urinary excretion (Table 41), along with the formation of faecal, biliary, and urinary metabolites (see 7.2.1.1), of ^{3}H-TCDD was studied in male C57BL/6, DBA/2, and

B6D2F1 mice after a single intraperitoneal dose of 10 µg ^{3}H-TCDD/kg body weight (Gasiewicz et al., 1983b). The principal tissue depot in C57BL/6 and B6D2F1 mice was the liver, followed by the adipose tissue. Most other tissues examined contained less than 1% of the administered dose. In DBA/2 mice, the adipose tissue contained more radioactivity than the liver. This difference may be due to the fact that these three strains of mice differ in their adipose tissue content, being 5.9, 11.5, and 5.0% of the body weight in C57BL/6, DBA/2, and B6D2F1 mice, respectively. The estimated half-lives of clearance of ^{3}H-TCDD from the liver of C57BL/6, DBA/2, and B6D2F1 mice were 17, 27, and 13 days, respectively, and the corresponding figures for the half-life in the adipose tissue were 11, 42, and 11 days. The cumulative faecal elimination 30 days after dosing was 59.3, 39.8, and 56.3% of the administered dose in C57B1/6, DBA/2, and B6D2F1 mice, respectively, and the corresponding figures for urinary elimination were 20.5, 16.8, and 20.5%.

Birnbaum (1986) studied in mice the distribution and excretion of a single intraperitoneal dose of 500 ng (45 µCi) ^{3}H-TCDD/kg body weight for up to 42 days after treatment. Two sets of congenic strains of mice were used, i.e., male C57B1/6 and female DBA/2 mice, where within each congenic pair the mice differed only at the Ah locus (or at a limited number of genes closely linked to the Ah locus). The mice were bred and phenotyped by zoxazolamine paralysis time. The results, some of them summarized in Tables 47 and 48, suggested that, at the dose level studied, the distribution and excretion of TCDD were primarily governed by the total genetic background rather than by the allele present at the Ah locus.

When male ICR/Ha Swiss mice (27 - 35 g) were given a single oral dose of 135 µg ^{14}C-TCDD/kg body weight, about 71% and 1-2%, respectively, of the administered dose was eliminated via faeces and urine within the first 24 h (Koshakji et al., 1984). During the following 10 days, an additional 7% and 2% of the administered radioactivity were recovered in faeces and urine, respectively. Based on the estimated body burden of radioactivity, a whole-body half-life of 20 days was calculated.

The distribution of ^{3}H-TCDD in the skin of hairless (SKH:HR-1) mice after a single intraperitoneal dose of 6.3 µg TCDD/kg body weight was examined for up to 14 days (Puhvel et al., 1986). Most of the ^{3}H-TCDD in skin was localized in the dermis, although the concentration of ^{3}H-TCDD was consistently higher in the epidermis.

Table 43. Tissue content of TCDD-derived ^{14}C (% of dose/g tissue)[a] in guinea-pigs following a single dose of ^{14}C-TCDD[d]

Tissue	Days after exposure					
	1	3	5	7	11	15
Perirenal adipose	3.2±1.0	4.1±0.4	2.1±0.4	1.3±0.2	2.1±0.2	
Epididymal adipose	1.5±0.8	3.8±0.5	3.4±0.7	3.2±0.1	3.9[b]	2.5±1.1
Adrenal	1.4±0.3	1.4±0.2	0.9±0.1	1.2±0.3	2.1±0.9	1.7±0.2
Liver	1.1±0.4	1.5±0.4	1.3±0.2	1.1±0.2	2.2±0.2	3.2±0.3
Liver[c]	11.4±3.3	15.5±3.3	14.0±2.3	12.0±1.9	21.2±2.3	29.6±2.7
Spleen	0.7±0.3	0.5±0.3	0.2±0.1	0.4±0.2	0.4±0.2	0.5±0.1
Duodenum	0.4±0.2	0.2±0.1	0.2±0.1	0.2±0.1	0.2±0.1	0.3±0.1
Pancreas	-	-	0.2±0.1	0.5±0.3	0.4±0.3	0.3±0.1
Stomach	0.2±0.1	0.3±0.1	0.1±0.1	0.2±0.1	0.3±0.1	0.3±0.1
Testes	0.2±0.1	0.3±0.1	0.2±0.1	0.3±0.1	0.3±0.1	0.2±0.1
Kidneys	0.3±0.1	0.3±0.1	0.2±0.1	0.4±0.1	0.8±0.4	0.7±0.1
Bone marrow	0.3±0.1	0.5±0.1	0.2±0.1	0.4±0.1	0.4[b]	0.2±0.1
Lungs	0.3±0.1	0.2±0.1	0.2±0.1	0.4±0.1	0.5±0.2	0.6±0.1
Skin[c]	13.8±0.7	16.3±0.3	15.8±2.4	6.5±0.8	6.5±0.7	6.7±0.6
Brain, heart, skeletal muscle	<0.25					

[a] Mean ± standard error for three animals, unless indicated otherwise.
[b] Mean of two animals.
[c] Percentage of dose/tissue.
[d] From: Gasiewicz & Neal (1979).

6.1.3 Studies on guinea-pigs

The retention of a single intraperitoneal dose of 2 µg ^{14}C-TCDD/kg body weight in various tissues of male Hartley guinea-pigs was determined 1, 3, 5, 7, 11, and 15 days after exposure (Table 43) (Gasiewicz & Neal, 1979). Three animals died and all animals lost 24 to 35% of the body weight during the study. The highest amount of radioactivity per tissue was found in the liver and skin. The radioactivity in the liver increased with time, concomitant to the depletion of adipose tissues. Radioactivity in the skin decreased also with time. No signs of toxicity were seen when the cumulative excretion of a single i.p dose of 0.5 µg ^{3}H-TCDD/kg body weight in male Hartley guinea-pigs was studied (Gasiewicz & Neal, 1979). The faecal and urinary excretion of radioactivity was linear throughout the 23-day study. Approximately 1.4% of the administered dose was excreted daily during that period, and the faeces contained 94% of the excreted radioactivity.

The microsomal fraction of the liver in male Hartley guinea-pigs contained 40.7 to 47.4% of the hepatic radioactivity 1 day after a single ip dose of 0.3, 2.0, or 7.0 µg of ^{3}H- or ^{14}C-TCDD/kg body weight (Gasiewicz & Neal, 1979). Corresponding values for the crude nuclear fraction, the mitochondrial fraction, and the soluble fraction were 20.1-35.6%, 9.5-12.9%, and 7.6-26.4%, respectively. The subcellular distribution was similar 1 and 6 days after the low dose but, following the high dose, more radioactivity was present in the microsomal fraction and less was recovered in the crude nuclear and soluble fractions on day 6 after exposure.

Olson (1986) followed the distribution, elimination and metabolism (see section 6.2.1.1) of a single ip dose of 0.56 µg ^{3}H-TCDD/kg body weight in adult (335 to 625 g) male Hartley guinea pigs for 45 days. One of seven animals died on day 27, but the remaining animals gained weight and exhibited no gross signs of toxicity. At termination the body composition was normal, and 61% of the administered radioactivity was recovered in the twelve investigated tissues at the end of the study. The adipose tissue contained 36% of the dose; liver, pelt, and skeletal muscle plus carcass contained each 7% of the dose; the gastrointestinal tract contained about 2% of the dose, and remaining tissues contained less than 0.5% of the dose. Urinary and faecal elimination followed apparent first-order kinetics, with half-lives of 82.5 ($\pm$ 22.4) and 94.4 ($\pm$ 14.7) days, respectively.

6.1.4 Studies on hamsters

In studies by Olson et al. (1980a), Golden Syrian hamsters absorbed about 73.5% of a single oral dose of 650 µg ^{3}H-TCDD/kg body weight, a dose that produced thymic atrophy and body weight loss in several of the animals. The distribution of radioactitivity in various tissues 1, 3, 10, and 20

Table 44. Tissue distribution of TCDD-derived radioactivity in Golden Syrian hamsters at 1, 3, 10, and 20 days following a single oral dose of 650 µg ^{3}H-TCDD/kg body weight[a]

	Tissue content of ^{3}H (% of dose/g tissue)[b]			
Tissue	Day 1	Day 3	Day 10	Day 20
Liver	4.03±1.00	5.32±.82	3.19±.93	0.86±0.09
Liver[b]	12.74±3.21	20.44±3.45	9.69±0.99	3.70±0.29
Perirenal adipose	2.93±0.87	3.48±0.56	1.38±0.28	0.32±0.03
Adrenals	1.56±0.52	1.12±0.14	0.47±0.08	0.10±0.01
Pancreas	0.39±0.20	0.61±0.13	0.62±0.26	0.21±0.04
Kidneys	0.60±0.16	0.64±0.11	0.60±0.32	0.12±0.03
Spleen	0.30±0.08	0.24±0.05	0.43±0.26	0.07±0.02
Thymus	0.49±0.14	0.34±0.11	-	0.05±0.02
Skin	0.84±0.26	0.31±0.07	0.56+0.18	0.03±0.01
Stomach	0.34±0.07	0.55±0.09	0.65±0.39	0.16±0.06
Duodenum	0.51±0.13	0.47±0.09	0.55±0.28	0.07±0.02
Jejunum	0.59±0.15	0.71±0.20	0.39±0.16	0.08±0.02
Ileum	0.41±0.12	0.35±0.05	0.37±0.21	0.06±0.02
Colon	0.92±0.27	0.60±0.14	0.34±0.07	0.06±0.01
Caecum	0.39±0.11	0.41±0.10	0.28±0.12	0.05±0.01
Lungs	0.38±0.09	0.37±0.05	0.41±0.25	0.07±0.03
Skeletal muscle	0.20±0.07	0.15±0.05	0.15±0.03	0.04±0.02
Heart	0.14±0.03	0.13±0.02	0.15±0.08	0.03±0.01
Testes	0.10±0.04	0.32±0.13	0.13±0.04	0.03±0.01
Blood	0.12±0.02	0.14±0.03	0.12±0.06	0.02±0.01
Brain	0.03±0.01	0.05±0.01	0.06±0.02	0.01

[a] From: Olson et al. (1980a).
[b] All values are the mean (± standard error) of four hamsters.
[c] Percentage of dose/liver.

days after administration is given in Table 44. The principal depots were the liver and adipose tissue. A similar pattern of distribution was obtained when the same dose was given intraperitoneally. The elimination of radioactivity in faeces and urine was followed for 35 days after a single intraperitoneal (ip) or oral dose of 650 µg/kg body weight

(Olson et al., 1980a). The half-life for elimination was 12.0 (± 2.0) days and 15.0 (± 2.5) days for the ip and oral routes, respectively. Of the excreted radioactivity 41% occurred in urine and 59% in faeces.

The hepatic retention of PCDDs and PCDFs from dietary intake of HCl-pretreated fly ash from a municipal incinerator was studied in male Golden syrian hamsters (van den Berg et al., 1986b). The livers were analysed for tetra-, penta-, and hexaCDDs and PCDFs after feeding the diet, which contained 25% fly ash, for 34, 58, and 95 days. No detectable hepatic retention was observed after 34 days. The highest retention after 95 days was 8.4% for 2,3,4,7,8-pentaCDF, but the retention was generally below 5% of the total dose. With the exception of 2,3,4,6,7-pentaCDF, only 2,3,7,8-substituted PCDDs and PCDFs were retained. Constant relative concentrations were found for the 2,3,7,8-substituted PCDDs and PCDFs at the time points studied.

6.1.5 Studies on monkeys

Van Miller et al. (1976) gave three adult female rhesus monkeys and four male infant rhesus monkeys a single intraperitoneal dose of 400 µg ^{3}H-TCDD/kg body weight in corn oil. This dose resulted in a loss of body weight: 10.8% for adults and 20.7% for infants, and light microscopic changes in the liver. Over a 7-day period the adult monkeys excreted 1.06% of the dose in the urine and 3.75% in the faeces. During the same period the infant monkeys excreted approximately 2% of the administered dose in urine and about 1.26% in the faeces. The authors questioned the accuracy of these figures owing to the difficulty of separating the two types of excreta from infant monkeys. The total tissue concentrations of radioactivity 7 days after dosing are given in Table 45. The principal tissue depots of radioactivity in adult monkeys were adipose tissue, skin, liver, and muscle; they contained 16.2, 13.1, 10.4, and 8.6% of the administered dose, respectively. The distribution in infant monkeys was 35.6% in muscle, 22.7% in skin, and only 4.5% of the dose in the liver.

The concentration of TCDD in samples of faeces, urine, and fat were measured by GC-MS at intervals after dosing up to 715 days in an adult female rhesus monkey (Macaca mulatta) given a single oral dose of 1 µg TCDD/kg body weight (McNulty et al., 1982b). During the 3 months after dosing the monkey lost 50% of its body weight but then began to gain weight again. The level of TCDD in faeces was high for 4 days and then fell to very low or undetectable levels. TCDD in urine was very low at all time points. The apparent half-life of TCDD in adipose tissue was about 1 year.

Table 45. Tissue distribution of TCDD-derived radioactivity in adult and infant rhesus monkeys 7 days following a single intraperitoneal dose of 400 µg ^{3}H-TCDD/kg body weight[a]

Tissue	(% of dose/tissue) Tissue content of ^{3}H[b]	
	Adult	Infant
Liver	10.4±6.9	4.51±1.60
Brain	0.58±0.34	1.41±1.40
Spleen	0.028±0.013	0.026±0.004
Small intestine	0.87±0.39	1.47±0.64
Large intestine	1.29±0.12	0.64±0.24
Muscle[c]	8.62±2.39	35.6±14.4
Skin	13.1±4.9	22.7±8.8
Adipose tissue[d]	16.2±5.8	

[a] From: Van Miller et al. (1976).
[b] Mean (± standard deviation) of three adults or four infants.
[c] Total muscle was taken as 40% of body weight.
[d] Quantities in infant monkey were insignificant. For adult monkeys, the calculation was based on an estimate of 300 g mesenteric fat.

There were no significant time-dependent changes in TCDD-derived radioactivity found in the tissues investigated from marmosets during the 3-week-period following subcutaneous treatment with 5 µg ^{14}C-TCDD/kg body weight, except for a minor decrease in levels found in the adipose tissue (Krowke, 1986). The data thus indicate a long half-life for TCDD in marmosets.

6.1.6 Studies on dogs

A one-year-old male beagle dog received a total dose of 5.4 mg of TCDD enterally by direct introduction into the duodenal lumen in four portions of 1-2 mg, with intervals of 2-7 days between treatments (Poiger et al., 1982). Severe toxic symtoms preceeded the death of the animal 17 days after the first dose. The excretion of radioactivity in the bile reached a maximum on day 1 or day 2 following administration. Significantly more biliary radioactivity was found after administration of doses 3 and 4 than after the administration of doses 1 and 2, suggesting that TCDD-administration stimulated its own metabolism. It was later demonstrated in a 18-months-old male boxer that TCDD-pretreatment (10 µg/kg body weight) stimulated the biliary excretion of ^{3}H-labelled TCDD

(32.8 ng/kg body weight), whereas phenobarbital-pretreatment had no effect when compared to the biliary excretion without pretreatment (Poiger & Schlatter, 1985). All the experiments were carried out in the same animal, which had enough time between treatments for the radioactivity to return almost to the background level.

6.1.7 Studies on cows

The major routes for elimination of ^{3}H-TCDD in Holstein cows (500-650 kg) after oral doses of 0.05 µg (two cows) or 7.5 µg (one cow) TCDD/kg body weight were faeces > milk > urine (Jones et al., 1987). Fifty percent of the administered dose was eliminated in faeces, the major part in the first few days after treatment. Three lactating Holstein cows received commercial technical grade pentachlorophenol orally by gelatine capsule at a dose rate of 10 mg/kg body weight twice daily for 10 days and once daily for the following 60 days (Firestone et al., 1979). One cow served as a control and received gelatine capsules containing only ground corn. The pentachlorophenol composite used contained ten PCDD congeners (0.1 to 690 mg/kg) and eight PCDF congeners (0.9 to 130 mg/kg). Faeces collected on day 28 of the treatment period contained three hexaCDDs (0.05 to 0.63 µg/kg), two heptaCDDs (21.3 to 33.1 µg/kg), and octaCDD (290 to 429 µg/kg). Faeces also contained hexa-, hepta-, and octaCDF. Milk, body fat, and blood contained only three of the PCDD congeners present in the pentachlorophenol composite, namely 1,2,3,6,7,8-hexaCDD, 1,2,3,4,6,7,8-heptaCDD, and octaCDD. Milk samples also contained hexa-, hepta-, and octaCDF. The average concentrations of 1,2,3,6,7,8-hexaCDD, 1,2,3,4,6,7,8-heptaCDD, octaCDD, and octaCDF in the composite milk fat at the end of the treatment period were 20, 40, 25, and 2 mg/kg respectively. Similar concentrations were found in body (shoulder) fat at the end of the treatment period (13, 24, and 32 mg/kg, respectively, of 1,2,3,6,7,8-hexaCDD, 1,2,3,4,6,7,8-heptaCDD, and octaCDD). Levels of dioxins in the blood were approximately 1000 times below the values in milk or body fat. The average daily excretion of 1,2,3,6,7,8-hexaCDD, 1,2,3,4,6,7,8-heptaCDD, and octaCDD in the milk during days 40-70 was about 20, 40, and 23 µg, corresponding to 33, 3, and 0.6% of the daily intake of PCDDs. One hundred days after the cessation of treatment, the average values for 1,2,3,6,7,8-hexaCDD, 1,2,3,4,6,7,8-heptaCDD, and octaCDD in shoulder fat and milk fat were 2.5, 6.6, 5.6 mg/kg and 4.3, 6.9, 3.0 mg/kg, respectively.

6.1.8 In vitro studies

The uptake of ^{3}H-TCDD in human fibroblasts was less efficient when the TCDD was associated with the high density lipoprotein (HDL) than with the low density lipoprotein (LDL), and even less when associated with serum (Shireman & Wei, 1986). From studies in mutant human fibroblasts lacking the normal LDL cellular receptor, the authors concluded that the LDL receptor pathway was involved in the cellular uptake of TCDD. The uptake from LDL was time, temperature, and concentration dependent.

6.2 Metabolic Transformation

6.2.1 Studies on mammals

6.2.1.1 In vivo studies

The possible existence of a urinary metabolite of TCDD was first suggested by the finding of Allen et al. (1975) that the radioactivity in urine of 14C-TCDD treated rats was highest from week 2 to 3. Later both Poiger & Schlatter (1979) and Ramsey et al. (1982) presented evidence for the *in vivo* biotransformation of TCDD in the rat. Male Sprague Dawley rats were given two, four, or six daily oral doses of approximately 15 µg ^{14}C-TCDD/kg body weight, and the bile was collected for 24 h following the last dose (Ramsey et al., 1982). Using high pressure liquid chromatography, at least eight metab olites of TCDD were found in the bile from these rats. Incubation of the bile with β-glucuronidase indicated the presence of glucuronide conjugates among the metabolites. Poiger & Schlatter (1979) incubated similarly the bile or the dialysate with glucuronidase/arylsulfatase, and the dichloro methane-extractable radioactivity increased from 1.5% to 75%. Their results indicate the elimination of TCDD-metabolites in the form of water-soluble sulfate and glucuronide conjugates. ^{3}H-TCDD metabolites extracted from the bile of one-year-old beagle dogs with ethanol (Poiger et al., 1982) were given to bile-duct-cannulated female Sprague Dawley rats (250 g) as single oral doses of 7.8-20.8 µg ^{3}H-TCDD-metabolites/kg body weight (Weber et al., 1982b). The mean 24-h elimination of radioactivity was 86.7 (± 6.7)% of the dose, 8.2% occurring in urine, 31.3% in bile, and 46.9% in faeces. A delay in the excretion of radioactivity in rats whose bile ducts were not cannulated suggested an enterohepatic circulation in the rat of the ^{3}H-TCDD-metabolites from the dog. The radioactive material in the rat bile seemed to be conjugated forms of the metabolites from the dogs. A metabolic breakdown scheme of TCDD in the rat and dog (Fig. 3) was proposed by Poiger &

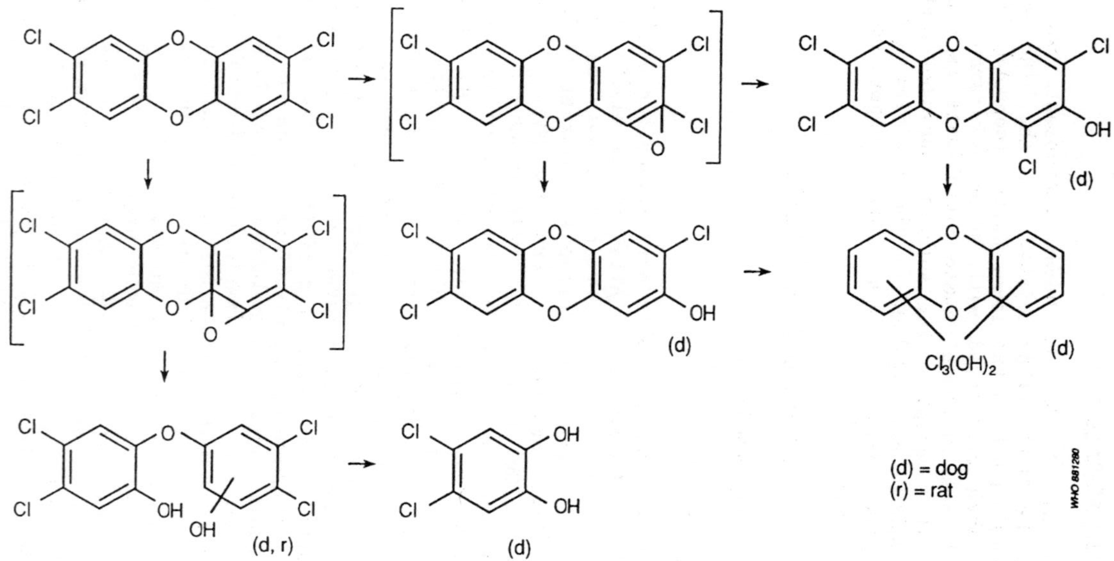

Fig. 3. Proposed metabolic breakdown scheme for TCDD. From: Poiger & Buser (1983).

Buser (1983). The major metabolite seems to be formed via cleavage of an ether bond.

The metabolic fate of a single ip dose of 10 µg, 500 µCi TCDD/kg body weight in male C57Bl/6, DBA/2, and B6D2F1 mice was studied by Gasiewicz et al. (1983b). Samples of urine, bile, and faeces, collected on days 5 to 8, 8, and 7 after treatment, respectively, were extracted and analyzed for metabolites of TCDD by HPLC. Unmetabolized TCDD was detected in faeces but not in urine or in bile. More than 85% of the total radioactivity eliminated was present as metabolites of TCDD in all three mouse strains. Metabolites in the bile appear to be less polar than in urine. Qualitatively the elution profiles for urine, bile, and faeces from all three strains appeared to be quite similar.

A dose of ^{3}H-TCDD (0.56 µg/kg body weight) that produced no gross toxicity was given ip in olive oil to six adult male Hartley guinea-pigs (Olson, 1986). Metabolites of TCDD were found in organic extracts of the liver, kidney, perirenal adipose tissue, and skeletal muscle in amounts corresponding to 13, 4, 8, and 28%, respectively, of the recovered radioactivity in these organs 45 days after dosing. These figures suggest that TCDD-metabolites are not efficiently eliminated from tissues in guinea-pigs. All radioactivity in urine and bile represented metabolites of TCDD, whereas in faeces most (70-90%) contained unchanged TCDD. Of the radioactivity administered, 73.4% was eliminated as unchanged TCDD in faeces and 25.7% as metabolites of TCDD in urine and faeces. The presence of TCDD in faeces and its absence in bile suggest that direct elimination of TCDD from the blood to the intestinal lumen may occur. The HPLC elution profiles for metabolites were similar, although not identical, for bile, urine, and tissues. Taken together, the data by Olson (1986) indicate that metabolism does not appear to have a major role in the ultimate elimination of TCDD in the guinea-pig.

Olson et al. (1980a) collected bile and urine from Golden Syrian hamsters that had been treated with a single ip dose of 650 µg ^{14}C-TCDD/kg body weight 7 days earlier. By means of HPLC, one major and several minor metabolites of ^{14}C-TCDD were demonstrated both in bile and urine. No metabolites of ^{14}C-TCDD were detectable in liver and adipose tissue, thus suggesting a rapid clearance of biotransformed products of TCDD.

A one-year-old beagle dog was cholecystectomized and a Thomas cannula was implanted about 3 months before the first dose of TCDD (Poiger et al., 1982, Poiger & Buser, 1983). A total dose of 5.4 mg was administered enterally in four portions of 1.8, 1.08, 1.08, and 1.44 mg on days 0, 2, 7, and 13. Five phenolic metabolites of TCDD excreted in dog bile were identified by combined gas chromatography-mass spectrometry. Severe toxic symptoms preceded the death of the dog 17 days after the first dose. A metabolic breakdown scheme of TCDD in the dog (Fig. 3) was proposed by Poiger & Buser (1983), lateral hydroxylation of TCDD seeming to be the major route of metabolism.

6.2.1.2 In vitro studies

Although there is evidence of different metabolites of TCDD and the possibility of its metabolic transformation was suggested as early as 1975 (Allen et al., 1975; Rose et al., 1976), it was only in 1982 that specific metabolites were identified by Sawahata et al. (1982). They incubated TCDD with isolated rat hepatocytes at 37 °C for 8 h, and the resulting incubation mixture was subjected to HPLC. The major peak of radioactivity not corresponding to TCDD was incubated with β-glucuronidase in order to split the possible glucuronide conjugate(s) of TCDD or its metabolite(s). They found that 4,5-dichlorocatechol and 4,5-dichloroguaiacol are potential metabolites of TCDD, but due to the limited amount of material the identity of these metabolites was not confirmed by gas chromatography-mass spectrometry. Two other metabolites of TCDD, namely 1-hydroxy-2,3,7,8-tetrachloro-dibenzo-p-dioxin and 8-hydroxy-2,3,7-trichlorodibenzo-p-dioxin, were isolated by means of HPLC, and were identified by mass spectrometry.

Primary hepatocytes from Sprague Dawley rats and Hartley guinea-pigs have been used to study the metabolism of ^{14}C-TCDD (Wroblewski & Olson, 1985). The overall metabolism was 2.8 times greater in rats than in guinea-pigs. The metabolism of ^{14}C-TCDD was increased 3.2-fold in rats pretreated with TCDD (5 µg TCDD/kg body weight ip 72 h prior to isolation of hepatocytes), but no effect was found in similarly TCDD-pretreated guinea-pigs, or in phenobarbital- pretreated rats (80 mg/kg body weight ip for 3 days, beginning 4 days prior to isolation of hepatocytes). Hepatocytes from TCDD-pretreated rats metabolized TCDD 9 times more rapidly than similarly pretreated guinea-pig hepatocytes. TCDD may be metabolized by an inducible form of cytochrome P448 which is expressed in rats but not guinea-pigs. These differences in metabolism may play a major role in explaining the differences in species susceptibility to the acute effects of TCDD.

6.3 Transfer Via Placenta and/or Milk

The transplacental passage of ^{14}C-TCDD has been studied by Khera & Ruddick (1973). Pregnant Wistar rats were given ^{14}C-TCDD in a single oral dose of 200 µg/kg body weight on gestation days 16, 17, or 18 and were killed 6 h after dosing.

^{14}C-activity was detected in maternal tissues and also in the fetuses and the placenta. Assuming that all the ^{14}C-activity found in the samples was present as ^{14}C-TCDD, the following levels (ng/gram tissue) were found for gestation days 16, 17, and 18 respectively: maternal liver 339 (± 15), 339 (± 19), and 275 (± 20); maternal blood 25 (± 11), 19 (± 9), and 10 (± 3); placenta 25 (± 6), 38 (± 4), and 41 (± 3); and fetus 11 (± 3), 15 (± 1), and 16 (± 1). Studies by Moore et al. (1973) indicated that the passage of TCDD or its metabolites into milk could be of importance, as TCDD-related effects were observed in sucklings, nourished by lactating mothers given, after delivery, a single oral dose of 1 or 3 µg/kg body weight.

The TCDD concentration in livers of pregnant NMRI mice, at a given dose, was significantly lower than in livers of non-pregnant mice (Krowke 1986). The concentration of TCDD in the liver of non-pregnant mice was about 5 times higher than in pregnant mice 7 days after a s.c. dose.

Nau & Bass (1981) studied the transfer of ^{14}C-TCDD to embryos and fetuses in NMRI mice. The animals were given a single dose of 5, 12.5, or 25 µg TCDD/kg body weight by gavage or by s.c. or ip injection at day 16 of gestation to study the transfer of TCDD to the fetus. The animals were killed two days later and various tissues were analyzed for radioactivity. No evidence was found to indicate a major first pass effect following oral administration. Maternal livers contained the highest levels of TCDD, 4.1 to 10.5% of the radioactive dose administered, which was about one order of magnitude higher than in extrahepatic maternal tissues, including placenta. Fetal liver and extrahepatic tissues contained low levels of radioactivity corresponding to 0.09 to 1.41% and 0.05 to 0.14%, respectively, of the dose administered to the dams. More radioactivity was recovered in the placenta and fetus when TCDD was given either as a single ip dose of 25 µg/kg body weight on day 10 of gestation or as 5 daily ip doses of 5 µg/kg body weight on days 7 to 11, when compared to a single i.p. dose of 25 µg/kg body weight on gestation day 7. Oral dosing of 30 µg ^{14}C-TCDD (0.332 µCi/µg)/kg body weight to pregnant C57Bl/6 mice on gestation day 11 resulted in 0 to 14% embryomortality on gestation days 12 to 14 (Weber & Birnbaum, 1985). About 0.03% of the radioactive dose was contained in the embryo and in the placenta on days 12 to 14 of gestation. The maternal liver contained 67.4, 67.9, and 50.6% of the administered radioactive dose on gestation days 12, 13, and 14, during which days the cumulative elimination of radioactivity in urine and faeces was 2.4 and 53.3% of the dose, respectively.

The transfer of ^{14}C-TCDD via placenta and milk and the distribution of the transformed TCDD between various embryonic and fetal tissues were studied in NMRI mice (Nau et al., 1986). Dams were given a single dose of 25 µg ^{14}C-TCDD (45 mCi/mmol)/kg body weight either orally, subcutaneously, or intraperitoneally. To differentiate between postnatal and *in utero* exposure, the experimental design included cross fostering. Depending on the route of administration, from 0.02 to 0.07% of the administered radioactivity was found in the liver of the fetus at birth. The highest levels were noted after ip administration and the lowest after oral intubation. The corresponding values one week after birth were 0.05 to 0.20%. The hepatic radioactivity in the neonate reached a peak 1 week after birth and then decreased slowly throughout and after lactation. The levels of TCDD-derived radioactivity in extrahepatic tissues of the offspring were approximately one order of magnitude lower than the hepatic levels. Very little radioactivity was found in the stomach filled with milk, indicating that TCDD ingested from milk was rapidly absorbed in the stomach.

Arstila et al. (1981) studied the excretion of TCDD in goat milk after a subchronic administration of 200 ng TCDD per day for 2 months in the first experiment and of 400 ng TCDD per day for one month in the second experiment. The minimal detectable concentration in this study was declared to be below 5 ng/litre. The maximum concentration of TCDD in milk in the first experiment was 20.8 (± 6.6) ng/litre and in the second experiment 19.3 (± 6.6) ng/litre. After 18 weeks feeding with TCDD the levels had dropped to 4.2 and 3.6 ng/litre, respectively.

The secretion of TCDD in milk and cream has also been studied in lactating dairy cows kept on a diet containing 10, 30, 100, 300, or 1000 mg/litre 2,4,5-T, corresponding to TCDD levels of 5, 15, 50, 150, and 500 ng/litre (Jensen & Hummel, 1982). This resulted in levels of TCDD in the excreted milk of below detection limit, 3, 10, 16-22, and 42-89 ng/litre, respectively, indicating that about 10-20% of the dose given was eliminated in the milk. The levels in cream were about ten times higher than those in milk.

One lactating Holstein cow, receiving commercial technical-grade pentachlorophenol containing several PCDDs and PCDFs orally in gelatine capsules at a dose rate of 10 mg/kg body weight twice daily for 10 days and once daily for the following 60 days, calved 151 days after treatment was stopped (Firestone et al., 1979). The PCDD content of blood, body fat (shoulder from the cow and hind quarter of the calf), and milk fat was determined 14 days later. The detected congeners were 1,2,3,6,7,8-hexaCDD, 1,2,3,4,6,7,8-heptaCDD, and octaCDD and their levels were 12, 13, 20 ng/litre and 27, 14, 6 ng/litre in the blood of the cow and calf, respectively. Corresponding values for body fat were 4.8, 11.1, and 6.1 µg/kg in the cow and 2.3, 1.9, and 0.5 µg/kg in the calf. The milk fat from the cow contained 2.2, 4.4, and 3.3 µg/kg of the respective congeners.

6.4 Matrix Effects on the Uptake ("Bio-availability")

Uptake of TCDD and other PCDD congeners is highly dependent upon the formulation in which it is applied. Although conflicting results have been obtained from studies where TCDD in soil was administered (McConnell et al., 1984; Umbreit et al., 1985, 1986a, 1986b), most available data support the idea that mixing TCDD with soil or activated carbon results in the adsorption of TCDD to the soil particles, thus reducing the availability of TCDD. Contact time of TCDD with soil seem to influence the availability, probably because the binding of TCDD to soil particles becomes strengthened (Poiger & Schlatter, 1980). Studies elucidating the matrix effects of various soils or activated carbon on the TCDD-responses in several animal species are summarized in Table 46.

Poiger & Schlatter (1980) showed decreasing hepatic recovery of TCDD in rats 1 day after dosing using suspensions of ethanol, soil, or activated carbon as vehicles. About 50% lower hepatic retention of TCDD was obtained in the rat, 6 days after dosing, when Minker stout site soil was the vehicle as compared to corn oil (Lucier et al., 1986). However, in this study hepatic enzyme-induction (AHH and UDPGT) was similar in the two vehicle groups.

The bioavailability of TCDD from environmentally contaminated soil samples has been studied in young guinea-pigs after intragastric administration (McConnell et al., 1984). Groups of six animals each were given soil samples corresponding to doses of approximately 1, 3, or 10 µg TCDD per kg body weight. The doses were based on analyses of soil siftings (60-gauge mesh) from the Times Beach and Minker Stout sites, which indicated concentrations of 770 and 880 µg TCDD/kg, respectively. Controls received soil samples in which no TCDD, PCBs, or PCDFs were detected. For comparison, pure TCDD in corn oil was given at either 0, 1, or 3 µg/kg. The observation time was 30 days. LD_{50} values calculated in this study were 1.75 µg/kg for TCDD in corn oil, 7.15 µg/kg for Times Beach soil, and 5.50 µg/kg for the Minker Stout site soil. An exact percentage for bioavailability was not calculated in this study, but the TCDD content of the livers of exposed guinea-pigs indicated a highly efficient absorption of TCDD from soil.

TCDD in contaminated soil from a 2,4,5-T manufacturing plant and from a metal salvage yard (Newark, New Jersey, USA) had a low bioavailability (0.5% and 21.3%, respectively) in guinea-pigs (Umbreit et al., 1985, 1986a). The soils were

Table 46. Matrix effects of various soils on TCDD-responses, as related to the estimated bioavailability of TCDD given orally to different species.

Species/ Length of study (days)	Vehicle/matrix	Dose of TCDD[c]	Lethality	Hepatic recovery of TCDD[e]	Estimated "bio-availability"	Reference
Rat 1 day	50% ethanol	14.7 ng		36.7[f]		Poigner & Schlatter (1980)
	recontaminated soil[a]	12.7, 22.9 ng		24.1[f]		
	recontaminated soil[b]	21.2, 22.7 ng		16.0[f]		
	activated carbon	14.7 ng		< 0.07[f]		
Rat 6 days	corn oil	1.0, 5.0		7.6 and 40.8		Lucier et al. (1986)
	Minker Stout site soil	1.1, 5.5		1.8 and 20.3	50%	
Guinea-pig 30 days	corn oil	1, 3	1/6, 6/6	1.6, 13.3		McConnell et al. (1984)
	Times Beach site soil	1.3, 3.8, 12.8	0/6, 1/5, 5/5	< 1.0-34.3	Efficient absorption from soil (85%)	
	Minker Stout site soil	1.1, 3.3, 11.0	0/6, 2/6, 6/6	< 1.0-25.7		
	recontaminated soil	10.0	6/6	45.4		
Guinea-pig 60 days	corn oil	6	5/8			Umbreit et al. (1985, 1986a)
	2,4,5-T-manufacturing site soil (Newark, New Jersey, USA).	3, 6, 12	0/8, 0/7, 0/7	0.09 (high dose)	0.5%	
	Metal salvage yard soil (Newark)	0.32		0.23	21.3%	
	recontaminated soil	6	6/7	18		

Table 46 (contd).

Species/ Length of study (days)	Vehicle/matrix	Dose of TCDD[c]	Lethality	Hepatic recovery of TCDD[e]	Estimated "bio-availability"	Reference
Guinea-pig 60 days	2,4,5-T-Manufacturing site soil, (Newark)	3, 5, 10	0/18, 1/20, 1/18			Umbreit et al. (1986b)
	Times Beach site soil	1, 3, 10	2/19, 2/20, 8/14			
	recontaminated soil	6	19/20			
Rabbit 7 days	corn oil	20, 40, 80[d]		0.26-2.7		Bonaccorsi et al. (1984)
	Seveso soil	80, 160[d]		0.88-2.2	> 32%	
	recontaminated soil	20, 40, 80[d]		0.26-1.5	> 66-100%	

a Contact time = 10-15 h.
b Contact time = 8 days.
c µg/kg body weight, unless otherwise stated.
d ng/kg body weight per day.
e µg/kg liver, unless otherwise stated.
f % of dose.

given as single oral doses in a 10% aqueous suspension in 5% gum acacia. The bioavailability was judged by the hepatic concentration of TCDD 60 days after dosing in guinea-pigs receiving site soils, decontaminated soil, and TCDD-recontaminated soil.

The difference in bioavailability of TCDD from 2,4,5-T-manufacturing site soil in Newark (New Jersey) and from Times Beach Site soil (Missouri) when given orally to guinea-pigs was confirmed by Umbreit et al. (1986b).

Bonaccorsi et al. (1984) gave to rabbits seven daily doses of TCDD in corn oil, TCDD-contaminated Seveso soil, or recontaminated soil. Taking the hepatic recovery of TCDD in the corn oil group as 100% "bioavailability", the decrease in "bioavailability" of TCDD from Seveso soil was 68%. The decrease in "bioavailability" of recontaminated soil varied from 0 to 44% with the doses used.

Considerably lower hepatic levels of PCDDs and PCDFs were observed in rats fed a diet containing fly ash from municipal incinerators compared with those fed a diet containing extracts from the same fly ash (van den Berg et al., 1983).

Dietary intake of soot-containing TCDD produced 60% mortality in male and female guinea-pigs on days 46 and 60, respectively, at which time the estimated TCDD-consumption was 1.3 µg/kg body weight for males and 1.9 µg/kg body weight for females (DeCaprio et al., 1983, see also section 8.2.3). These data thus suggest a high uptake of TCDD from the soot matrix.

7. EFFECTS OF TCDD AND OTHER PCDDs ON EXPERIMENTAL ANIMALS AND IN VITRO TEST SYSTEMS

7.1 Acute Toxicity

7.1.1 In vivo studies on mammals

The range of doses required to cause death varies considerably between species, as well as between strains of species, and with sex, age, and route of administration within a single strain (Table 47). More than an 8000-fold difference exists between the dose of TCDD reported to cause 50% lethality to male Hartley guinea-pigs, the most sensitive species tested (Schwetz et al., 1973), and the corresponding dose for male Golden Syrian hamsters (Henck et al., 1981). The rat seems to be the second most sensitive species, although there is a more than 200-fold variability in LD_{50} values between different strains. The oral LD_{50} value was 22 µg TCDD/kg body weight for male Sherman rats (Schwetz et al., 1973), whereas Walden & Schiller (1985) found LD_{50} values ranging from 164 to 340 µg TCDD/kg body weight when male Fisher 334 N rats from three different suppliers were tested. The Han/Wistar-strain of rat has been demonstrated to be particularly resistant to TCDD-exposure (Pohjanvirta & Tuomisto, 1986). Among the five rats per dose group (0, 1500, 2000, 2500, or 3000 µg TCDD/kg body weight) only one animal died within the 39-40 days observation period.

Monkeys (McConnell et al., 1978a), New Zealand rabbits (Schwetz et al., 1973), C57B1/6 mice (Chapman & Schiller, 1985; Jones & Greig, 1975; McConnell et al., 1978b; Smith et al., 1981; Vos et al., 1974), DBA/2-mice (Chapman & Schiller, 1985), and B6D2F1-mice (Chapman & Schiller, 1985) gave oral LD_{50} values of 70, 115, 114, 2570, and 296 µg TCDD/kg body weight, respectively. The difference in sensitivity towards TCDD among various strains of mice has been claimed to depend on a genetic variability in the Ah and/or hr-locus (see section 7.8.1).

Male Sherman rats were found to be more sensitive to TCDD than were females (Schwetz et al., 1973), whereas Beatty et al. (1978) reported that male Sprague Dawley rats were more resistant to TCDD than were females. Smith et al. (1981) found adult female C57BL/10 mice to be more resistant to TCDD than adult males of the same strain. No differences in sensitivity to TCDD between sexes were recorded for guinea-pigs (McConnell et al., 1978b; Silkworth et al., 1982) or hamsters (Olson et al., 1980b). Thus data on sex differences in sensitivity to lethal effects of TCDD are conflicting.

Table 47. Single lethal dose values for TCDD[a]

Species/strain (Reference)	Sex/No/ group	Age/weight	Route/vehicle	Dose tested (μg/kg)	Duration of observation	LD_{50} (μg/kg)	Time to death (days)
Rats							
Porton (Greig et al., 1973)	F/5-12	8-9 weeks/ 170-200 g	oral/DMSO	0 30 48 75 120 190 300	90 days	NR	40
Porton (Greig et al., 1973)	F/6	9-10 weeks/ 170-200 g	oral/arachis oil	0 126 199 315 500	90 days	NR	40
Sherman (Schwetz et al., 1973)	M/5-10	NR	oral/corn oil acetone (9:1)	8 16 32 63	2-8 weeks	22	9-27
Sherman (Schwetz et al., 1973)	F/NR	NR	oral/corn oil acetone(9:1)	NR	2-8 weeks	45	13-43

Table 47 (contd).

Rats (contd)							
Sprague Dawley (Beatty et al., 1978)	M/6	adult/NR	ip/olive oil	4 doses 20-80	20 60	60	NR
Sprague Dawley (Beatty et al., 1978)	F/6	adult/NR	ip/olive oil	4 doses 10-60	20	60	NR
Sprague Dawley (Beatty et al., 1978)	M/6	25 days/NR	ip/olive oil	4 doses 5-50	20	25	NR
Fisher 334N (Walden & Shiller, 1985)	M/7	11-12 weeks/ 230-280 g	oral/corn oil	0 75 150 225 275 325 375	30 days	340[b] 303[c] 164[d]	28[b] 26[c] 25[d]
CD (Walden & Shiller, 1985)	M/7	10-11 weeks/ 350-370 g	oral/corn oil	0 75 150 225 275 325 375	30 days	297[d]	25[d]

Table 47 (contd).

Species/strain (Reference)	Sex/No/ group	Age/weight	Route/vehicle	Dose tested (µg/kg)	Duration of observation	LD_{50} (µg/kg)	Time to death (days)
Rats (contd)							
Han/Wistar (Pohjanvirta & Tuomisto, 1986)	M/5	NR/300-350	oral/corn oil	1500 2000 2500 3000	39-40 days	> 3000	NR
Mice							
C57BL/6 (Vos et al., 1974)	M/14	3 months/ 23.6-30.8 g	oral/corn oil acetone (6:1)	0 100 150 200	2 months	114	15-30
C57BL/6 (Jones & Greig, 1975)	M/NR	7-15 weeks/ 14-30 g	oral/arachis oil	NR	35 days	126	21±1.6
C57BL/6 (McConnell et al., 1978[b])	M/8	9 weeks/ 21-25 g	oral/corn oil	NR	30 days	284	22-25
C57BL/6J (Gasiewicz et al., 1983b[d])	M/NR	NR	ip/olive oil	NR	30 days	132	NR

Table 47 (contd).

<u>Mice</u> (contd)							
C57BL/6J (Chapman & Schiller, 1985)	M/10-15	10-12 weeks/ 22-32 g	oral/corn oil	95 145 190 285	30 days	182	24
C57BL/10 (Smith et al., 1981)	M/5	42-121 days/NR	oral/arachis oil	85 107 135 170 213	45 days	146	22-38
C57BL/10 (Smith et al., 1981)	F/5	42-121 days/NR	oral/arachis oil	85 107 135 170 213 269 338 426 536	45 days	> 450	22-38
DBA/2J (Gasiewicz et al., 1983b[e])	M/NR	NR	ip/olive oil	NR	30 days	620	NR
DBA/2J (Chapman & Schiller, 1985)	M/10-15	10-12 weeks/ 22-32 g	oral/corn oil	1370 1870 2610 3500 4470	30 days	2570	21

Table 47 (contd).

Species/strain (Reference)	Sex/No/ group	Age/weight	Route/vehicle	Dose tested (μg/kg)	Duration of observation	LD_{50} (μg/kg)	Time to death (days)
Mice (contd)							
B6D2F_1/J (Gasiewicz et al., 1983e	M/NR	NR	ip/olive oil	NR	30 days	300	NR
B6D2F_1J (Chapman & Schiller, 1985)	M/10-15	10-12 weeks/ 22-32 g	oral/corn oil	170 220 265 325 425 450	30 days	296	25
Guinea-pigs							
Hartley (Schwetz et al., 1973)	M/NR	NR	oral/corn oil	NR	2-8 weeks	0.6	5-34
Hartley (Schwetz et al., 1973)	M/NR	NR	oral/corn oil acetone (9:1)	NR	2-8 weeks	2.1	9-42
Hartley (McConnell et al., 1978b)	M/6	3-4 weeks/ 200-250 g	oral/corn oil	NR	30 days	2	17-20

Table 47 (contd).

<u>Guinea-pigs</u> (contd)							
Hartley (Silkworth et al., 1982)	F/6	NR/500-600 g	oral/corn oil	0.1 0.5 2.5 12.5 20.0	42 days	2.5	32-42
Hartley (Silkworth et al., 1982)	F/6	NR/500-600 g	oral/methyl-cellulose	0.1 0.5 2.5 12.5 20.0	42 days	19	12-42
<u>Rabbits</u>							
New Zealand (Schwetz et al., 1973)	M, F/NR	NR	oral/corn oil acetone (9:1)	NR	2-8 weeks	115	6-39
New Zealand (Schwetz et al., 1973)	M, F/NR	NR	dermal/acetone	31.6 63 126 252 500	3 weeks	275	12-22
New Zealand (Schwetz et al., 1973)	M, F/5	NR	ip/corn oil	31.6 63 126 252 500	4 weeks	NR	6-23

Table 47 (contd).

Species/strain (Reference)	Sex/No/ group	Age/weight	Route/vehicle	Dose tested (μg/kg)	Duration of observation	LD_{50} (μg/kg)	Time to death (days)
Hamsters							
Golden Syrian (Olson et al., 1980b)	M/5-6	NR/50-80 g	ip/olive oil	0 500 1000 2000 3000	50 days	> 3000	
Golden Syrian (Olson et al., 1980b)	F/5	NR/50-80 g	ip/olive oil	0 500 1000 2000 3000	50 days	> 3000	14-32
Golden Syrian (Olson et al., 1980b)	M/5	NR/50-80 g	oral/olive oil	500 1000 2000 3000	50 days	1157	2-47
Golden Syrian (Henck et al., 1981)	M/6	NR/70-120 g	oral/corn oil acetone (9:1)	0 300 600 1000 3000 6000	55 days	5051	9-43

Table 47 (contd).

Monkeys							
Macaca mulatta	F/3	juvenile/ 2.1-2.6 kg	oral/corn oil	0 70 350	47 days	< 70	14-34
(McConnell et al., 1978a)							
Dogs							
Beagle	M/2	NR	oral/corn oil acetone (9:1)	300 3000	2-8 weeks	NA	9-15
(Schwetz et al., 1973)							
Beagle	F/2	NR	oral/corn oil acetone (9:1)	30 100	2-8 weeks	NA	all animals survived
(Schwetz et al., 1973)							
Chickens							
Leghorn	NR	4-6 weeks/NR	oral/NR	NR	NR	25-50	12-21
(Grieg et al., 1973)							

[a] M = male, F = female, NR = not reported, NA = not applicable, ip = intraperitoneal, DMSO = dimethyl sulfoxide.
[b] supplied by Harlan.
[c] supplied by Frederick.
[d] supplied by Charles River.
[e] based on unpublished studies by Gasiewicz et al., 1983.

Data on the effect of age at exposure to TCDD on the sensitivity of acute response are scarce, and comparisons are hampered by the absence of information, or incomplete information, on the age and/or body weight of the tested animals. However, Beatty et al. (1978) found that weanling male Sprague Dawley rats were more sensitive to TCDD than were adult males. A dose of 25 μg TCDD/kg body weight caused, after 35 days, a cumulative lethality of 62% in weanling Sprague Dawley rats and 25% in young adults (Christian et al., 1986a). When weanling and mature adults were exposed to a similar toxic dose of TCDD (LD_{62} and LD_{60}, respectively), onset of death occurred 9 days later in the adults (Christian et al., 1986a).

Schwetz et al. (1973) found LD_{50} values in rabbits of 115 μg TCDD/kg body weight after oral exposure, as compared to 275 μg TCDD/kg body weight after dermal exposure. C57B1/6-mice seem to be more sensitive to ip administration of TCDD (Gasiewicz et al., 1983b) than to oral administration (McConnell et al., 1978b). The LD_{50} value in guinea-pigs was increased from 2.5 μg/kg body weight to 19 μg/kg body weight when the vehicle for the oral administration of TCDD was changed from corn oil to methyl cellulose (Silkworth et al., 1982). Umbreit et al. (1985) compared mortality, and time to death, among guinea-pigs given single oral doses of TCDD in corn oil, TCDD in a suspension of cleaned soil, from an industrial site, or TCDD-contaminated soil from the same industrial site. Animals treated with corn oil, cleaned soil and contaminated site soil survived the 60-day study without any sign of TCDD intoxication. Among animals that received 6 μg TCDD/kg body weight either in corn oil or mixed with cleaned soil, only 3/8 and 1/7 survived, respectively. Deaths occurred between days 9 to 31 and 15 to 25, respectively. These results are different from those reported by McConnell et al. (1984) where TCDD-contaminated soils from Times Beach and Minker Stout were highly toxic to guinea-pigs. LD_{50} values calculated in this study were 1.75 μg/kg for TCDD in corn oil, 7.15 μg/kg for TCDD in Times Beach soil, and 5.50 μg/kg for TCDD in Minker Stout site soil. The Minker Stout site soil was also potent in inducing AHH-activity in female Sprague Dawley rats. The different results may be due to the vehicle used and/or to the presence of other substances in the soils that may potentiate or retard the TCDD-induced toxicity (Umbreit et al., 1986a). In section 6.4, the results from McConnell et al. (1984) and Umbreit et al. (1985, 1986a) are further discussed from the viewpoint of the "bioavailability" of TCDD in soils (Table 46).

Despite similar routes and vehicles for the administration of TCDD to Golden Syrian hamsters, LD_{50} values varied between 1157 μg/kg body weight (Olson et al., 1980b) and 5051 μg/kg body weight (Henck et al., 1981). A possible explanation for this difference could be the spontaneous occurrence of ileitis observed in the former study, which might have increased the susceptibility of those hamsters to TCDD toxicity.

TCDD affects a variety of organ systems in different species. The organ primarily affected in rodents and rabbits is the liver. In guinea-pigs atrophy of the thymus and lymphatic tissues seems to be the main effect, while dermal effects are prominent signs in non-human primates. Generally it is not possible to specify a single organ whose dysfunction is responsible for death. Overall, TCDD seems to have a predilection for causing pathological changes in epithelial tissues, both cutaneous and internal. This is particularly apparent in non-human primates (Macaca mulatta), and is noteworthy that the lesions mimic to some degree the effects in human beings. The histopathological alterations in tissues include hyperplastic and/or metaplastic alterations as well as hypoplastic responses. The toxic responses of various species to TCDD are summarized in Table 48, adapted from Poland & Knutson (1982). In all animal species studied, death occurred after a time lapse ranging from several days to more than one month after exposure. The delay was dependent on dose but not on species (Table 48). Progressive loss of body weight was a characteristic sign observed in animals given a lethal dose of TCDD. The weight loss became manifest usually within a few days after exposure and resulted in a substantial reduction of the adipose tissue observed at autopsy. At sublethal doses of TCDD a dose-dependent decrease in body weight gain occurred. This TCDD-induced wasting syndrome has been thoroughly investigated in several studies discussed more fully in section 7.4.1.

The greatest difference between species at necropsy, both in gross and histological effects, concerns pathological alterations in the liver. As discussed in detail in section 7.4.2, a dose of TCDD lethal to guinea-pigs did not result in liver damage comparable to the liver lesions described in rabbits and rats or to liver changes observed in mice dying after doses higher than those needed to cause death in these species. In the hamster, frank liver lesions do not occur even after fatal doses.

Chloracne-like lesions can be induced by topical application and/or systemic administration of TCDD in rabbits, non-human primates, and hairless mice. These lesions are further discussed in section 7.4.4.

Severe thymus atrophy was also found at autopsy in all animal species given lethal doses of TCDD. Histological examinations revealed lymphoid cell depletion in thymus cortex, spleen, and lymph nodes. These consistent findings in TCDD

Table 48. Specific differences in toxic responses following exposure to 2,3,7,8-TCDD[a, b]

	Monkey	Guinea-pig	Cow[c]	Rat	Mouse	Rabbit[c]	Chicken[c]	Hamster
<u>Hyperplasia and/or metaplasia</u>								
Gastric mucosa	++	0	+	0	0			0
Intestinal mucosa	+							++
Urinary tract	++	++	++	0	0			
Bile duct and/or gall bladder	++	0	+		++			0
Lung: focal alveolar				++				
Skin	++	0	+[d]	0	0	++		0
<u>Hypoplasia, atrophy, or necrosis</u>								
Thymus	+	+	+	+	+		+	+
Bone marrow	+	+			±		+	
Testicle	+	+		+	+			
<u>Other responses</u>								
Liver lesions	+	+		++	+	++	+	±
Porphyria	0	0		+	++		+	0
Oedema	+	0		0	+		++	+

a References: monkey (Norback & Allen, 1973; Allen et al., 1977; McConnell et al., 1978a), guinea-pig (McConnell et al., 1978b; Moore et al., 1979; McConnell, 1980; Turner & Collins, 1983), cow (McConnell, 1980), rat (Kociba et al., 1978; Kociba et al., 1979a; McConnell, 1980), mouse (Vos et al., 1973; Schwetz et al., 1973; McConnell et al., 1978b), rabbit (Vos & Beems, 1971; Schwetz et al., 1973), chicken (Allen & Lalich, 1962; Vos & Koeman, 1970; Norback & Allen, 1973; Schwetz et al., 1973), hamster (Olson et al., 1980b; Henck et al., 1981).

b Symbols: 0 = lesion not observed, + = lesion observed (number of "+" denote severity), ± = lesion observed to a very limited extent, blank = no evidence reported in literature.

c Responses followed exposure to 2,3,7,8-TCDD or structurally related chlorinated aromatic hydrocarbons.

d Skin lesions in cattle have been observed, but they differ from the skin lesions observed in other species.

poisoning will be discussed in detail in section 7.4.5 together with the other lymphoid tissue-related effects.

There are also substantial interspecies differences in the effects observed in other organs of animals given lethal doses of TCDD. Icterus was reported in rats (Buu-Hoi et al., 1972a; Gupta et al., 1973), hepatic porphyria occurred in mice and rats (see section 7.4.3), and ascites with subcutaneous oedema and hydrothorax appeared in mice (Jones & Greig, 1975; Vos et al., 1974) and monkeys (Allen et al., 1977). The accumulation of serous fluid in the pericardial sac occurred in chickens after a single lethal dose of TCDD (see section 7.1.4). Haemorrhages were frequently observed in many organs following lethal doses in monkeys (Allen et al., 1977), rats, and guinea-pigs (Gupta et al., 1973). In mice, death was frequently attributed to terminal haemorrhages (Vos et al., 1974).

When administered in doses sufficient to cause overt toxicity, TCDD causes testicular atrophy and degeneration characterized by reduced spermatogenic activity in mice (McConnell et al., 1978b), rats (Kociba et al., 1976; Van Miller et al., 1977), and guinea-pigs (McConnell et al., 1978b). The same symptoms were present in monkeys fed dioxin-containing toxic fat (Allen & Carstens, 1967; Norback & Allen, 1973). The decreases in male sex organ weights (seminal vesicles, ventral prostate, testes, and caput epididymis) were dose-dependent. ED_{50} values were around 15 µg TCDD/kg body weight in Sprague Dawley rats 7 days after TCDD-treatment when compared to pair-fed control rats (Moore et al., 1985). Shrunken, hyperchromatic nuclei in the two layers of seminiferous tubules closest to the basement membrane were observed in testes of young Sprague Dawley rats 90 h after a single ip dose of 5 µg TCDD/kg body weight (Mittler et al., 1984). Epididymal lesions (Khera & Ruddick, 1973) and decreased amounts of secretory material within the accessory sex glands (Kociba et al., 1976) have been reported in TCDD-treated rats. Reduced prostate weights, both absolute and relative, were found in Han/Wistar rats at non-lethal doses of TCDD (Pohjanvirta & Tuomisto, 1986).

Reduced relative uterine weight, accompanied by decreased mucosa, stroma, and glands, occurred in young C57Bl/6 mice dosed with 6 µg TCDD/kg body weight three times a week for 1 month, but there was no effect on the ovaries (Gallo et al., 1986). TCDD had no effect on the uterine weight in 25 day-old Long Evans rats 2 - 10 days after treatment with single ip doses of 20 or 80 µg/kg body weight (Romkes et al., 1987). However, the increase in uterine weight induced by estradiol treatment was counteracted by simultaneous TCDD-treatment.

Proliferative lesions of the gastrointestinal tract have been found primarily in non-human primates (Allen et al.,

1977; McConnell et al., 1978a) whereas proliferative changes of the transitional epithelium in the urinary tract have been found in both guinea-pigs (Gupta et al., 1973; McConnell et al., 1978b) and monkeys (Norback & Allen, 1973).

Reduced or unaffected spleen weight and slight to moderate loss of lymphocytes from spleen germinal centers have been common findings in laboratory animals exposed to sublethal to lethal doses of TCDD (Gasiewicz et al., 1980; Greig et al., 1973; Kociba et al., 1978; McConnell et al., 1978a; Olson et al., 1980b; Vos et al., 1973, 1974). Spleen cellularity in C57BL/6 mice was decreased 14 and 21 days after treatment with 30 µg TCDD/kg body weight (Chastain & Pazdernik, 1985), but not in B6C3F1 or DBA/2 mice 7 days after oral doses of up to 10 µg TCDD/kg body weight (Luster et al., 1984).

The thyroid weight, both absolute and relative to body weight, of the rat has been found to be increased by TCDD-treatment (Bastomsky, 1977; Potter et al., 1983, 1986b). Degenerative changes in the epithelial cells of the thyroid gland were observed in rats after 31 daily oral doses of 1 µg TCDD/kg body weight (Gupta et al., 1973) and 7 days after a single ip dose of 150 µg TCDD/kg body weight (Rozman et al., 1986). However, Potter et al., (1986b) found no consistent changes in follicle size or colloid content, variation in follicle size, height of follicular epithelium, or resorption of colloid at the periphery of follicles in rats one week after an oral dose of TCDD in the range 6.25 to 100 µg/kg body weight.

Histological changes in the pancreas and in the interscapular brown adipose tissue have been found in Sprague Dawley rats exposed to single ip doses of 150 µg TCDD/kg body weight (Rozman et al., 1986).

Lesions of the adrenal glands have been observed in mice and guinea-pigs treated with (Gupta et al., 1973; McConnell et al., 1978b).

Acute exposure to lethal doses of TCDD has produced minor haematological alterations in all species studied. Anaemia was not observed in mice or guinea-pigs (Zinkl et al., 1973), but a moderate anaemia and leukocytosis occurred in rats (Buu-Hoi et al., 1972a) and monkeys (McConnell et al., 1978a). On the contrary, haemoconcentration was observed in rats after exposure to a somewhat lower but still lethal dose of TCDD (Greig et al., 1973; Zinkl et al., 1973). Thrombocytopenia and clotting abnormalities were observed in rats after acute exposure to lethal levels of TCDD (Weissberg & Zinkl, 1973). Hypocellularity of the bone marrow was found in guinea-pigs (McConnell et al., 1978b), rhesus monkeys (Allen et al., 1977; McConnell et al., 1978a), and mice (McConnell et al., 1978b). However, in these studies decreased bone marrow cellularity, as judged by histological examination, appeared only at doses high enough to cause severe toxicity in the experimental animals. More recent studies (Chastain & Pazdernik, 1985; Luster et al., 1980, 1985) have demonstrated that collection and enumeration of bone marrow cells in suspension provides a more sensitive and quantitative method than histological preparation for assessing bone marrow cellularity. Decreased bone marrow cellularity was found in adult male C57B1/6 mice 3 days after exposure to 120 µg TCDD/kg body weight (Chastain & Pazdernik, 1985), and in female B6C3F1 mice 5 days after exposure to 10 µg TCDD/kg body weight (Luster et al., 1985), but not in female DBA/2 mice, even at a dose of 50 µg TCDD/kg body weight (Luster et al., 1985). The myelotoxic potential of TCDD is described in section 7.4.6.

Changes in clinical chemistry, including serum enzyme activities, serum protein concentrations, and lipid levels, observed in animals after acute exposure to TCDD, primarily reflect damage to other organ systems, mainly the liver (McConnell et al., 1978a; McConnell & Moore, 1979; Olson et al., 1980b). Liver-related enzyme activities in serum are affected in those animal species where liver damage is a prominent sign of TCDD toxicity. In those animal species where hepatotoxicity is not as apparent, such as monkeys and guinea-pigs, these enzyme activities are essentially normal. Also the TCDD-related decrease in serum albumin seems to be secondary to the hepatotoxic effect, since the decrease is less evident or non-existent in those animals that show little liver damage. Generally serum triglycerides and free fatty acid levels are increased after TCDD exposure, while that of serum cholesterol is decreased. However, marked species differences exist and again these effects seem to be secondary to liver damage. For further details on hyperlipidaemia, see section 7.4.7.

Indicators of renal damage such as blood urea nitrogen, creatinine, and blood electrolytes are usually within normal limits after TCDD exposure.

In view of the interspecies differences in the organ distribution of TCDD and the variability in the effects on various organs in the different species, the effects of TCDD in non-human primates are of particular interest. Nine female juvenile rhesus monkeys (Macaca mulatta) were divided into three groups of three and given TCDD in a single oral dose of 0, 70, or 350 µg per kg/body weight (McConnell et al., 1978a). The first indication of a toxic effect of TCDD, at day 3, was weight loss, followed by periorbital oedema, conjunctivitis, and thickening of the Meibomian glands on day 12. Subsequently, the eye lashes, facial hair, and toe and finger nails were lost. Monkeys given the highest dose showed a moderate absolute lymphopenia and thrombocytopenia. Serum cholesterol levels dropped, while the serum triglyceride levels increased. Alkaline phosphatase and total bilirubin were normal, but glutamic oxalic transaminase and aldolase were increased. A decrease in the albumin fraction of the total serum protein was noticed. The three monkeys given TCDD in a dose of 350 µg/kg body weight died or became moribund between days 28 and 34 after administration. One of the monkeys given TCDD in a dose of 70 µg/kg body weight died 14 days after administration. At autopsy body fat was almost completely absent in all treated monkeys. Ascites was noticed in two animals and all monkeys had markedly distended and thickened bile ducts and gall-bladders. Small focal ulcerated areas in the fundus of the stomach were observed in two monkeys. Microscopic examination showed that the Meibomian glands were dilated and filled with keratinaceous debris. Squamous metaplasia of the glandular portion, with atrophy of sebaceous cells, was present. Occasional scattered necrotic hepatocytes were noted in the liver on microscopic examination. The gastric ulcers that were found extended into the lamina propria.

Schwetz et al. (1973) reported that no signs of toxicity were observed in four male mice and two female rats given single oral doses of respectively 2 and 1 g 2,7-diCDD/kg body weight (purity 99.6-99.8%). For octaCDD (purity 98.86%), oral doses of 1 g/kg body weight to five female rats and 4 g/kg body weight to four male mice did not cause any toxic symptoms. A sample containing two different isomers of hexaCDD (purity > 99%, 89:11) killed 1 of 2 and 0 of 2 male rats when given as single oral doses of 100 and 10 mg, respectively. The only toxic sign observed among these rats was loss of body weight. These studies lasted for 2 to 8 weeks.

The toxicities of single oral doses of nine PCDDs, including TCDD, in C57BL/6J mice and Hartley guinea-pigs were compared by McConnell et al. (1978b) (Table 49). The purity of the various isomers tested exceeded 97%. Groups of eight male mice and of six male guinea-pigs were used for each dose of any of the tested compounds, and the animals were followed for 30 days after administration. The toxic effects observed after administration of the different PCDDs were similar, the only difference among the congeners being the amount needed to produce a given effect. Progressive decrease of body weight, more pronounced in guinea-pigs than in mice, was observed after a lethal dose of any of the congeners tested. Marked reduction in deposited adipose tissue deposits was a constant finding in animals given a lethal dose of any of the PCDDs. Reduction of muscle mass and severe dehydration were observed in guinea-pigs, and ascites, subcutaneous oedema, and hydrothorax in some of the treated mice. Decrease of thymus weight was a constant finding in both species, being more pronounced in mice and in the guinea-pigs that died. Histological exam-

Table 49. Estimated single oral LD_{50} values for some PCDDs[a]

Chlorination of PCDDs	Guinea-pigs (µg/kg)[b]	Mice (µg/kg)[b]
2,8	> 300 000	NR
2,3,7	29 444	> 3000
2,3,7,8	2	284
1,2,3,7,8	3	338
1,2,4,7,8	1125	> 5000
1,2,3,4,7,8	73	825
1,2,3,6,7,8	70-100[c]	1250
1,2,3,7,8,9	60-100[c]	> 440
1,2,3,4,6,7,8	> 600	NR

a From: McConnell et al. (1978b).
b Spearman-Karber method.
c Estimated range due to variability in replicates.
NR = not reported.

ination of the thymus of the guinea-pigs that died as early as 5 days after administration of PCDDs revealed scattered necrosis of lymphocytes throughout the cortex, with concomitant phagocytosis by macrophages. This was even more apparent in animals that died 14 days after administration, in which a noticeable decrease in the thickness of the cortex was observed. In the animals that had died by day 20 it was difficult to differentiate the cortex from the medulla, but little evidence of necrosis was present.

In guinea-pigs that survived 30 days after a lethal dose of any of the congeners, the thymus was reduced to one-fourth of its size in controls. However, thymus histology at this time was often comparatively normal. A reduction of the lymphoid follicles in the spleen and of the Peyer's patches in the intestine was observed with less conspicuous necrosis, which again was not evident in the 30-day survivors. Striking hypocellularity was found in the sternal bone marrow in the guinea-pigs that died, but was less obvious in survivors. Similar thymic and splenic changes were found in mice. However, bone marrow atrophy occurred only rarely in this species and then it was less pronounced than in guinea-pigs. In the guinea-pigs that died, and occasionally in survivors, a marked hyperplasia of the renal pelvis was observed, invariably extending into the ureter and at times involving the urinary bladder mucosa. Gastrointestinal haemorrhages and occasional microscopic dilatation of crypts in the glandular portion of the gastric mucosa were observed in dead PCDD-treated animals of both species. Retro-orbital haemorrhages with exophthalmus and haemorrhages with detachment of the retina were seen in mice that died after a lethal dose of any of the congeners tested. Adrenal haemorrhages and moderate atrophy of the zona glomerulosa were seen in guinea-pigs that died. These changes were not observed in mice or in surviving guinea-pigs. In guinea-pigs, primarily in animals that died during the observation period, changes in the spermatogenic epithelium were observed, with testicular tubules containing only spermatogonia and Sertoli cells in severely affected animals. Reduced spermatogenesis, necrotic spermatocytes, and spermatozoa within the lumen of the testicular tubules and in the epididymis, and multi-nucleated giant cells within the seminiferous tubules, were found in the mice that died but not in those that survived. On the other hand, liver lesions were observed with the same frequency and degree of involvement in all the mice given the same dose, whether they died or survived. Minimal liver changes were detected in guinea-pigs, changes largely confined to central congestion with occasional degeneration of hepatocytes in dead animals. Fluorescence, as an indication of porphyria, was found only in mice, particularly in the liver but also in the incisors, cranial bones, costochondral junction, and stifle joint. It was dose related and detectable at doses several times less than the LD_{50}.

Haemolysis and hyperproteinaemia were found in dying animals of both species. In mice surviving 30 days, but not in guinea-pigs, the blood α-globulin level was decreased, with a resultant increase in the albumin/globulin ratio.

With all PCDDs for which it was possible to establish an LD_{50} values were in the range 10 to 100 times lower in guinea-pigs than in mice. To produce the greatest toxicity the lateral positions 2,3,7, and 8 must be fully chlorinated. With 2,3,7-triCDD or 2,8-diCDD the LD_{50} values were in the range 1000 to 100 000 times higher than with TCDD. The addition of a chlorine atom at an <u>ortho</u>-position, e.g., 1,2,3,7,8-pentaCDD, resulted in only a minor reduction of toxicity. An additional chlorine atom further reduced the toxic potency but the LD_{50} values of 1,2,3,4,7,8-hexaCDD and 1,2,3,6,7,8-hexaCDD remained comparatively low. The toxicity of 1,2,3,4,6,7,8-heptaCDD was further reduced. A reduction in the rate of weight gain was observable in guinea-pigs given doses of this compound exceeding 200 μg/kg body weight. However, no deaths were observed during the experiment even at doses as high as 600 μg/kg body weight.

The acute oral toxicities of soot and benzene extracts of soot, containing PCDDs and PCDFs from a fire in a PCB-containing transformer (Binghamton, New York, USA) were determined to be 410 mg/kg body weight and 327 mg equivalents/kg body weight, respectively, in female Hartley guinea-pigs (Silkworth et al., 1982). The observation period was 42 days.

The test substances were given in 0.75% aqueous methyl cellulose and the doses used were 250, 500, 750, 1000, and 1250 mg soot/kg body weight and benzene extracts corresponding to 4, 20, 100, 500, and 1000 mg soot/kg body weight. An extensive investigation, including pathology, haematology, and serum chemistry alterations, in groups of six male and female Hartley guinea-pigs, 42 days after single oral doses of 1, 10, 100, or 500 mg Binghamton soot/kg body weight in 0.75% methyl cellulose, was reported by Silkworth et al. (1982). Control animals received 500 mg activated carbon/kg body weight in the same vehicle. No treatment-related differences were observed at 1 and 10 mg soot/kg body weight. Decreased body weight gain occurred in both sexes at 100 and 500 mg/kg, and decreased thymus weight occurred at 500 mg/kg for males and at 100 and 500 mg/kg for females. The kidney weight was decreased only in males at 100 and 500 mg/kg. There were no treatment-related alterations in haematological values. Male guinea-pigs had significantly increased serum triglyceride levels at 100 and 500 mg/kg and females at 500 mg/kg only. Elevated aspartate amino transferase (at 100 and 500 mg/kg) and decreased γ-glutamyltransferase (at 500 mg/kg) were observed in the serum of female guinea-pigs. The only clearly dose-related microscopical findings in soot-exposed guinea-pigs were metaplasia of salivary gland interlobular duct epithelium and goblet cell hyperplasia of pancreatic interlobular ducts. These lesions occurred only in males at doses of 100 or 500 mg soot/kg body weight. Microscopic lesions, which tended to be more frequent and/or severe in treatment groups than in controls, included bile duct hyperplasia, hepatocellular cytoplasmic inclusions, vacuolation of the adrenal cortex, and focal lacrimal adenitis.

7.1.2 In vitro studies on mammalian cells

Over 30 cell types, including primary cultures and cells from established and transformed cell lines derived from various tissues of at least six animal species, have been examined for their response to TCDD (Beatty et al., 1975; Knutson & Poland, 1980a; Niwa et al., 1975; Yang et al., 1983). The effects studied were viability, growth rate, and morphological alterations. No toxic effects were observed except in one rat hepatoma cell line in which Niwa et al. (1975) reported decreased viability after exposure for 72 h to TCDD at a concentration of 300 nmol/litre. This concentration is high when compared to the LD_{50} in rats and mice. No effect on these cells was observable at 30 nmol/litre.

The biochemical responses found in primary hepatocytes from rats exposed to 10 µg TCDD/kg body weight in vivo was not present when the hepatocytes were exposed in vitro to TCDD at 50, 100, or 200 nmol/litre for 48 h (Yang et al., 1983a).

7.1.3 Studies on birds

Chick oedema disease first gained attention in the United States in 1957. An extensive outbreak among chickens occurred in that year in Georgia (Firestone, 1973; Sanger et al., 1958; Simpson et al., 1959). The cause of the disease was traced to the presence in the feed of toxic components later identified as chlorinated dibenzo-*p*-dioxins. TCDD was identified as one of the isomers in the mixture of chlorinated dibenzo-*p*-dioxins capable of producing chick oedema (Flick et al., 1973).

Clinical signs of chick oedema disease consist of dyspnea, reduced body weight gain, stunted growth, subcutaneous oedema, pallor, and sudden death. In young chickens gasping was the first noticeable sign, followed by a waddling gait. Gross inspection of the birds at autopsy revealed an increased amount of fluid in the pericardial sac and pale livers with a mottled and irregular granular surface. In advanced stages the chickens developed a distended abdomen filled with fluid. Endotheliosis of the vascular system was observed at microscopic examination, as well as pronounced proliferation of the endothelium of the glomerular capillaries and necrosis of the liver cells. Diseased chickens developed pulmonary oedema and perivascular lymphocyte infiltration, as well as oedema of the cardiac muscle with interstitial lymphocytic infiltration (Allen, 1964; Allen & Lalich, 1962, McCune et al., 1962; Simpson et al., 1959).

Experimentally, chick oedema has been produced with a single dose of 25 to 50 µg TCDD/kg body weight (Greig et al., 1973). When mixtures of tri- and tetraCDDs were fed at dietary concentrations of 0.01 µg/kg, the chickens developed oedema and 83% of them died (Flick et al., 1972).

Potency for inducing chick oedema was compared for three different PCDDs: TCDD (purity 91% and > 99%), hexaCDD (purity > 99%, two isomers), and octaCDD (purity 98.86%) (Schwetz et al., 1973). In the experiments, 3-day-old white Leghorn cockerels were exposed for 20 to 21 days to one of these congeners at several dose levels. Chick oedema occurred in birds given oral doses of 1 or 10 µg TCDD/kg per day, or of 10 or 100 µg hexaCDD/kg per day. Chick oedema was not observed in chicks maintained on a diet containing 0.1 or 0.5% octaCDD. The weight of the Bursa of Fabricius was significantly decreased in 2-week-old white Leghorn cockerels decapitated 2 days after three daily ip doses of 10 µg TCDD/kg body weight (Sawyer et al., 1986).

7.1.4 Toxicity of metabolites

Not only has identification of several in vivo metabolites been achieved, but the acute oral toxicity of TCDD metabolites excreted in the bile of dogs has been studied in the guinea-pig (Weber et al., 1982a). ^{3}H-labelled TCDD was administered directly into the duodenal lumen of two 1-year-old Beagle dogs in four portions of 1 to 2 mg at time intervals of 2 to 7 days. Excretion of radioactive material from pooled bile samples collected daily for 4 or 7 days, and thereafter in pooled samples of 2 or 3 days, was performed with a method yielding about 50% of the total radioactivity of the bile. The extracts containing the metabolites were concentrated and dissolved in 1,3-propanediol for administration. Male Pirbright guinea-pigs were used in a 5-week toxicity study. Five animals in each of four dose-groups were given a single oral dose via gastric intubation. The amount of TCDD metabolites was calculated by means of radioactivity measurements to be 0.6, 6.0, 30.0, or 60.0 µg/kg body weight. Three animals, one control and two in the high-dose group, died within 48 h after administration. One death in the high-dose group was due to gastric perforation during dosing. The other animals which died exhibited histological lesions which, according to the authors, were due to material coextracted from bile together with the metabolites. The light microscopic examination of the liver, spleen, pancreas, thymus, kidneys, lungs, and adrenals revealed no histological changes, and no other toxic effects due to the metabolites of TCDD could be recorded in this study. The authors concluded that TCDD metabolites from the dog are at least 100 times less toxic to male guinea-pigs than TCDD itself.

When the metabolites 2-hydroxy-3,7,8-triCDD and 2-hydroxy-1,3,7,8-tetra CDD were given as single ip injections of 100, 1000, or 5000 µg/kg body weight to young male Wistar rats, no decrease in body weight gain was noted and thymic atrophy was not seen 14 days later (Mason & Safe, 1986). When compared to TCDD, 1-hydroxy-3,7,8-triCDD was at least 3 orders of magnitude less effective in inducing hepatic AHH and EROD activities, whereas 2-hydroxy-1,3,7,8-tetra CDD was inactive at all dose levels tested.

7.1.5 Modulation of the acute toxicity

Several studies have been performed which attempt to modify the acute toxicity of TCDD. Manara et al. (1984) studied the effect of activated charcoal or cholic acids in the diet on the mortality after 60 days and mean time to death in mice, rats, and guinea-pigs exposed to TCDD. Dietary levels of charcoal (2.5%), cholic acid (0.25%), and dehydrocholic acid (0.5%) decreased the mortality induced in C57Bl/6 mice by a single sc dose of 110 μg TCDD/kg body weight from 93% to 53, 21, and 53%, respectively. The mean time to death was prolonged from 29 days with a normal chow diet to 35-48 days with the above dietary additives. In CD rats the addition of charcoal (2.5%) and cholic acid (0.15%) decreased mortality from 80% to 50 and 70% respectively. The mean time to death was not affected. Charcoal (5%) added to guinea-pig chow decreased TCDD induced mortality from 64% to 29% and reduced the mean time to death from 29 to 14 days. These additions to the diet did not prevent body weight loss or liver enlargement in the mice or guinea-pigs (Manara et al., 1984), but 5% charcoal in the diet protected against TCDD-induced thymus athrophy in C57Bl/6 mice 14 days after a single oral dose of 10 μg TCDD/kg body weight (Manara et al., 1982). The addition of 5% _n_-hexadecane in the diet increased the TCDD induced mortality from 60% to 100% and the mean time to death, within the 50 day study, from 19.8 to 28.8 days in Sprague Dawley rats treated with a single ip dose of 60 μg TCDD/kg body weight (Rozman, 1984). _N_-hexadecane itself did not affect animal viability.

Increased survival times have been demonstrated in mice receiving daily injections of triiodothyronine (T_3) after TCDD treatment (Neal et al., 1979) and in rats thyroidectomized before TCDD treatment (Rozman et al., 1984). Although thyroidectomy increases the mean time to death, it does not prevent TCDD-related mortality in rats (Rozman et al., 1985a). Thyroidectomy has been demonstrated to counteract TCDD-induced decreases in thymus weight and to reduce the spleen plaque-forming cell response (Pazdernik & Rozman, 1985). A number of hepatic enzyme activities were induced by TCDD to an equal magnitude in thyroidectomized and normal rats (Rozman et al., 1985b). It has been suggested that TCDD-treatment of rats leads to hypothyroidism, a possible protective mechanism against TCDD toxicity (Pazdernik & Rozman, 1985). However, available data on changes in T_3, thyroxine (T_4), and thyroid-stimulating hormone (TSH) levels in TCDD-treated rats are not sufficient to state whether the animals are functionally hypothyroid, euthyroid, or hyperthyroid. Results presented by Potter et al. (1986b) (see section 8.4.9) suggest that TCDD-treated rats remain essentially euthyroid and that the altered thyroid status is neither a major contributor to TCDD toxicity nor a key response to TCDD exposure.

Daily injections of butylated hydroxyanisole protected against TCDD-induced lethality in female Sprague Dawley rats, whereas vitamins E and A, two other antioxidants, did not (Hassan et al., 1985a,b). Dietary selenium, if given in an optimal dose, provides partial protection from the lethal effects of TCDD in female Sprague Dawley rats (Hassan et al.,

1985c). None of these treatments could counteract the TCDD-induced body weight loss (Hassan et al., 1985a,b,c).

7.2 Short-term Toxicity

7.2.1 Studies on rats

Data from the earliest subchronic laboratory study, in which rats were exposed to daily and/or weekly doses of TCDD, were reported in four separate papers (published simultaneously) covering general effects (Harris et al., 1973), pathology (Gupta et al., 1973), haematological and clinical chemistry changes (Zinkl et al., 1973), and immuno-biological effects (Vos et al., 1973). Female CD rats were given TCDD by gavage in daily doses of 0.1, 1, or 10 μg/kg body weight for 31 days. The body weight of animals exposed to the highest dose started to decrease within the first week of exposure and 15/16 animals died or became moribund 17 to 31 days after administration of the compound began. Pathological changes were comparable to those observed in rats given a single lethal dose, and included severe thymic atrophy and liver damage, icterus, haemorrhages in various organs, and the depletion of lymphoid organs. Weight gain was also reduced at the daily dose level of 1 μg/kg body weight. However, there were no deaths and in the animals that were killed moderate thymic atrophy, slight to moderate liver damage, and, in some of the animals, degenerative changes in the kidneys and in the thyroid gland were reported. The weight gain was not affected and significant histopathological changes were not found in rats that received 0.1 μg/kg body weight per day. A decrease in thymic weight that was significant on day 24, was observed at the lowest exposure level (Gupta et al., 1973; Harris et al., 1973). Blood samples were collected 3, 6, 10, 13, 17, 24, and 31 days after administration of TCDD began. Serum enzyme activities related to liver damage began to increase after 10 days of exposure and remained high until death occurred in the 10 μg TCDD/kg per day group. This group of animals also exhibited increased serum bilirubin levels commencing on day 13. These parameters were only slightly affected in rats receiving 1 μg TCDD/kg per day. Thrombocytopenia occurred at all dose levels. After 3 days of treatment with either 1 or 10 μg/kg per day, animals had depressed platelets counts that remained low throughout the study. In the low-dose rats, platelets were significantly decreased by day 17. No significant leukocytopenia or lymphocytopenia occurred in rats at any dose level. These results are in good agreement with the results from a more detailed haematological study on female CD rats given daily oral doses of 10 μg TCDD/kg body weight for 10 and 14 days (Weissberg & Zinkl, 1973).

When oral doses of 0.02, 1.0, or 5.0 µg TCDD/kg body weight were given weekly to groups of 10 female CD rats for 6 weeks, all the animals survived (Harris et al., 1973). However, body weight gain decreased in the 5.0 µg/kg group during the exposure period, and at the end of this period the thymus/body weight ratio was approximately 50% of the ratio found in the controls. Liver damage was reported as slight at this dose level. No effect on body or thymic weight and no significant histopathological changes were observed in rats given 1 µg/kg body weight or less.

Adult male and female Sprague Dawley rats, in groups of 12, were given 0, 0.001, 0.01, 0.1, and 1.0 µg TCDD/kg body weight by gavage, 5 days per week for 13 weeks (Kociba et al., 1976). At the end of the treatment period, five rats of each sex were killed for histopathological examination, while the remaining animals were retained for post-exposure observation. Doses of 1 µg TCDD/kg body weight per day caused five deaths in females, with three occurring during treatment and two after treatment, and two deaths in males, both occurring in the post treatment period. Decreased body weights and food consumption were found at the two highest dose levels both in males and females. Decreased relative thymus weight and increased relative liver weight occurred only in the males given the highest dose but in both the 0.1 and 1.0 µg/kg female groups. Male rats had significantly depressed haematological values (packed cell volume, red blood cell count, and haemoglobin) in the two high-dose groups, while these values were normal in all female rats. Gross, as well as histological, examination revealed treatment-related effects only in the high-dose groups with some minor findings in the 0.1 µg/kg group. Subcutaneous oedema, decreased sizes of testes and uteri, and a decreased number of corpora lutea were found at necropsy. Histological findings were limited to lymphoid tissues, liver, and epithelial linings. The lymphoid tissues, including thymus, were depleted of lymphocytes. The liver of both male and female rats showed pleomorphic and multinucleated hepatocytes. Foci of necrosis, with focal reticulo-endothelial aggregations in the areas of parenchymal cell necrosis, were observed. Hyperplasia of Kupffer cells and an increased amount of a golden-brown pigment were noted. The hepatic changes were more pronounced near the periphery of the lobules. Slight hyperplasia of bile ducts and ductular epithelium was present. The uterus was lined by cuboidal epithelium in the female rats. The rats given 0.01 µg TCDD/kg did not differ from the controls in any of these parameters, except for a slight increase in the mean liver to body weight ratio.

Goldstein et al. (1982) exposed groups of eight female Sprague Dawley rats to 16 weekly oral doses of 0, 0.01, 0.1,

1.0, and 10.0 µg TCDD/kg body weight in a study (further discussed in section 8.4.3) primarily aimed at investigating TCDD-induced porphyria. All animals given the highest dose died, or were moribund after eight to twelve doses and were killed. A decrease in body weight gain was seen in this group within one week of treatment. Decreased body weight gain was observed also in the 1.0 µg TCDD/kg per week group, but not until several weeks after the start of treatment. Hepatic porphyria was found in 7 out of 8 animals receiving weekly doses of 1.0 µg TCDD/kg body weight, in 1 out of 8 receiving 0.1 µg/kg per week, and in none of the animals receiving 0.01 µg/kg per week or the lethal dose of 10.0 µg/kg per week. Porphyria was not reversed after six months recovery from a 16-week exposure to 1.0 µg/kg body weight per week.

Feeding male Wistar rats (110 g) 0, 0.2, or 1.0 µg octaCDD/kg diet for two weeks, resulting in a total intake of 0, 22.7 (± 1.0) or 120.7 (± 2.8) µg octaCDD, had no effect on body weight gain, feed consumption, or tissue weights (liver, thymus, testes, heart, and kidney) (Williams et al., 1972). Congestion of the liver occurred in the high-dose group.

Daily doses of 100 µg octaCDD for 21 days produced no effects on appearance, activity, or eating habits in male Sprague Dawley rats, but slightly increased relative liver weight. A moderate increase in the hepatic smooth endoplasmic reticulum was noted (Norback et al., 1975).

7.2.2 Studies on mice

Oral doses of 0.2, 1, 5, or 25 µg TCDD/kg body weight were given in corn oil to male C57Bl/6 mice weekly for four weeks (Harris et al., 1973; Vos et al., 1973). One animal of the 25 µg/kg group died after 24 days. Significant weight loss was observed only in the high-dose group. Thymic atrophy, characterized by nearly complete loss of cortex, occurred in the 5 and 25 µg TCDD/kg body weight groups.

7.2.3 Studies on guinea-pigs

All 10 female Hartley guinea-pigs that received weekly oral doses of 1 µg TCDD/kg body weight died, or were killed when moribund, between days 24 and 32 after the first dose (Gupta et al., 1973; Harris et al., 1973; Vos et al., 1973). Light microscopic findings of moribund or dead animals revealed severe atrophy of the cortex of the thymus with destruction of lymphocytes. There was lymphoid cell depletion in spleen and lymph nodes. Haemorrhages, mitotic figures, and loss of lipid vacuoles were observed in the adrenals. Liver effects were restricted to diffuse single-cell necrosis, predominantly in the periportal area. Haemorrhages were found in the urinary bladder and gastrointestinal tract. The lymphocyte count was decreased at all doses, whereas total leukocyte values were decreased at doses > 0.04 µg/kg. Animals that received eight weekly doses of 0.008, 0.04, or 0.2 µg TCDD/kg body weight all survived. At the 0.2 µg/kg dose level, decreased body weight gain and decreased relative thymus weight were observed.

A 90-day feeding study of TCDD in male (250-370 g) and female (230-340 g) Hartley guinea-pigs was performed by DeCaprio et al. (1986) and included extensive pathology, haematology, and serum chemistry on surviving animals. The diets contained 0, 2, 10, 76, or 430 ng TCDD/kg. Animals that received the highest dose exhibited severe body weight loss, decreased feed consumption, and mortality. When 60% mortality was reached, on day 46 for males and day 60 for females, the remaining animals in these groups were sacrificed. The estimated total TCDD consumption at that time was 1.3 and 1.9 µg TCDD/kg body weight for males and females, respectively. No treatment-related mortality was observed at the 76 ng/kg dose level, which corresponded to a total estimated intake of 0.44 µg TCDD/kg body weight over the 90 days. Decreased body weight gain and increased relative liver weight were seen in both sexes, whereas reduced relative thymus weight occurred in males only. At doses of 2 and 10 ng/kg diet, no dose-related alterations were observed. The only treatment-related effect on haematology and serum chemistry parameters was the elevation of serum triglycerides for male guinea-pigs at the 76 ng/kg dose level. The presence of hepatocellular cytoplasmic inclusion bodies in female guinea-pigs was the only significant microscopical finding, except for thymus atrophy. Based on this study, a no-observed-effect level of 0.6 ng TCDD/kg body weight per day in guinea-pigs was estimated.

DeCaprio et al. (1986) also followed the body weight changes and mortality during and after feeding male Hartley guinea-pigs (250-360 g) a diet containing 430 ng TCDD/kg. The diet was fed for 11, 21, or 35 days and was then withdrawn during a 79, 69, or 55-day recovery period. The rate of change of weight per day was the same as that of animals on a control diet, after an initial weight loss of approximately 10% during the first 5 days. When animals were fed the TCDD-diet for 21 and 35 days, a significant mortality, 10% and 70%, respectively, was apparent. Both body weight gain and absolute body weight were severely depressed in surviving animals throughout the study. Animals destined to die generally lost more than 20% of the original weight, whereas less pronounced weight losses were usually followed by increases in body weight during the recovery period.

A PCB-containing transformer fire at the State office building, Binghamton, New York, USA, resulted in contamination of the building with soot-like material containing various PCDDs and PCDFs (see section 4.5.10). This soot, mixed with diet, was fed to groups of 10 male (250-350 g) and female (200-350 g) Hartley guinea-pigs for 90 days (0, 0.2, 1.9, 9.3, and 46.3 mg soot/kg diet) or 32 days (231.5 mg soot/kg diet) (DeCaprio et al., 1983). The total intake of soot during the study corresponded to approximately 0.3, 3, 13, 67, and 100% of the LD_{50} dose of Binghamton soot in guinea-pigs (Silkworth et al., 1982) (see section 8.1.1.1). A dose-related decrease in body weight gain occurred at 9.3 and 46.3 mg soot/kg diet. Body weight loss and decreased feed intake was evident in the animals given 231.5 mg soot/kg diet. Three male and three female guinea-pigs given 46.3 mg soot/kg died. Seven animals in the highest-dose group died within 28 to 31 days and the remaining moribund animals were killed on day 32. Gross pathology revealed no effects at 0.2 mg soot/kg diet. Thymic atrophy occurred only in males at 1.9 mg soot/kg diet, but in both sexes at higher doses. The relative spleen weight was significantly increased at 46.3 mg TCDD/kg in both sexes. Treatment-related microscopical findings included metaplasia of salivary gland epithelia (> 1.9 mg soot/kg diet), increased number of goblet cells in pancreatic ducts (> 46.3 mg soot/kg diet for males), focal lacrimal gland adenitis (> 9.3 mg soot/kg diet for males and > 46.3 mg soot/kg diet for females), depletion of haematopoietic cells from the bone marrow (> 46.3 mg soot/kg diet for females, > 231.5 mg soot/kg diet for males), and hepatocellular cytoplasmic inclusion bodies (9.3 and 46.3 mg soot/kg diet in both sexes). Fatty infiltration of the liver, reduced thickness of thymic cortex, and degenerative changes of the stomach and intestine were observed only in high-dose animals. Haematological alterations were observed only in animals at the 46.3 mg soot/kg diet dose level, whereas alterations in serum chemistry values were found also at lower levels. Toxic effects of feeding Binghamton soot for 90 days were similar to the effects occurring after acute exposure (Silkworth et al., 1982) (see section 8.1.1.1), but the effects were seen at a lower total dose after subchronic exposure than after acute dosing. The effect seen at the lowest level in this study was thymic atrophy at 1.9 mg soot/kg diet, which was equivalent to 7.8 ng TCDD/kg body weight per day. A comparison between the effects of feeding pure TCDD and TCDD-contaminated soot to guinea-pigs (DeCaprio et al., 1986) demonstrated that pure TCDD produced less variability of alterations and gave a steeper dose-response relationship for many effects. Exposure to Binghamton soot characteristically resulted in salivary gland duct metaplasia and decreased serum sodium and potassium levels (DeCaprio et al., 1983).

When male guinea-pigs (200 g) were fed a diet containing 2.5% HCl-pretreated fly ash from a municipal incinerator (Zaanstad, The Netherlands) for up to 95 days, the animals exhibited progressive weight loss, hair loss, and increased relative liver weight (van den Berg et al., 1986b). One animal died on day 76.

7.2.4 Studies on hamsters

No toxic effects were reported in male Golden Syrian hamsters (50-70 g) given a diet containing 2.5% HCl-pretreated fly ash from a municipal incinerator in Zaanstad, The Netherlands for up to 95 days (van den Berg et al., 1986b).

7.2.5 Studies on monkeys

A cumulative dose of 0.2 µg TCDD/kg body weight, divided into nine oral doses given three times per week, produced no clinical toxicity in female rhesus monkeys (*Macaca mulatta*) (McNulty, 1984). However, clearly toxic signs did occur in those monkeys that received cumulative doses of 1.0 and 5.0 µg TCDD/kg body weight over the same time period. The first signs were thickening and reddening of the eyelids, followed by weight loss, dryness and granularity of the skin, and loss of hair, and in some cases anaemia, purpura, and bleeding from the nose and mouth. Animals that died showed squamous metaplasia of the sebaceous glands, mucous metaplasia of the gastric mucosa, hyperplasia of biliary ductal epithelium, gingivitis, and hypoplasia of the bone marrow. The times to death after dose were 65 and 116 days at 5 µg/kg and 130 to 211 days at 1 µg/kg.

7.3 Long-term Toxicity

Chronic toxicity studies performed on laboratory animals exposed to TCDD are summarized in Table 50. Studies on carcinogenicity are presented in section 7.7.

7.3.1 Studies on rats

In studies by Van Miller et al. (1977), male Sprague Dawley rats were maintained in groups of 10 on diets containing 0, 1, 5, 50, 500, 1000, 5000, 50 000, 500 000, and 1 000 000 ng TCDD/kg for 65 weeks and survival was monitored. At the five highest dose levels, all animals died before the study was completed. The first deaths in these treated groups occurred by weeks 31, 31, 3, 2, and 2 of treatment, respectively. Groups receiving 50, 500, or 1000 ng TCDD/kg in the diet died from acute toxic effects including severe liver

Table 50. Studies on long-term exposure (excluding cancer studies) to TCDD in laboratory animals

Species/Strain	Sex/number/ group[d]	Doses tested	Treatment schedule	Parameters monitored
Rats				
Sprague Dawley[a]	M/10	0 ng/kg 1 ng/kg 5 ng/kg 50 ng/kg 500 ng/kg 1000 ng/kg 5000 ng/kg 50 000 ng/kg 500 000 ng/kg 1 000 000 ng/kg	in diet continuously for 65 weeks	survival
Sprague Dawley[b]	M and F/10	0.001 µg/kg per day 0.01 µg/kg per day 0.1 µg/kg per day	in diet continuously for 2 years	extensive histopathology, haematology and clinical chemistry
Mice				
Swiss	M/38-44	0 µg/kg/week 0.007 µg/kg per week 0.7 µg/kg per week 7.0 µg/kg per week	by gavage weekly for 1 year	histopathology
Monkeys				
Macaca mulatta[c]	F/8	500 ng/kg	continuous in the diet for 9 months	extensive histopathology, haematology and clinical chemistry

[a] Van Miller et al. (1977). [b] Kociba et al. (1978, 1979a,b). [c] Allen et al. (1977).
[d] M = male; F = female.

necrosis, bile duct hyperplasia and oedema, atrophy of spleen and thymus, and gastrointestinal haemorrhages.

Groups of 50 male and 50 female Sprague Dawley rats were fed diets providing daily doses of 0.001, 0.01, and 0.1 µg TCDD/kg body weight for 2 years (Kociba et al., 1978, 1979a, b). Control rats, 86 males and 86 females, received diets to which the vehicle acetone had been added. The dose levels corresponded to a dietary content of 22, 208, and 2193 ng TCDD/kg feed. Increased mortality was observed in females given 0.1 µg/kg per day, while no increased mortality was observed in male rats at this dose or in animals receiving doses of 0.01 or 0.001 µg/kg per day. From month 6 to the end of the study the mean body weights of males and females decreased at the highest dose and to a lesser degree in females given 0.01 µg/kg per day. During the course of the study, subnormal body weights were occasionally also recorded in the low-dose group, although during the last quarter of the study the body weights were similar to those of the controls.

Increased urinary coproporphyrin and uroporphyrin were noted in females, but not in males, given TCDD at a dose rate of 0.01 and 0.1 µg/kg per day. Analyses of blood serum collected at terminal necropsy revealed increased enzyme activities related to impaired liver function in female rats given 0.1 µg TCDD/kg per day. Necropsy examination of the rats surviving TCDD exposure to the end of the study revealed that liver effects constituted the most consistent alteration in both males and females. Histopathological examination revealed multiple degenerative inflammatory and necrotic changes in the liver that were more extensive in females. Multinucleated hepatocytes and bile duct hyperplasia were also noted. Liver damage was dose-related and no effect was observable at the lowest dose studied.

7.3.2 Studies on mice

Weekly oral doses of 0, 0.007, 0.7, and 7.0 µg TCDD/kg body weight for 1 year resulted in amyloidosis and dermatitis in male Swiss mice (Toth et al., 1979). The incidence of these lesions was 0/38, 5/44, 10/44, and 17/43 in the control, low-, medium-, and high dose groups, respectively.

7.3.3 Studies on monkeys

In a study by Allen & Carstens (1967) groups of four to five rhesus monkeys were fed diets containing 0, 0.125, 0.25, 0.5, 1.0, and 10.0% of fat (which had been shown to be toxic to chickens) until death. The "toxic fat" was later demonstrated to contain various PCDDs, of which 65% by mass of the total PCDDs present was TCDD (Norback & Allen, 1973). The survival time became shorter with increasing doses of "toxic fat". Mean time to death was 445 days for the low dose and 91 days for the high dose. Decreased food consumption and progressive body weight loss, compared with controls, were noted. Both clinical and histological changes near the time of death appeared similar regardless of dose. The monkeys developed subcutaneous oedema, progressing from the eyelids and face, ascites, and hydropericardium. Characteristic skin changes were observed as well as anaemia, leukopenia, and hypoproteinaemia. The bone marrow was hypoplastic. Centrilobular necrosis, bile duct hyperplasia, and multinucleated hepatocytes were found in the liver. In more than half of the animals, there was marked hypertrophy of the gastric mucosa, with crypts and mucin-containing cysts penetrating into the submucosa. Ulcerations in the fundic and pyloric regions were observed.

Allen et al. (1977) fed eight adult female rhesus monkeys a diet containing 500 ng TCDD/kg for 9 months. Thereafter, surviving animals were removed from the TCDD diet and were observed for another 4 months. No control animals were included, and so data were compared with pre-exposure values where possible. During the first 3 months of exposure animals developed periorbital oedema, acne, and loss of facial hair and eyelashes. By 6 months these changes were quite prominent in six out of eight monkeys, and a decrease in haemoglobin haematocrit was noticed. The animals lost weight even though their food intake was unaltered. Two animals died within the 9-month exposure period and three monkeys continued to develop toxic symptoms and died after 3 months on a TCDD-free diet. The three surviving animals continued to experience periorbital oedema and loss of hair. The total intake of TCDD over the 9-month period was calculated to be 2-3 μg/kg body weight. Death was preceded by severe anaemia, a decreased white blood cell count, and severe thrombocytopenia. Autopsy findings included haemorrhage into a variety of organs, ascites, and subcutaneous oedema. Hypertrophy, dilatation, oedema, and hydropic degeneration of the myocardium were noted in all animals. The biliary ducts showed marked dilatation. Moderate hyperkeratosis of the skin, with cystic keratosis of the hair follicles, was noted, and hypocellularity of the lymphoid tissue and the bone marrow were observed. The hyperplastic mucous-secreting cells of the gastric epithelium had invaded the submucosa, and ulceration and mucinous cysts were common in the modified gastric mucosa. Hypertrophy and hyperplasia of the epithelial lining of the biliary system were present. The bronchial epithelium, salivary glands, bile ducts, and pancreatic ducts showed metaplastic changes. Death was attributed to complications from the severe pancytopenia.

The same pattern of morphological changes were reported to occur in a similar study performed by Barsotti et al. (1979).

Similar, though less severe, effects were observed in four adult female rhesus monkeys fed a diet of 50 ng TCDD/kg for 20 months (Schantz et al., 1978).

7.4 Effects Detected By Special Studies

7.4.1 Wasting syndrome

TCDD causes a starvation-like or wasting syndrome in several animal species. In young animals, or following a sublethal dose in adults, this response is manifested as a cessation of weight gain. Early studies suggested that acute or chronic treatment with TCDD decreased food consumption, but insufficiently to account for the weight loss (Allen et al., 1975, 1977; Greig et al., 1973; Harris et al., 1973; Kociba et al., 1976; McConnell et al., 1978a, b). To elucidate whether malabsorption could explain the wasting syndrome, the transfer of a number of nutrients has been studied with everted intestinal sacs from TCDD-treated rats. A transient increase in the serosal transfer of ^{59}Fe in Sprague Dawley rats was reported by Manis & Kim (1979). Absorption of glucose (Ball & Chabra, 1981; Madge, 1977) and lipids (Shoaf & Shiller, 1981) was decreased by TCDD treatment. The absorption of cobalt, galactose, and proline (Manis & Kim, 1977) as well as of D-galactose, L-arginine, L-histidine (Madge, 1977), and penicillin (Manis & Apap, 1979) was reported to be unaffected by TCDD treatment. Leucine transport was depressed in Sprague Dawley rats 4 h after a single oral dose of 100 µg TCDD/kg body weight (Ball & Chabra, 1981), whereas no effect was observed in Fisher rats 7 days after exposure to 80 µg TCDD/kg body weight (Schiller et al., 1982). Neal et al. (1979) found normal absorption and intermediary metabolism of glucose, L-alanine, and oleate in guinea-pigs treated with a single oral dose of 2 µg TCDD/kg body weight. Apparently there was no generalized impairment of intestinal absorption. The effects reported may well be secondary to decreased food consumption which by itself causes structural changes in the intestine (Steiner et al., 1968) as well as impaired absorption of nutrients (Esposito et al., 1967).

The connection between the wasting syndrome and the lethal effect of TCDD has been investigated in pair-feeding and forced nutrition studies. Courtney et al. (1978) fed TCDD-treated female Wistar rats a normal pelleted diet *ad libitum*. Supplementation with water, electrolyte solution, or liquid diet, administered by gavage, could not reverse or change the pattern or extent of TCDD-induced weight loss or mortality.

To bypass gastrointestinal absorption, Gasiewicz et al. (1980) fed rats intravenously with total parenteral nutrition (TPN). Rats that had received a single ip dose of 100 µg TCDD/kg body weight gained weight similarly to their TPN-fed controls, yet still died at days 13 to 17 following treatment. TCDD-treated rats fed a chow diet ad libitum lost weight progressively (as compared to pair-fed controls that maintained their starting weight) and died at days 11 to 20. In TPN-fed TCDD-treated rats, liver damage was more severe and fat depots were increased as compared to chow-fed TCDD-treated animals. Similar results were obtained with TPN-fed male Hartley guinea-pigs treated with a single ip dose of 2 µg TCDD/kg body weight in olive oil, when compared to TPN-fed control guinea-pigs (Lu et al., 1986). Similar signs of toxicity were present in TPN- and ad libitum-fed TCDD-treated guinea-pigs. In contrast to TPN-fed rats (Gasiewicz et al., 1980), TCDD-treatment in TPN-fed guinea-pigs only produced mild hepatic changes, including increased liver lipid and cytochrome P 450 content, but no morphological changes (Lu et al., 1986).

Seefeld et al. (1984a) suggested that TPN-fed TCDD-treated rats might have suffered from overnutrition and, secondary to that, enhanced hepatotoxicity, as compared to chow-fed, TCDD-treated rats. These same investigators have presented a heuristic model for the TCDD-induced wasting syndrome based on the assumption that body weight in rats is regulated around an internal standard or set point (Keesey et al., 1976). Prevailing weight at a given age is constantly being compared to this set point value and if differences occur, feed consumption is adjusted so as to raise or lower body weight to match the set point level. If TCDD lowers this setpoint, reduction in food consumption would result, as the rat attempts to reduce its weight to a new lower level of regulation determined by the dose of TCDD administered. This hypothesis has been tested in several experiments under carefully controlled feeding procedures.

Repeated studies have demonstrated that reduction of feed intake, due to increased food spillage, is sufficient to account for the loss of body weight in TCDD-treated Sprague-Dawley rats (Seefeld & Peterson, 1983, 1984; Seefeld et al., 1984a, b). TCDD-treated rats maintain and defend their reduced weight level with the same precision as control rats (fed ad libitum) defend their normal weight level (Seefeld et al., 1984b). The percentage of the daily feed intake that is absorbed by the gastrointestinal tract of TCDD-treated and control rats is similar (Potter et al., 1986a; Seefeld & Peterson, 1984). Water intake, resting and total oxygen consumption, carbon dioxide production, respiratory quotient, and spontaneous motoractivity were decreased in a dose-dependent manner by TCDD-treatment (Potter et al., 1986a;

Seefeld & Peterson, 1983; Seefeld et al., 1984a). Urine output was unaffected by TCDD-treatment, despite decreased water intake, whereas urinary excretion of energy and urea were decreased and urinary ammonia was increased (Potter et al., 1986a).

Hypophagia was the major cause of the loss of adipose and lean tissue in male Fisher F-344 rats, C57Bl/6 mice, and albino guinea-pigs when exposed to a calculated LD_{80} dose of TCDD (Kelling et al., 1985). Body weight loss followed a similar time course in TCDD-treated and pair-fed control animals of all three species. Lethalities for TCDD-exposed rats, mice, and guinea-pigs were 95%, 69%, and 81%, respectively, compared to lethalities in the appropriate pair-fed controls of 48, 14, and 64%, respectively (Kelling et al., 1985).

Lethality and body weight loss followed almost identical time-course-curves in Sprague Dawley rats that received a single oral dose of 75 µg TCDD/kg body weight and in pair-fed controls (Christian et al., 1986a). Thus the contribution to lethality made by body weight loss seems to depend on the species and strain. Weight loss appears to play a greater role in causing death in Sprague Dawley rats and guinea-pigs than in Fisher F-344 rats and C57Bl/6 mice. Christian et al. (1986a) demonstrated differences in organ weights and histopathology in TCDD-treated and pair-fed animals, despite similar time-courses and magnitude of body weight loss and lethality. Pair-fed animals exhibited lesions in the gastro-intestinal tract, which were absent in TCDD-treated rats, that may have contributed to death. The hepatic carbohydrate, protein, and lipid metabolism was affected differently in TCDD-treated and pair-fed Sprague Dawley rats (Christian et al., 1986b). To distinguish direct effects of TCDD from effects secondary to hypophagia, the studies by Christian et al. (1986a,b) and Potter et al. (1986a) were performed with schedule-fed animals. The reason for this was the finding that the 24-h feeding pattern for TCDD-treated rats was different from the feeding pattern for pair-fed controls, although it was similar to that of control rats fed ad libitum. Decreased feed consumption did not contribute to weight loss in C57BL/6 mice exposed to TCDD until the animals were moribund (Chapman & Schiller, 1985).

Besides being typical signs of TCDD toxicity, loss of body weight and appetite are also prominent signs of thyroid dysfunction (see section 8.4.9). Serum glucose levels were also decreased by TCDD independently of hypophagia, whereas the decrease in serum insulin appeared to result from hypophagia, since it was seen in both TCDD-treated and pair-fed controls. These results indicate that the effect of TCDD on thyroid hormones cannot explain the TCDD-induced decrease in body weight gain.

An interesting biochemical effect in TCDD-induced wasting is the ability of TCDD to decrease hepatic vitamin A storage in rats (see section 8.4.10). It has long been known that vitamin A is necessary for growth and that vitamin A deficiency will result in depressed body weight gain as well as in reduced food intake. However, the animal continues to eat and grow though body weight gain is less than normal (Brown & Morgan, 1948; Coward, 1947; Hayes, 1971; Orr & Richards, 1934; Patterson et al., 1942).

The effect of chemical structure on the ability of several PCDDs to cause body weight loss in rats has been investigated (Mason et al., 1986). Of the congeners studied, 2,3,7,8-TCDD was the most active. Those congeners fully substituted in the 2,3,7, and 8 positions but containing additional chlorosubstituents in the non-lateral 1,4,6, and 9 positions were less active.

7.4.2 Hepatotoxicity

TCDD produces hepatomegaly, due to hyperplasia and hypertrophy of parenchymal cells, in all species that have been investigated, even at sublethal doses. However, there is considerable variation between species in the extent of this lesion. Other liver lesions are more species specific.

Liver lesions alone cannot explain lethality following TCDD administration, though it may be a contributing factor at least in the rat and rabbit.

The morphological changes in the liver are accompanied by impaired liver function, characterized by liver enzyme leakage, increased microsomal monooxygenase activities, porphyria, impaired plasma membrane function, hyperlipidaemia, and increased regenerative DNA synthesis.

7.4.2.1 Morphological alterations

In Charles River rats given single oral sublethal doses of TCDD (5 or 25 µg/kg body weight) a dose-related increase was observed 3 days after dosing in the amount of hepatic smooth endoplasmatic reticulum (SER) around the periphery of cells, particularly in the areas around bile canaliculi. The effect progressed by days 6 and 9, when an increased amount of rough endoplasmatic reticulum (RER) was also present. By day 28 these changes had returned essentially to normal levels (Fowler et al., 1973).

The livers of CD rats given high sublethal doses of TCDD (5.0 mg/kg body weight per week) for six weeks showed transient degenerative changes, followed by megalocytosis, regeneration, and the occurrence of multinucleated giant hepatocytes (Gupta et al., 1973). They also showed that the hepatotoxic reaction in rats given lethal doses of TCDD (10 µg/kg body weight per day for 16-31 days) was characterized by degenerative and necrotic changes, with the appearance of mononuclear cell infiltration, multinucleated giant hepatocytes, increased numbers of mitotic figures, and pleomorphism of cord cells. These lesions were considered severe enough to be a contributing factor to death.

Parenchymal cell necrosis was observed by Greig et al. (1973) in Porton rats 3 weeks after exposure to an LD_{50} dose of TCDD. The necrosis, which was located in the centrilobular zone close to the central vein, became more severe with time.

Jones & Butler (1974) further investigated the time course of the TCDD-induced liver lesions appearing in the centrilobular zone. They confirmed the transient degenerative and inflammatory lesions previously reported (Greig et al., 1973; Gupta et al., 1973). At the ultrastructural level, consistent changes occurred in the cytoplasm whereas normal nuclear morphology and division were found throughout the study. Two weeks after a single oral dose of 200 µg TCDD/kg body weight to Porton rats, extensive fusion of parenchymal cell plasma membranes in the centrilobular zone was replaced by a diffuse zone with islands of normal membrane occurring at intervals. Normal tight and gap junctions were present in control animals and in periportal areas of the test animals. These findings suggest that the multinucleated cells occurring in TCDD-treated rats might form by coalescence of parenchymal cells. The effect of TCDD on plasma membranes demonstrates a specific subcellular site of action, which might be involved in the toxic action of TCDD. This lesion was, however, not observed until 2 weeks after treatment and thus could not explain the immediate effects on, for instance, food intake, body weight gain, and general health.

The time course for liver lesions in male Sprague Dawley rats (200 g) given a single ip dose of 20 µg TCDD/kg body weight was followed for up to 32 weeks by Weber et al. (1983). The lesions became progressively worse up to the 16th week after injection, and thereafter appeared to regress slowly. The lesions were almost identical to those reported previously (Fowler et al., 1973; Jones & Butler, 1974). The histological findings were accompanied by hyperbilirubinaemia, hypercholesterolaemia, hyperproteinaemia, and increased serum glutamic-oxaloacetic transaminase and serum glutamic-pyruvic transaminase activities, further indicating decreased liver function (Greig et al., 1973; Zinkl et al., 1973).

Fewer studies of liver lesions produced by TCDD have been made in other species than in the rat.

In C57BL/6 mice given single oral doses of 100, 150, or 200 µg TCDD/kg body weight (Vos et al., 1974) and 250 µg TCDD/kg body weight (Jones & Greig, 1975), centrilobular degenerative and necrotic changes were present but multinucleated parenchymal cells were not seen. Proliferation of the bile ducts and bile duct epithelial cells, as well as lipid accumulation, have been observed, with a substantial increase in the hepatic levels of esterified fatty acids and cholesterol. Only slight damage, hepatocellular swelling, was reported in CD-1 mice 21 days after a single dose of 50 µg TCDD/kg body weight, and no histological changes were detected 7 or 35 days after administration (Gupta et al., 1973).

The guinea-pig, while being very sensitive to TCDD, as indicated by LD_{50} data, shows less severe morphological alterations in the liver than do other species. No manifest liver lesions at the light microscopical or ultrastructural levels has been found (Gupta et al., 1973; McConnell et al., 1978b; Moore et al., 1979; Turner & Collins, 1983).

The hamster is very resistant to TCDD toxicity (Table 47) and exhibits no manifest liver damage even after a fatal dose (Henck et al., 1981; Olson et al., 1980b). However, Gasiewicz et al. (1986) found bile duct hyperplasia, numerous inflammatory cells, and increased number of multinucleated cells in the livers of male Golden Syrian hamsters 35 days after they received a single ip dose of 500 µg TCDD/kg body weight in olive oil.

7.4.2.2 Hepatic plasma membrane function

The morphological impairment of hepatic plasma membranes in the centrilobular parenchymal cells of TCDD-treated Porton rats was demonstrated histochemically to be preceeded by a loss of ATPase activity (Jones, 1975). The effect occurred 3 days after treatment in an area five to six cells deep around the central vein along the canalicular borders, and became more severe with time. At the end of the study (day 42 post-treatment) the ATPase activity was completely abolished around the central vein, including the mid-zonal region, and encroached on the periportal area in moribund animals. The loss of ATPase activity was related to the clinical state of the animal. Thus animals displaying minimal signs of intoxication retained the normal distribution of ATPase in the periportal zone. In animals killed 9 months after treatment, partial restoration of the normal liver architecture and the ATPase activity were evident.

Biochemical studies of isolated heptatic plasma membranes from Holtzman rats treated with 10 or 25 µg TCDD/kg body weight revealed depressed ATPase activities (Peterson et al., 1979a). The activity of Na/K-ATPase was depressed to the same extent for both doses from day 2 to 40 after treatment, while a similar depression of Mg-ATPase activity was observed only in the high-dose group. The Mg-ATPase activity tended to recover by day 40, whereas Na/K-ATPase activities did not. A pair-feeding experiment demonstrated that these effects were independent of the TCDD-induced decrease in food consumption. In vitro incubation of plasma membranes indicated that ATPase inhibition did not occur by direct interaction with TCDD. Greig & Osborne (1981) demonstrated a decrease in K/Mg-ATPase activity, but not in the Na/K-ATPase or 5'-nucleotidase activities of hepatic plasma membranes prepared from female Porton rats 6 and 11 days after a dose of 200 μg TCDD/kg body weight.

Many physiological homeostatic mechanisms are dependent on proper plasma membrane function and composition. Matsumura et al. (1984) reported that a single ip dose of 25 μg TCDD/kg body weight to male Sprague Dawley rats had reduced hepatic plasma membrane ATPase-activities by 40% 10 days after treatment. The marker enzyme for putative preneoplastic hepatocytes, glutamyl transpeptidase, was reduced, while protein kinase (both c-AMP-stimulated and c-AMP-nonstimulated) was increased (Matsumura et al., 1984). Both c-AMP-dependent and c-AMP-independent protein kinase, in hepatic plasma membranes from male Sprague Dawley rats treated with an ip dose of 25 μg TCDD/kg body weight, were maximally increased on day 20 after treatment (4.5- and 12-fold, respectively). The induction was measurable within 2 days after the administration and was still persistent after 40 days (Bombick et al 1985). Protein kinase C was significantly increased in hepatic plasma membranes from Sprague Dawley rats but not from guinea-pigs 10 days after single ip doses of 25 and 1 μg TCDD/kg body weight, respectively (Bombick et al., 1985). TCDD treatment in vivo also affected the in vitro binding of concanavalin A, epidermal growth factor, and insulin to their cell surface membrane receptors.

The binding of glucagon and prostaglandin E were not affected by a dose of 25 μg TCDD/kg body weight (Matsumura et al., 1984). Studies with Sprague Dawley rats demonstrated that the TCDD-induced decrease in epidermal growth factor binding (EGF) was observable within 2 days after dosing, reached its maximum by day 20, and was still significant 40 days after dosing. The decrease was observable after a single ip dose of 0.1 μg TCDD/kg body weight (Madhukar et al., 1984). The relative doses of TCDD needed to suppress EGF binding to 50% of the control level were 1, 14, and 32 μg/kg body weight for the guinea-pig, the Sprague Dawley rat, and the Golden Syrian hamster, respectively (Madhukar et al., 1984). A single ip dose of 115 μg TCDD/kg body weight had decreased the EGF binding 10 days after treatment by 93.1, 97.8, and 46.0% in C57Bl/6, CBA, and AKR mice, respectively (Madhukar et al., 1984). The effect of daily sc injections of 2 ng EGF/kg body weight to newborn Balb/c-mice was compared with the effect of a single ip dose of 10 µg TCDD/kg body weight given to the dam of newborn Balb/c-mice within 3 h of delivery (Madhukar et al., 1984). The parameters studied, all well known in vivo effects of EGF, were: time for eyelid opening and tooth eruption; hair length and diameter on day 14; and body weight and thymus weight on day 22. All parameters were significantly reduced both by TCDD treatment and EGF treatment, as compared to controls.

Bombick et al. (1984) found that, 10 days after treatment, in vitro binding of ^{125}I-low density lipoprotein (LDL) to its receptor on hepatic plasma membranes was decreased by 73% in TCDD-treated guinea-pigs (1 µg TCDD/kg body weight) as compared to pair-fed controls. Primary hepatocytes from guinea-pigs treated in the same way had a reduced ability to internalize ^{125}I-LDL. The reduction of LDL receptors on hepatic plasma membranes might be responsible for the increase in plasma of very low density lipoproteins (VLDL) and LDL noted in TCDD-treated animals.

Quantitative changes in the protein composition of plasma membranes following TCDD treatment have been reported (Brewster et al., 1982; Matsumara et al., 1984). The membranes were isolated from male Sprague Dawley rats 10 days after an ip injection of 25 µg TCDD/kg body weight and analyzed by SDS-polyacrylamide gel electrophoresis. Some small proteins (14 000-30 000 daltons) were completely abolished by TCDD treatment. The effect was most pronounced 10 to 20 days after treatment.

7.4.2.3 Biliary excretion

The early proliferation of liver cells around bile canaliculi seen after TCDD treatment (Fowler et al., 1973) was suggestive of an effect on biliary excretion.

The cumulative biliary excretion of indocyanine green (ICG), an organic anion, was decreased in a dose-dependent manner by treatment with 5 or 25 µg TCDD/kg body weight in CD rats (Hwang, 1973). On the contrary, biliary excretion of the organic anions sulfobromophthalein and phenol-3,6-dibromophthalein was unaffected by treatment with 10 or 25 µg TCDD/kg body weight in Holtzman rats (Yang et al., 1977).

Biliary excretion of ouabain, a model compound for neutral non-metabolized substrates such as estradiol, progesterone, and cortisol, was depressed in male Holtzman rats in a dose-related manner by a single oral dose of 10 or 25 µg TCDD/kg body weight (Yang et al., 1977). The effect was detectable two days after treatment, reached a peak between 10 and 20 days, and recovery was only slight by day 40. Increased plasma concentration and decreased bilary excretion of ouabain was also measured in male Sprague Dawley rats 10 days after a single oral dose (25 µg/kg body weight) of TCDD, or 1,2,3,7,8,9-hexaCDD (Yang et al., 1983b). Two other congeners, 1,2,4,6,7,9-hexaCDD and 1,3,6,8-tetraCDD had no effect on these parameters.

When hepatocytes from TCDD-treated (10 µg/kg body weight) male Sprague Dawley rats were incubated with labelled ouabain or procaine amide ethobromide (PAEB) 10 days post-treatment, both the rate of uptake and the steady-state concentration of ouabain were decreased, whereas the uptake of PAEB was unaffected by TCDD (Eaton & Klaassen, 1979). The dose of TCDD was very small relative to ouabain (approximately 150 µmol/litre), so it is not likely that TCDD exerted its effect by competing with the drug for transport into bile. These data suggest that the hepatic membrane transport process for ouabain may be selectively damaged by TCDD.

Peterson et al. (1979a) observed a positive correlation between the levels of hepatic plasma membrane ATPase activities, biliary excretion of ouabain, and bile flow in vivo after TCDD treatment. However, in a further experiment, using perfused rat liver, Peterson et al. (1979b) demonstrated that biliary excretion of ouabain and liver membrane ATPase activities could be decreased independently. Therefore, ATPase activities cannot be directly responsible for the reduced ouabain excretion.

7.4.3 Porphyria

Chronic sublethal exposure to TCDD produces an accumulation of porphyrins in the liver and an increase in urinary porphyrin excretion. In stages of manifest porphyria, accumulation of porphyrins occurs not only in the liver but also in the kidney and spleen (Goldstein et al., 1982). It was demonstrated that mice respond to four weekly doses of 25 µg TCDD/kg body weight with hepatic porphyria, accompanied by an increase in aminolevulinic acid (ALA) synthetase activity, and liver lesions (Goldstein et al., 1973), whereas a single dose of 5, 25, or 100 µg TCDD/kg body weight did not induce porphyria nor ALA synthetase activity in the rat (Woods, 1973). The suggested species difference was later ruled out by Cantoni et al. (1981) and Goldstein et al. (1976, 1982). Chronic administration of 1 µg TCDD/kg body weight per week to rats for 16 weeks resulted in hepatic porphyria (Goldstein, 1976a,b, 1982). In contrast, single oral doses as high as 30 µg TCDD/kg did not produce porphyria either acutely or 16 weeks later. A 6-month recovery period following the final dose was not long enough to reverse the porphyria. Urinary porphyrins and hepatic ALA synthetase activity remained maximally elevated, while hepatic porphyrin levels decreased during this period. Failure to demonstrate porphyria in rats after chronic administration of TCDD for 13 weeks (Kociba et al., 1976) or 2 years (Kociba et al., 1978) was suggested to be the result of unsatisfactory porphyrin analysis (Goldstein et al., 1982).

To further characterize TCDD-induced porphyria, Cantoni et al. (1981) performed a 45-week study to follow the pattern of porphyrin excretion in rats exposed orally to 0.01, 0.1, or 1.0 µg TCDD/kg body weight/week. They found an increase in the coproporphyrin level in the initial phase of exposure, which remained the only sign of exposure in the lowest-dose group. A marked porphyric state appeared only in the 1.0 µg/kg dose group, commencing 8 months after dosing started. At that time urinary porphyrin excretion was 70 times higher than in control rats. The excretion pattern was characterized by increased levels of carboxylated porphyrins.

In attempts to elucidate the mechanism of TCDD-induced porphyria, the effects of TCDD on the enzymes involved in the synthesis and catabolism of porphyrins have been studied. TCDD was found to be a potent inducer of ALA synthetase, the initial and rate-limiting enzyme in haeme synthesis in the liver of chicken embryos (Poland & Glover, 1973b). Elevated ALA synthetase activity has since been demonstrated also in mice and rats (Goldstein et al., 1973, 1982; Kociba et al., 1976, 1978). However, the TCDD-induced increase does not appear after acute exposure and only after several weeks of chronic exposure to TCDD. Jones & Sweeny (1980) failed to demonstrate increased ALA activity in mice exposed to 25 µg TCDD/kg body weight per week for 11 weeks, although porphyria was evident. Thus, induction of ALA synthetase does not seem to be the primary event in TCDD-induced porphyria. Elder et al. (1976, 1978) suggested that decreased hepatic porphyrinogen decarboxylase is the primary event in porphyria induced by halogenated aromatics. TCDD depresses this enzyme activity in vivo in the liver of mice (Jones & Sweeny, 1980; Elder & Sheppard, 1982; Cantoni et al., 1984a,b) but not in vitro (Cantoni et al., 1984b).

A decrease in porphyrinogen decarboxylase activity was present one week after a single dose of 75 µg/kg body weight and continued to decrease with time, thus preceding the increase in hepatic porphyrins, which started to rise during the first 2 weeks after treatment (Smith et al., 1981). TCDD-induced depression of hepatic uroporphyrinogen decarboxylase activity occurs also in the newly regenerating liver, as demonstrated by Smith et al. (1985) in C57Bl/10 mice 10 days after partial (2/3) hepatectomy. The mice were treated with 75 µg TCDD/kg body weight orally 4 weeks before hepatectomy. Greig et al. (1984) demonstrated that pretreatment of five different strains of mice with 12.5 mg Fe^{2+} one week before the administration of 75 µg TCDD/kg body weight had a synergistic effect on porphyria assessed 5 weeks after dosing, expressed as increased hepatic porphyrin and decreased porphyrinogen decarboxylase activity. Iron alone did not increase hepatic porphyrin levels, nor did it affect hepatic porphyrinogen decarboxylase activity.

7.4.4 Epidermal effects

Chloracne and associated pathological changes in the skin are among the most sensitive and widespread responses to TCDD in humans. Similar skin toxicity is expressed only in a limited number of animal species, namely rabbits, monkeys, and hairless mice. To characterize the epidermal response and to elucidate the mechanism(s) of toxicity to epidermal cells, numerous studies have been performed both in vivo and in vitro.

7.4.4.1 In vivo studies

The acnegenic activity of TCDD and related compounds has been tested in the rabbit ear bioassay, first developed by Adams et al. (1941) for industrial applications. The test substance is applied to the inner surface of one of the ears, while pure vehicle is applied to the other. Responses indicative of acnegenic activity include comedo formation, increased ear thickness, and hyperkeratosis. Mild irritation, increased ear thickness, slight enlargement of follicular aperture, slight exfoliation and slight crust formation alone are not considered indicative of acnegenic activity. Microscopically there is conversion of sebaceous cells in the hair follicles into keratin-forming cells. A dose-dependent, positive response was found in this assay when a total dose of 1, 3, or 10 µg TCDD was applied on three successive days (Jones & Krizek, 1962). Also Schwetz et al. (1973) found a dose-dependent acnegenic response in the rabbit-ear bioassay after repeated applications of 4-40 µg TCDD/ear, five days per week for four weeks, corresponding to total doses of 80-800 µg. No response was obtained when the total application was 8 ng. Poiger & Schlatter (1980) applied a single dose of TCDD in various vehicles on the inner surface of the rabbit ear and followed the appearance of inflammation, hyperkeratosis, and chloracne. The minimum dose that induced skin lesions was around 1 µg TCDD/ear when the vehicle was acetone, vaseline, or polyethylene glycol 1500 with 15% water. When TCDD was mixed with soil-water (2:1), or activated carbon-water (1:8) before application, 2-3 and 160 µg TCDD/ear, respectively, were needed to induce lesions. Even 160 µg TCDD/ear produced very small changes on the skin surface when applied as an activated carbon-water paste.

Hairless mice constitute another in vivo model for studies of epidermal effects of TCDD. Puhvel et al. (1982) studied cutaneous changes induced by topical application of 0.1 µg TCDD, three times per week for four weeks, in two strains of hairless mice (Skh:HR-1 and HRS/J). Epidermal hyperplasia, hyperkeratinization, loss of sebaceous glands and follicles, and keratin build-up in the dermal cysts were noted in both strains of mice. Follicular keratosis, considered the pathognomonic lesion in human chloracne, did not appear within 4 weeks of application. In the same study, follicular keratosis did develop after topical application of 2 mg 3,4,3',4'-tetrachlorobiphenyl, five times per week for 8 weeks, suggesting that follicular keratosis is an extension of the epidermal response and, thus, not related to metabolic changes in sebaceous glands. The authors considered hairless mice a less sensitive model for the chloracnegenic response than the rabbit ear bioassay. Similar findings were obtained when HRS/J mice were exposed to TCDD topically applied two to three times per week for four weeks (Knutson & Poland, 1982; Poland & Knutson, 1982). They found, with a total applied dose of 1.2 µg TCDD, a moderate to severe response, including hyperplasia, hyperkeratosis of the interfollicular epidermis, squamous metaplasia of the sebaceous glands, and hyperkeratosis within the dermal cysts, but no keratosis in the sebaceous follicles.

Soot or a benzene extract of soot, containing PCDDs and PCDFs from a PCB-containing transformer fire (Binghamton, New York, USA), were applied to 64.5 cm^2 of the shaved, unabraded dorsal surface of (3 + 3) and (1 + 1) male and female New Zealand white rabbits (3.5 kg), respectively (Silkworth et al., 1982). The dose applied was 500 mg soot or benzene extract corresponding to 500 mg soot/kg body weight. Controls, one male plus one female, were exposed to activated carbon or benzene in corresponding amounts. Exposure lasted for 24 h and the observation period was 67 days. The soot produced no overt toxicity, no weight loss, and no histological findings in thymus, kidney, or skin, but hepatic centrilobular hypertrophy was found in both sexes. The soot extract gave rise to a reversible skin inflammation and hepatic centrilobular hypertrophy in the female only. No weight loss was recorded and the kidney, thymus, and skin were histologically normal at necropsy.

7.4.4.2 In vitro studies

Keratinocytes, the principal cell type of epidermis, form an in vitro model for studies of TCDD-induced hyperkeratosis both in human- and animal-derived cell cultures. The response is analogous to hyperkeratinization in vivo.

Newly confluent epidermal cell cultures exhibit proliferative properties, while the number of basal cells tends to decrease with increasing time of post-confluency growth. Thus, with the appropriate selection of culture medium and time of treatment, different aspects of TCDD toxicity in vivo can be modelled in vitro.

A TCDD-induced response of in vitro keratinization was first demonstrated in XB cell cultures, an established keratinocyte cell line derived from a mouse teratoma, plated at high density to avoid spontaneous keratinization (Knutson & Poland, 1980b). Keratinization was dose-related and histologically similar to that which occurs spontaneously when XB cells are plated at low density. The epidermal proliferation in XB cells produced by TCDD could not be biochemically related to the response produced by cholera toxin, epidermal growth factor, or 12-O-tetradecanoylphorbol-13-acetate, other compounds known to affect cell proliferation in XB cells (Knutson & Poland, 1984). Late passage XB cells, i.e. XBF cells, show increased cell density at saturation and a fusiform morphology at high density. Additionally, they have lost their ability to respond with keratinization upon TCDD treatment. Exposing XBF cells to TCDD concentrations in the range 10 to 11 X 10^{-8} mol/litre resulted in normal growth until confluency was reached by day 7. Thereafter TCDD-treated cultures showed a persistent decrease in cell growth and cell proliferation as well as changed morphology, whereas viability was unaffected (Gierthy & Crane, 1984). Reseeding these quiescent XBF cells, previously exposed to 10^{-9} mol/litre TCDD for 14 days, resulted in normal growth and proliferation until confluency. These TCDD-pretreated cells maintained their susceptibility to TCDD-induced changes in cell growth and morphology. Both XB cells (keratinization assay) and XBF cells (flat-cell-assay) have proved to be useful in vitro bioassays to measure "dioxin-like" activity of both environmental samples and of pure isomers (Gierthy et al., 1984; Gierthy & Crane, 1985a,b). Although XBF cells, a highly transformed variant of XB cells, seem to be less appropriate as a model for TCDD action on normal mammalian epithelial cell proliferation and differentiation, they seem to be more stable and easier to maintain than XB cells. Several continuous lines of human keratinocytes derived from neonatal foreskin (Milstone & Lavigne, 1984; Osborne et al., 1984) or squamous cell carcinomas (SCC) (Rice & Cline, 1984; Willey et al., 1984; Hudson et al., 1985, 1986) have been shown to respond to TCDD in nanomolar concentrations with a variety of signs that indicate alterations in the normal differentiation process. Stimulation of ^{3}H-thymidine incorporation was seen in post-confluent human epidermal cells derived from neonatal foreskin after exposure to TCDD (Milstone & Lavigne, 1984). Newly confluent human epidermal cells, derived from foreskin, responded to exposure for 4 days to 10 nmol TCDD/litre with decreased DNA synthesis, a decrease in the number of proliferating basal cells, decreased binding of epidermal growth factor (EGF), an increase in the number of differentiated cells, and increased envelope formation, i.e., a decrease in the proliferative capacity and an increase in the state of differentiation (Osborne & Greenlee, 1985). The decreases in small (basal) cell number and EGF binding were dose dependent, with EC_{50} values for TCDD of 2 and 1 nmol/litre, respectively. The responses were also obtained with TCDF but not with 2,4-diCDD.

The proliferation and differentiation of epidermal cells is normally regulated by several growth factors and hormones, e.g., EGF, vitamin A and hydrocortisone. Mouse hepatoma cells exposed to TCDD for 24 h showed 20% inhibition of EGF binding (Karenlampi et al., 1983).

Hudson et al. (1985, 1986) demonstrated that TCDD decreases, in a dose-dependent manner, the specific binding as well as the cellular uptake of EGF in cultures of human epidermal cells. The EC_{50} dose for inhibition was 1.8 nmol/litre. A similar inhibitory effect was obtained by TCDF, while 2,7-diCDD was inactive even at doses 100-fold greater. Maximal inhibition, almost 60%, of EGF binding in confluent SCC-12F cells exposed to 100 nmol TCDD/litre was obtained after a pretreatment period of 72 h. No effect was obtained when TCDD was added at the same time as EGF; thus TCDD did not compete for EGF-binding sites, neither did TCDD affect the process of internalizing the EGF. Further studies of the SCC-12F cell line revealed data suggesting that TCDD specifically reduces the high affinity EGF-binding sites in the basal cell population of this cell line (Hudson et al., 1986).

The addition of 10^{-6} mol hydrocortisone/litre to the medium antagonized the growth inhibition of SCC cells grown in 10^{-10} mol TCDD/litre (Rice & Cline, 1984). Hydrocortisone stimulated several aspects of keratinocyte differentiation. These stimulatory effects were abolished in the presence of 10^{-8} mol TCDD/litre, although TCDD alone had no effect on these parameters. The hydrocortisone level in the medium was unaffected by TCDD. TCDD, and even more so hydrocortisone, were able to stimulate stratification in SCC cultures held at confluence for extended periods. This effect was opposed by vitamin A (Rice & Cline, 1984).

Like TCDD, vitamin A suppressed the stimulation of keratinocyte differentiation by hydrocortisone. However, vitamin A had no effect on TCDD-induced growth inhibition or its reversal by hydrocortisone (Rice et al., 1983; Rice & Cline, 1984).

Epidermal transglutaminase (ETG) activity, the marker enzyme for terminal differentiation, was increased by treatment of basal keratinocyte cultures from neonatal BALB mice with 10^{-9} mol TCDD/litre for 5 to 12 days, although morphologically no signs of terminal differentiation were present. A parallel increase in ETG activity was present when these cells were grown in medium rich in Ca^{2+}, although these cells did stratify and differentiate (Puhvel et al., 1984).

7.4.5 Effects on the immune system

TCDD produces a pronounced atrophy of the thymus, spleen, and, to a lesser, extent the peripheral lymph nodes of most experimental animals. Since Buu-Hoi et al. (1972a) reported on TCDD-induced thymic atrophy, many studies in rats, mice, guinea-pigs, and monkeys have shown that the thymus is one of the organs most severely affected by TCDD. Lesions in the thymus appear at exposure levels well below those inducing lesions in other organs. Although there is species variation in the degree and severity of other organ effects, the effects of TCDD on lymphoid tissues is consistent in all species. Further investigations of the effect of TCDD on the immune system, which is a rapidly proliferating and differentiating organ system containing many cellular components in a highly organized and regulated network, have revealed that TCDD affects both the humoral-mediated (section 7.4.5.2) and the cell-mediated immune response (section 7.4.5.3). Also the complement system, a key component of the innate immunity, is affected by TCDD treatment (White et al., 1986). Damage to the thymus and to the cell-mediated immune system seems to be rather specific in that it occurs at doses considerably lower than those affecting other immune functions (Faith & Luster, 1979). Thymic involution is believed to be a direct effect on the gland, and not secondary to factors such as undernutrition (van Logten et al., 1980), altered levels of hormones including corticosteroids (Vos et al., 1973; van Logten et al., 1980), pituitary hormones (Vos et al., 1973), and thymosin (Vos et al., 1978a,b), or zinc deficiency (Vos et al., 1978a,b), or to a direct cytotoxic effect on lymphocytes (Vos et al., 1978a,b). A direct effect of TCDD on mouse fetal thymus organ cells grown *in vitro* was demonstrated at concentrations as low as 10^{-10} mol/litre (Dencker et al., 1985). Within the thymus, lymphocytes in the cortex, i.e., the immature T-cells, are more severely affected in TCDD-treated animals than are lymphocytes in the medulla, i.e., the mature T-cells. Thus, it seems that TCDD impairs the differentiation of thymocytes into immunocompetent T cells. Greenlee et al., (1985) obtained results demonstrating a direct effect of TCDD on thymus epithelial (TE) cells.

High levels of Ah receptors (section 7.8.1) have been found in the thymus (Carlstedt-Duke, 1979; Mason & Okey, 1982;

Gasiewicz & Rucci, 1984). Studies with C57Bl/6 mice (responsive to TCDD), DBA/2 mice (less responsive to TCDD), and B6D2F1 mice, hybrid mice from crosses between these strains, suggest that TCDD-induced thymic involution, as well as immunosuppression, segregates with the Ah locus in these strains of mice (Poland & Glover, 1980; Clark et al., 1983; Vecchi et al., 1983; Nagarkatti et al., 1984; Dencker et al., 1985). The most profound and persistent effect of TCDD on the immune system is found when TCDD is administered during pre- and/or immediate postnatal life. Contrary to other experimental animals investigated, rainbow trout (Salmo gairdneri) are relatively resistant to the immunosuppressive effects of TCDD (Spitzbergen et al., 1986). No humoral-mediated effects, and only minor cell-mediated effects, were present at doses which caused clinical toxicity.

7.4.5.1 Histopathology

Lymphoid organs, primarily thymus but also spleen and lymph nodes, have been found to be affected by TCDD over a wide spectrum of dose ranges in adult rats, guinea-pigs, and mice (Gupta et al., 1973; Vos et al., 1973; Vos and Moore, 1974; McConnell et al., 1978b). The marked reduction in the size of thymus has been referred to as atrophy (Gupta et al., 1973; Vos & Moore, 1974), regression (Allen et al., 1975), or involution (Kociba et al., 1976), though these terms do not clearly represent the pathogenesis of this lesion but are more a description of the final event. Toxic effects on thymus appeared in adult guinea-pigs, rats, and mice exposed to eight weekly doses of 0.2 µg TCDD/kg body weight, six weekly doses of 5 µg TCDD/kg body weight and four weekly doses of 5 µg TCDD/kg body weight respectively (Vos et al., 1973). The thymus from moribund animals, or from animals that died from TCDD exposure, showed a dose-dependent decrease in the number of cortical lymphocytes, markedly smaller thymic lobules, and loss of demarcation between the cortex and medulla. Guinea-pigs, the species most severely affected by TCDD, showed large cystic Hassall bodies, filled with polymorphonuclear leukocytes (Gupta et al., 1973; Vos et al., 1973). Guinea-pigs that received lethal doses of TCDD showed scattered necrosis of lymphocytes in the cortical region with concomitant phagocytosis by macrophages as early as 5 days post-exposure (McConnell et al., 1978b). The effect was more apparent at day 14, and by day 20 it was difficult to differentiate the cortex from the medulla. At day 20 little evidence of necrosis remained, though karyorrhectic debris and prominent phagocytosis indicated that this had occurred. Since the thymus from guinea-pigs surviving the TCDD dose for 30 days was usually normal microscopically (Vos et al., 1973; McConnell et al., 1978b), it seems that thymic necrosis must be an early event in the course of the toxic syndrome. Furthermore, in animals which survive, thymic regeneration seemed to be rapid. Decreased weight of thymus, loss of cortical cells, and cell necrosis have also been found in hamsters exposed to TCDD (Gasiewicz et al., 1986).

Depletion of lymphoid cells in the spleen, intestinal tract, and various lymph nodes observed in guinea-pigs, rats, and mice (Gupta et al., 1973; McConnell et al., 1978b) was less extensive than in the thymus. The major effect in the spleen of rats is the loss of the T-cell-dependent areas, namely the periarterial lymphoid sheet and the paracortical areas (Vos & Moore, 1974).

Depressed immunoglobulin levels were reported for 1- and 4-month-old C57B1/6 mice exposed to four and six weekly doses, respectively, of 25 µg TCDD/kg body weight (Vos & Moore, 1974). Feeding 10, 20, 50, or 100 µg TCDD/kg in the diet depressed dose-dependently the γ-globulin level in 7-week-old Swiss-Webster mice (Hinsdill et al., 1980).

Vos & Moore (1974) demonstrated a dose-related lymphocyte depletion of thymus cortex, spleen, and intestinal lymph nodes in maternally exposed pups of rats and mice. However, no effect on immunoglobulin levels was observed in 25-day-old rats maternally exposed (5 µg TCDD/kg body weight) on days 0, 7, and 14. The developing lymphoid tissues were found to be more sensitive to TCDD than were the lymphoid tissues of adults or young.

7.4.5.2 Humoral-mediated immunity

The humoral-mediated immunity (Tables 51 and 52) operates through antibody-producing cells and is transferable by serum. This system includes classical antibody-mediated protective immunity and immediate hypersensitivity reactions. Vos et al. (1974) reported a significant decrease in the α-, β-, and γ-globulin levels in C57BL/6 mice given non-toxic doses of TCDD. The effects of TCDD on specific humoral immunity responses in adult animals are summarized in Table 51. Feeding levels of 10 µg TCDD/kg body weight or more reduced the primary and secondary antibody response to both sheep red blood cells (sRBC) and tetanus toxin in male Swiss-Webster mice (Hinsdill et al., 1980). Weekly oral doses of 1 or 10 µg TCDD/kg body weight reduced both the primary and secondary serum antitetanus titres in male New Zealand rabbits (Sharma et al., 1984). The secondary, but not the primary, serum tetanus antitoxin level was decreased in Hartley guinea-pigs given eight weekly doses of 0.2 µg TCDD/kg body weight (Vos et al., 1973). Results presented by Vecchi et al. (1980, 1983) show that single doses as low as 1.2 µg TCDD/kg body

Table 51. Effects of TCDD on humoral-mediated immune responses in adult animals

Species/strain (reference)	Sex/age/weight[f]	TCDD exposure Frequency/route/dose	Parameter measured[e]
Mice			
Swiss-Webster (Hinsdill et al., 1980)	F/4-7 weeks/NR	fed 10, 20, 50, 100, or 500 µg/kg continuously in the diet for 5 weeks	primary and secondary sRBC[a] antibody level, primary and secondary serum tetanus antitoxin level
C57BL/6J (Vecchi et al., 1980)	M/6-8 weeks/NR	single ip dose of 1.2, 6, or 30 µg/kg body weight	anti-sRBC[a] plaque-forming spleen cells anti-SIII[b] plaque-forming spleen cells
C57BL/6J (Clark et al., 1981)	M/6-8 weeks/NR	four weekly ip doses of 0.1, 1, or 10 µg/kg body weight	anti-sRBC[a] plaque-forming spleen cells anti-TNP-BA[c] plaque-forming spleen cells
C57BL/6 C3H/HeN DBA/2 AKR $B6D2F_1$ (Vecchi et al., 1983)	M/8-10 weeks/NR	single ip dose of 1.2, 6, or 30 µg/kg body weight	anti-sRBC[a] plaque forming spleen cells
C57BL/6 (Chastain & Pazdernik, 1985)	M/6-8 weeks/NR	single ip dose of 30, 60, 90, or 120 µg/kg body weight	anti-TNP-LPS[d] plaque-forming spleen cells anti-TNP-LPS[d] plaque-forming bone marrow cells

Table 51 (contd).

Species/strain (reference)	Sex/age/weight[f]	TCDD exposure Frequency/route/dose	Parameter measured[e]
Mice (continued) DBA/2N (Luster et al., 1985)	F/6-8 weeks/ 18-21 g	single oral doses of 5, 10, or 50 μg/kg body weight	anti-sRBC[a] plaque-forming spleen cells
$B6C3F_1$ (Luster et al., 1985)	F/6-8 weeks/ 18-21 g	single oral doses of 0.2, 1, 2, 5, or 10 μg/kg body weight	anti-sRBC[a] plaque-forming spleen cells
Guinea-pigs Hartley (Vos et al., 1973)	F/NR/256 g	eight weekly oral doses of 0.008, 0.04, 0.2, or 1.0 μg/kg body weight	primary serum tetanus antitoxin level secondary serum tetanus antitoxin level
Rabbit New Zealand (Sharma et al., 1984)	M/Adult/3 kg	eight weekly oral doses of 0, 0.01, 0.1, 1.0, or 10.0 μg/kg body weight	primary and secondary serum tetanus antitoxin level

[a] sRBC = sheep red blood cell.
[b] SIII = type III pneumoccal polysaccharide.
[c] TNP-BA = trinitrophenylated *Brucella abortus*.
[d] TNP-LPS = trinitrophenylated lipolysaccharide.
[e] = all parameters measured were decreased except for primary serum tetanus antitoxin level in guinea-pigs (Vos et al., 1973).
[f] M = male; F = female; NR = not reported.

weight to C57BL/6 mice decreased the number of plaque-forming spleen cells in response to an injection of the thymus-dependent antigen sRBC. The response was dose dependent and lasted for at least 42 days. Luster et al. (1985) found a decrease in anti-sRBC plaque-forming spleen cell production in B6C3F1 and DBA/2 mice 5 days after single oral doses of 2 and 10 µg TCDD/kg body weight, respectively. A dose of 30 µg TCDD/kg body weight was needed to produce a significant antibody response to the thymus-independent antigen type III pneumococcal polysaccharide (sIII) in C57Bl/6 mice (Vecchi et al., 1980). With sRBC and the thymus-independent antigen trinitrophenylated Brucella abortus, Clark et al. (1981) found a depressed number of spleen plaque-forming cells in C57BL/6 mice only with a total dose of 40 µg/kg body weight given as four equal weekly doses. Chastain & Pazdernik (1985) demonstrated decreased numbers of plaque-forming spleen and bone marrow cells in response to the thymus-independent antigen trinitrophenylated lipopolysaccharide (LPS). Spleen and bone marrow cells were collected from male C57BL/6 mice 7 days after a single ip dose of 30, 60, 90, or 120 µg TCDD/kg body weight. The decrease occurred at lower doses in the spleen cell assay but was more pronounced at higher doses in the bone marrow cell assay. The number of antibody-producing cells, measured as plaque-forming cells, following immunization with either sRBC or LPS was reduced in B6C3F1 mice treated with 1 and 5 µg TCDD/kg body weight (Tucker et al., 1986).

Only minor effects on antibody responses have been reported in rodents maternally exposed to TCDD (Table 52). Single oral doses of 5 µg TCDD to pregnant Fisher-344 N (poor immunological responder) and Fisher-Wistar rats (good immunological responder) on gestation day 18 and/or postnatal days 0, 7, and 14 did not affect the antibody reponse to bovine gammaglobulin (BGG) in the offspring (Faith & Moore 1977; Faith & Luster, 1979).

Dietary exposure of female Swiss-Webster mice to 2.5 or 5 µg TCDD/kg for 4 weeks before mating and throughout gestation and lactation resulted in normal antibody production in the offspring but in a decrease in anti-sRBC plaque-forming spleen cells.

In vitro exposure of B6C3F1 spleen cells to 10^{-9} mol TCDD/litre decreased the production of anti-sRBC plaque-forming cells (Luster et al., 1984). The ED_{50} for this effect was found to be 7 nmol/litre when TCDD was present from the first day of culture (Tucker et al., 1986). Similar activity to that of TCDD was found with 2,3,7-triCDD and 1,2,3,7,8-pentaCDD, whereas 2,8-diCDD and octaCDD were without effect at concentrations up to 5×10^{-8} mol/litre (Tucker et al., 1986).

Table 52. Effects of TCDD on humoral-mediated immune responses in maternally exposed animals

Species/strain (reference)	Time of TCDD exposure	Route/dose	Parameter measured-response
Rats			
Fisher-344 N (Faith & Moore, 1977)	Prenatal day 18 and/or postnatal days 0, 7, and 14	oral/5 μg/kg body weight	primary and secondary BGG[a] antibody level - no effect
Fisher/Wistar (Faith & Luster, 1979)	Prenatal day 18 and/or postnatal days 0, 7, and 14	oral/5 μg/kg body weight	primary and secondary BGG[a] antibody level - no effect
Mice			
Swiss-Webster (Thomas & Hinsdill, 1979)	four weeks before mating, throughout gestation and lactation	in the diet/ 1, 2.5, 5, 10, or 20 μ/kg	primary and secondary sRBC[b] antibody level - no effect; primary anti sRBC[b] plaque forming spleen cells - decreased

a = BGG - bovine γ-globuline.
b = sRBC - sheep red blood cell.

The doses producing 50% suppression of splenic IgM response to sRBC in C57Bl/6 mice were 7.1 and 85 µg/kg body weight, respectively, for 1,2,3,6,7,8-hexaCDD and 1,2,3,4,6,7,8-heptaCDD given as single oral doses 2 days prior to sRBC challenge (Kerkvliet et al., 1985). OctaCDD had no effect even at doses of 100 and 500 µg/kg body weight.

Humoral immune responses of the rainbow trout (*Salmo gairdneri*) were not significantly impaired even at doses of TCDD that caused clinical toxicity (Spitsbergen et al., 1986).

7.4.5.3 Cell-mediated immunity

Cell-mediated immunity (CMI) operates through specifically sensitized lymphocytes and is transferred by these cells. Processes included in this system are classical cell-mediated protective immunity (which protects against fungi, bacteria, and viruses), delayed type hypersensitivity, rejection of tumors and foreign tissues such as transplants, and graft versus host response. Many assays, both *in vivo* and *in vitro*, have been developed to test CMI functions. Besides a reduction in the number of immunologically competent cells after TCDD exposure (Gupta et al., 1973; Vos et al., 1973; Zinkl et al., 1973) TCDD has been demonstrated to induce a decreased CMI response in adults (Table 53) and even more in maternally exposed animals (Table 54). Delayed hypersensitivity response, correlating with decreased host resistance to infectious agents in man, was depressed in rodents exposed to low levels of TCDD (Vos et al., 1973; Faith & Moore, 1977; Sharma et al., 1978; Faith & Luster, 1979; Thomas & Hinsdill, 1979; Hinsdill et al., 1980; Clark et al., 1981). TCDD-exposure also adversely affects host susceptibility to bacteria, viruses, tumor cells and endotoxins (Thigpen et al., 1975; Thomas & Hinsdill, 1979; Hinsdill et al., 1980; Luster et al., 1980; Clark et al., 1983).

Depressed graft versus host response was reported in 2-month-old C57BL/6 mice exposed to 4 weekly oral doses of 5 µg TCDD/kg body weight (Vos et al., 1973), whereas no effect was seen in a subsequent study on 1- and 4-months old C57BL/6Sch mice (Vos & Moore, 1974). In the same study, Fisher-344 rats maternally exposed to TCDD showed decreased graft versus host response and prolonged allograft-rejection time. The latter effect was also demonstrated in maternally TCDD-exposed C57BL/6Sch mice (Vos et al., 1973). Proliferative responses of spleen and/or thymus lymphocytes, stimulated by mitogens specific for the generation of B-lymphocytes and/or T-lymphocytes from TCDD-exposed animals, were depressed both in adults (Vos & Moore, 1974; Sharma et al., 1978) and maternally exposed rodents (Vos & Moore, 1974; Faith & Moore, 1977; Vos et al., 1978; Faith & Luster, 1979; Luster et al.,

Table 53. Effects of TCDD on cell-mediated immunity responses in adult animals

Species/strain (reference)	Sex/age/weight[d]	TCDD exposure Frequency/route/dose	Parameter measured-response[d]
Rats			
CD (Vos et al., 1973)	F/NR/185 g	six weekly oral doses of 0.2, 1.0, or 5.0 µg/kg body weight	delayed hypersensitivity to tuberculin - NE
Mice			
C57BL/6 (Clark et al., 1981)	M/6-8 weeks/NR	four weekly ip doses of 0.1, 1.0, or 10.0 µg/kg body weight	delayed hypersensitivity to sRBC[a] - Dec; delayed hypersensitivity to oxazalone - Dec; generation of alloantigen-specific cytotoxic T-cells - Dec
C57BL/6 (Clark et al., 1983)	M/NR/NR	four weekly ip doses of 0.001, 0.01, 1.0, or 10.0 µg/kg body weight	resistance to Herpes virus challenge - Dec; generation of alloantigen-specific cytotoxic T-cells - Dec
DBA/2 (Clark et al., 1983)	M/NR/NR	four weekly ip doses of 0.001, 0.01, 0.1, 1.0, or 10.0 µg/kg body weight	generation of alloantigen-specific cytotoxic T-cells - Dec
Swiss-Webster (Hinsdill et al., 1980)	F/4-7 weeks/NR	five weeks feeding of diets containing 10, 50, or 100 µg/kg body weight	resistance to *Salmonella typhimurium* challenge - Dec; resistance to *Listeria monocytogenes* challenge - Dec; contact sensitivity to 2,4-dinitro-1-fluorobenzene - Dec

Table 53 (contd - 2)

Mice (continued)			
C57BL/6J (Mantovani et al., 1980)	M/6-8 weeks/NR	single ip doses of 1.2, 6 or 30 µg/kg body weight	number of peritoneal macrophages - Dec; number of splenic natural killer cells - Dec; macrophage mediated cytolysis - NE; macrophage mediated cytostasis - NE
C57BL/6 DBA $B6D2F_1$ (Nagarkatti et al., 1984)	M/NR/NR	four weekly ip doses of 0.001 µg/kg body weight	generation of allospecific cytotoxic T-cells - Dec - NE - Dec
CD-1 (Sharma & Gehring, 1979)	M/NR/28	two, four, or eight weekly doses of 0.01, 0.1, 1.0, or 10.0 µg/kg body weight	lymphoproliferative response of PHA[b]- and PWM[c]-stimulated splenic cells - Dec
C57BL/6Jfh (Thigpen et al., 1975)	M/4 weeks/NR	four weekly oral doses of 0.5, 1.0, 5.0, 10.0, or 20.0 µg/kg body weight	resistance to *Salmonella bern* challenge - Dec; resistance to Herpes virus challenge - NE
C57BL/6 (Vos et al., 1973)	M/2 months/ 24.4 g	four weekly oral doses of 0.2, 1.0, 5.0, or 25.0 µg/kg body weight	graft versus host activity - Dec
C57BL/6Sch (Vos & Moore, 1974)	M/1 month/NR	four weekly oral doses of 1.0, 5.0, or 25.0 µg/kg body weight	lymphoproliferative response of PHA[b]-stimulated spleen cells - Dec; graft versus host activity - NE

Table 53 (contd - 3)

Species/strain (reference)	Sex/age/weight[d]	TCDD exposure Frequency/route/dose	Parameter measured-response[d]
Mice (continued)			
C57BL/6Sch (Vos & Moore, 1974	M/4 months/NR	six weekly oral doses of 1.0, 5.0, or 25.0 µg/kg body weight	lymphoproliferative response PHA-stimulated spleen cells - NE graft versus host activity - NE
Swiss (Vos et al., 1978a)	M/3-4 weeks/NR	four or five weekly oral doses of 50 µg/kg body weight	resistance of *Listeria monocytogenes* - NE; number of peritoneal macrophages - NE; macrophage reduction of nitroblue tetrazodium - NE
Guinea-pigs			
Hartley (Vos et al, 1973)	F/NR/256 g	eight weekly oral doses of 0.008, 0.04, 0.2, or 1.0 µg/kg body weight	delayed hypersensitivity to tuberculin - Dec
Rabbits			
New Zealand (Sharma et al., 1984)	M/adult/3 kg	eight weekly oral doses of 0.01, 0.1, 1.0, or 10.0 µg/kg body weight	delayed hypersensitivity to tuberculin - Dec

[a] sRBC = sheep red blood cells.
[b] PHA = phytohaemagglutinin.
[c] PWM = poke weed.
[d] NR = not reported; NE = no effect; Dec = decreased; M = male; F = female.

Table 54. Effects of TCDD on cell-mediated immunity responses in maternally exposed animals

Species/strain (reference)	TCDD exposure Frequency/route/dose	Age when tested[g]	Parameter measured - response[f]
Rats			
Fisher/Wistar (Faith & Luster, 1979)	5 µg/kg body weight on gestation day 18 and on postnatal days, 0, 7, and 14, or 5 µg/kg body weight on postnatal days 0, 7, and 14	25 days	lymphoproliferative response of PHA[a]- and ConA[b]-stimulated spleen and thymus cells - Dec; delayed hypersensitivity to tuberculin - Dec
Fisher-344 (Faith &Moore, 1977)	5 µg/kg body weight on gestation day 18 and on postnatal days 0, 7, and 14, or 5 µg/kg body weight postnatal days 0, 7, and 14	25 days	lymphoproliferative response of PHA[a]- and Con[b]-stimulated spleen and thymus cells - Dec; delayed hypersensitivity to oxazolone - Dec
Fisher 344 (Vos & Moore, 1974)	1 µg/kg body weight on gestation days 11 and 18 and on postnatal days 4, 11 and 18 or 5 µg/kg body weight on postnatal days 0, 7 and 14	25 days	lymphoproliferative response of PHA[a]-stimulated spleen cells and of PHA[a]- and ConA[b]-stimulated thymus-cells - Dec
Mice			
B6C3F1 [c] (Luster et al., 1980)	1, 5, or 15 µg/kg body weight on gestation day 14 and on postnatal days 1, 7, and 14	NR	lymphoproliferative response of mitogen-stimulated spleen cells: PHA[a] - Dec; ConA[b] - Dec; LPS[d] - NE; Macrophage proliferation - NE; Phagocytizing ability - NE; Resistance to *Listeria monocytogenes* - Dec; Resistance to PYB6 tumor cells - Dec

Table 54 (contd).

Species/strain (reference)	TCDD exposure Frequency/route/dose	Age when tested[g]	Parameter measured - response[f]
Mice (continued)			
Swiss-Webster (Thomas & Hinsdill, 1979)	Feeding 1, 2.5, or 5 μg TCDD/kg 4 weeks before mating, throughout gestation, and 3 weeks postnatally	5-6 weeks	Contact sensitivity to 2,4-dinitro-1-fluorobenzene - Dec; lymphoproliferative response of PHA[a]- and ConA[b]-stimulated spleen and thymus cells - NE; Resistance to *Salmonella typhimurium* endotoxin - Dec; Resistance to *Listeria monocytogenes* - NE
C57BL/6Sch (Vos et al., 1974)	2 or 5 μg/kg body weight on gestation days 14 and 17 and on postnatal days 1, 8, and 15	23 days	Skin graft assay - prolonged skin graft rejection time
Swiss (Vos et al., 1978a)	10 μg/kg body weight on postnatal days 1, 4, 8, 11, 15, and 18	22 days	lymphoproliferative response of PHA[a]-, ConA[b]- & PWM[e]-stimulated thymus cells - Dec

a PHA = phytohaemagglutinin.
b ConA = concanavalin A.
c $B6C3F_1$ = progeny to female C57BL/6N and male C3H mice.
d LPS = lipopolysaccharide.
e PWM = poke weed.
f Dec = decreased, NE = no effect.
g NR = not recorded.

1980). However, Thomas & Hinsdill (1979) found no effect on the lymphoproliferative response in offspring from Swiss-Webster mice fed with up to 5 µg TCDD/kg diet 4 weeks before mating and throughout gestation and lactation. Depressed lymphoproliferative response is regarded as an extremly sensitive indicator of immunotoxicity, rather than as a predictor of immune dysfunction. Cytotoxic T-cell generation in response to allogeneic antigens has been demonstrated in male DBA/2, C57Bl/6, and B6D2F1 mice given four weekly ip injections of 1 ng/kg body weight (Clark et al., 1981, 1983). At this dose no effects were seen on delayed hypersensitivity, antibody response, thymus cellularity, or enzyme induction. The adverse effect of TCDD on CMI function seems to be an age-related phenomenon in rodents. In order to obtain a complete and persistent immune suppression, TCDD exposure must occur during ontogenesis of the immune system. In the initial experiments on the developing immune system, Vos & Moore (1974) exposed Fisher-344 rats to 1 µg TCDD/kg body weight on gestation days 11 and 18 and on postnatal days 4, 11, and 18, or to 5 µg TCDD/kg body weight on postnatal days 0, 7, and 14. CMI functions adversely affected included in vitro immune competence of spleen and thymus lymphoid cells, delayed hypersensitivity reaction, prolonged allograft-rejection times and reduced graft versus host activity. The immune suppression demonstrated persisted throughout the study, i.e., for 145 days. The depression of T-cell-dependent immune functions appeared to occur without helper-cell function being affected (Faith & Moore 1977).

Attempts to study direct effects of TCDD on lymphocytes in vitro were previously hampered by the low solubility of TCDD in physiological buffers (Matsumura & Benezet, 1973). Vos & Moore (1974) obtained no lymphoproliferative response in unstimulated or PHA- or concanavalin-A-stimulated rat thymus organ cells and mouse spleen cells when cultured in the presence of up to 20 ng TCDD/ml. Dencker et al. (1985) demonstrated that mouse fetal thymus cells cultured in vitro in the presence of TCDD gave a similar response similarly to that occurring in vivo, i.e., with a dose-dependent inhibition of the time-dependent increase in the number of lymphoid cells ($EC_{50}=10^{-10}$ mol TCDD/litre). It could not be determined with certainty whether the decreased cell number caused by TCDD was due to reduced cell proliferation or to increased cell death. The TCDD-induced suppression of mitogen-stimulated lymphoproliferation has recently been demonstrated to be mediated by thymus epithelial cells (Greenlee et al., 1985).

7.4.5.4 Macrophage function

The primary pathway of endotoxin detoxification is thought to be macrophage-dependent. Thus the increased sensitivity to endotoxin following TCDD treatment (Vos et al., 1978; Thomas & Hinsdill, 1979) was suggestive of macrophage dysfunction. However, the number of peritoneal macrophages, as well as their capacity to mediate cytolytic and cytostatic effects, was not adversely affected by single ip doses of 1.2, 6 or 30 µg TCDD/kg body weight to male C57Bl/6J mice (Mantovani et al., 1980), nor was the ability of macrophages to reduce nitroblue tetrazolium affected by four to five weekly oral doses of 50 µg TCDD/kg body weight in Swiss-Webster mice (Vos et al., 1978a). Macrophage function does not appear to be altered by TCDD.

7.4.6 Myelotoxicity

TCDD treatment inhibits the bone marrow haematopoiesis in mice, both *in vivo* and *in vitro*, by directly altering colony growth of stem cells (Luster et al., 1980, 1985; Chastain & Pazdernik, 1985). The bone marrow granulocyte-macrophage progenitor cell (CFU-GM) production was reduced in B6C3F1 mice, receiving 1 µg TCDD/kg body weight, but was unaffected in DBA/2 mice, even at a dose of 50 µg TCDD/kg body weight (Luster et al., 1985). Chastain & Pazdernik (1985) used the B-lymphocyte colony-forming unit assay to demonstrate reductions in spleen and bone marrow B-cell function of C57BL/6 mice exposed to single ip doses of TCDD in the range 30 to 120 µg TCDD/kg body weight. Bone marrow B-cells tended to be more suseptible to TCDD than spleen B-cells. A maternal oral dose of 5 µg TCDD/kg body weight on the 14th day of gestation and postnatal days 1, 7, and 14 resulted in a weak normocytic anaemia indicative of depressed erythrogenesis, decreased bone marrow cellularity, and decreased stem cell proliferation in B6C3F1 offspring, assessed 7 days after weaning (Luster et al., 1980). *In vitro* exposure of B6C3F1 bone marrow cells to 10^{-9} mol TCDD/litre resulted in decreased CFU-GM development and decreased number of erythrocyte colony-forming units. The decrease in CFU-GM occurred 1 day post-treatment and remained below control values until 10 days post-treatment (Luster et al., 1985).

7.4.7 Effects on the intermediary metabolism

Changes in intermediary metabolism have been demonstrated in TCDD-treated experimental animals. The circulating concentration of glucose in TCDD-treated rats was decreased relative to *ad libitum*-fed (Zinkl et al., 1973; Schiller et al., 1985) and pair-fed (Gasiewicz et al., 1980; Potter et al., 1983) control rats. TCDD-treated and pair-fed controls (both groups were schedule fed) had similar concentrations of serum glucose (Christian et al., 1986b). The TCDD-induced hypoglycaemia was not caused by altered pancreatic function, as judged by insulin and glucagon levels (Potter et al., 1983).

Reduced hepatic glycogen content, compared to the value in control rats, was reported in Sprague Dawley rats 16 days after a single ip dose of 20 μg TCDD/kg body weight (Weber et al., 1983). However, in studies by Christian et al. (1986b), compared to pair- and schedule-fed control rats, TCDD-treated (75 μg/kg body weight daily) Sprague Dawley rats had significantly increased hepatic glycogen levels but unaffected cardiac and muscle (gastrocnemius) levels of glycogen 2-8 days post-treatment.

TCDD-treated rats maintained a normal overall nitrogen balance, as judged by urinary urea, creatinine, and ammonia levels, but exhibited changes in certain plasma protein levels (Christian et al., 1986b).

Elevated circulating cholesterol levels were found in TCDD-treated rats (Albro et al., 1978; Poli et al., 1980; Schiller et al., 1985), whereas circulating free fatty acids and triacylglycerols were decreased in TCDD-treated rats, when compared to pair- and schedule-fed control rats (Christian et al., 1986b).

A marked accumulation of hepatic lipid has been found in rats after single doses of TCDD (Cunningham & Williams, 1972; Gupta et al., 1973; Albro et al., 1978; Schiller et al., 1985). At a sublethal dose of TCDD, hepatic triglyceride and free fatty acid levels were elevated already one day after dosing. Abnormal lipid deposition patterns persisted for at least 2 months (Albro et al., 1978). The increased level of triglycerides in the liver (Schiller et al., 1985; Christian et al., 1986b) of TCDD-treated rats was not accompanied by increases in cardiac or muscle (gastrocnemius) triacylglycerol levels (Christian et al., 1986b). Hepatic lipid synthesis in Wistar rats, measured as the 1-h incorporation of ^{3}H-acetate, was not affected by TCDD treatment when studied 7 days after exposure to 10 μg TCDD/kg body weight (Cunningham & Williams, 1972).

Mice (both C57BL/6 and DBA/2 strains) responded to TCDD treatment with dose-dependent decreases in serum levels of glucose, cholesterol, and triglycerides, and increases in hepatic triglycerides, whereas serum glycerol and free fatty acid levels were unaffected (Chapman & Schiller, 1985).

Hartley guinea-pigs given a lethal ip dose of 2 μg TCDD/kg body weight had significantly increased circulating levels of cholesterol esters, triglycerides, and phospholipids but a normal free fatty acid level 7 days post-treatment. The increase in serum lipids was accompanied by a pronounced increase in low density lipoproteins, particularly the very low density lipoprotein fraction (Swift et al., 1981). The plasma cholesterol and triglyceride levels were elevated also when

TCDD-treated guinea-pigs were compared to pair-fed controls (Gasiewicz & Neal, 1979).

A TCDD-induced increase in plasma triglyceride levels was also noted in New Zealand rabbits, fed 20 µg TCDD/kg body weight, whereas plasma cholesterol was unaffected 12 weeks after dosing (Lovati et al., 1984). TCDD treatment did not alter the liver lipid levels (free and esterified cholesterol, triglycerides, and phospholipids), but the triglyceride level was significantly increased. These results were valid both for rabbits fed normal chow and those fed a cholesterol-rich (0.5%) diet. Golden Syrian hamsters exposed to 1000 µg TCDD/kg body weight, orally or ip, had elevated plasma cholesterol levels until 20 days after exposure but normal levels on day 50, whereas serum triglyceride levels were normal until day 20 and then became significantly lower than those of controls (Olson et al., 1980b).

7.4.8 Enzyme induction

Primarily, TCDD has been found to increase enzyme activities although observations on enzyme inhibition have also been made. Since the first reports of enzyme systems as targets for TCDD (Buu-Hoi et al., 1971a, 1972b; Greig, 1972; Poland & Glover, 1973b,c), enzyme induction has become the most extensively studied biochemical response produced by TCDD. The mixed function oxidase system (MFO), capable of metabolizing both endogenous and foreign lipophilic compounds to more polar products, has been the most thoroughly investigated one, and arylhydrocarbon hydroxylase (AHH) and 7-ethoxyresorufin O-deethylase (EROD) are the most frequently assayed enzyme activities in this system. TCDD has also been reported to affect UDP-glucuronosyl transferases (UDPGT) (Thunberg et al., 1980, 1984) and glutathione-S-transferases (GT) (Manis & Apap, 1979), which are multifunctional enzyme systems involved in conjugating a wide variety of compounds.

Most studies have been performed with microsomal enzymes, but TCDD has also been found to have effects on enzymes in the cytosolic fraction. It seems that TCDD produces organ-specific effects, and although, quantitatively, hepatic enzyme induction is of more concern than extrahepatic enzyme effects, the latter may qualitatively be as important. Studies in different species have revealed that enzyme induction due to TCDD exposure also is a species-specific phenomenon.

Time course studies have shown that maximal increases in enzyme activities are reached within 3 to 4 days post-treatment. After a lag period of about 2 to 3 weeks, enzyme activities begin to return to normal levels (Hook et al., 1975a,b; Lee & Suzuki, 1980; Lucier et al., 1973; Poland & Glover, 1973a).

According to Kitchin & Woods (1979), TCDD-induced AHH activity did not reach the normal level until 6 months after rats were exposed to a single daily dose of 2 µg/kg body weight.

Hook et al. (1975a) found no apparent dependence on age when studying AHH induction in CD rats which were 10 to 335 days old at the time of exposure to 25 µg TCDD/kg body weight.

Several investigators have studied the relative potency of various PCDDs and PCDFs to induce AHH and/or EROD activities (Bradlaw et al., 1980; Poland et al., 1976; Bandiera et al., 1984a,b; Sawyer & Safe, 1985; Mason et al., 1986). They found an apparent structure-activity relationship between the location of the halogen atoms on the dibenzo-p-dioxin molecule and the ability to induce AHH activity both *in vivo* and *in vitro*. Isomers with halogens at the four lateral ring positions produced a greater biological response than those with halogens at three lateral ring positions, while two lateral halogen atoms seemed to be insufficient to produce a biological response. TCDD was the most potent enzyme inducer of the compounds tested.

On a molecular basis TCDD is the most potent MFO-inducing compound known and MFO induction seems to be the most sensitive biochemical response produced by this chemical. According to Kitchin & Woods (1979), induction in the rat takes place after a single daily dose of only 0.002 µg TCDD/kg body weight. In the guinea-pig (the animal most sensitive to TCDD toxicity), MFO induction has been observed, but the induced activities were low even at lethal doses (Hook et al., 1975a). Neither is there a correlation in cell cultures between induction of MFO and toxicity. Furthermore, it is known that metabolites of TCDD are less toxic and more readily excreted than the parent compound (see section 8.1.5). Thus, TCDD-induced MFO activities represent a detoxification process rather than one leading to toxic effects.

However, induction of MFO activities might potentiate the toxicity of other foreign compounds requiring metabolic transformation by the MFO system before they can exert their toxic effect. A number of studies have shown that induction of MFO activities alters the metabolism of the model xenobiotic, benzo(a)pyrene by increasing the rate of microsomal metabolism, changing the metabolic profile to more toxic metabolites, and increasing the extent of covalent binding to liver microsomes (Berry et al., 1976, 1977; Uotila et al., 1978). TCDD, applied topically or subcutaneously increased the carcinogenicity of 3-methyl cholanthrene (MC) in DBA/2 mice (Kuori, 1978), but decreased the carcinogenicity of 7,12-dimethylbenz(a)anthracene (DMBA) in CD-1 mice (DiGiovanni et al., 1979a). These authors suggested that TCDD induces the

MFO system and thus increases activation of MC to the ultimate carcinogen, as well as inactivation of DMBA, which would explain these effects.

Furthermore, increased MFO activities might adversely affect important metabolic pathways of endogenous compounds. The effects of TCDD on enzyme activities, both MFO and others, involved in such biological pathways as keratinization, steroid metabolism, lipid metabolism, plasma membrane function and porphyrin metabolism, are discussed under separate sections. The minute quantities of TCDD required for maximal enzyme induction or suppression, the long duration of the effect, and the stereospecific requirements suggest a specific interaction of TCDD with a cellular species, possibly at the gene level. Accordingly considerable research has been directed toward the study of the genetic regulation of AHH induction by TCDD. A hepatic cytosolic species that bound TCDD has been suggested as the receptor for the hepatic AHH activity. Numerous studies of this cytosolic receptor in several species and tissues have been performed and it seems that there is a structural gene, the Ah locus, for this receptor, which is responsible for the expression of various enzyme activities (see sections 7.8 and 7.8.1).

7.4.8.1 Studies on rats

The effect of TCDD on enzyme activities has been most extensively investigated in the rat. In the liver, TCDD has been shown to increase both the content of cytochrome P-450 (Lucier et al., 1973, 1986; Poland & Glover, 1974a, b; Hook et al., 1975a; Aitio & Parkki, 1978; Kitchin & Woods, 1979; Madhukar & Matsumura, 1981; Goldstein & Linko, 1984) and cytochrome b5 (Lucier et al., 1973; Hook et al., 1975a), as well as the microsomal enzyme activities involved in the oxidative transformation and conjugation of xenobiotics, e.g., aniline hydroxylase, arylhydrocarbon hydroxylase (AHH), biphenyl hydroxylase, 7-ethoxycoumarin-O-deethylase (ECOD), EROD, and UDPGT. These enzyme activities have been investigated in a vast number of studies, some of them quoted in Table 55. Goldstein & Linko (1984) demonstrated that TCDD induced two isozymes of cytochrome P-450 (P-448) in the liver but only one of these in extrahepatic tissues of young Sprague Dawley rats 2 days after a single oral dose of 25 µg/kg body weight.

Microsomal glutathion-s-transferase (GT) did not respond to TCDD (Aitio & Parkki, 1978; Mukitari et al., 1981; Baars et al., 1982), but cytosolic GT was induced both by a single dose of 17 µg TCDD/kg body weight 2 days post-treatment (Manis & Apap, 1979), and by near lethal or lethal doses 1 and 6 days after dosing (Mukitari et al., 1981; Baars et al., 1982; Hassan et al., 1983). Glutathione reductase was also

Table 55. Studies demonstrating in vivo induction of mixed function oxidases and UDP-glucuronosyltransferases in TCDD-exposed strains of rats

Enzyme activity	Rat strain	Reference
Aniline hydroxylase	SD	Beatty et al. (1978)
	CD	Lucier et al. (1973); Hook et al. (1975a)
Aryl hydrocarbon hydroxylase	SD	Poland & Glover (1973a, 1974a); Beatty et al. (1978); Manis & Apap (1979); Haaparanta et al. (1983); Thunberg et al. (1984); Lucier et al. (1986); Ahlborg et al. (1987)
	CD	Lucier et al. (1973); Hook et al. (1975a); Kitchin & Woods (1979)
	Wistar	Nagayama et al. (1983); Keys et al. (1985); Bannister et al. (1986); Farrell & Safe (1986); Mason et al. (1986); Tsyrlov et al. (1986)
Biphenyl hydroxylase	CD	Hook et al. (1975a,b,); Kitchin & Woods (1979)
7-Ethoxycoumarin-*O*-deethylase	Wistar	Aitio & Parkki (1978)
7-Ethoxyresurofin-*O*-deethylase	SD	Haaparanta et al. (1983)
	CD	Kitchin & Woods (1979)
	Wistar	Keys et al. (1985); Bannister et al. (1986); Farrell & Safe (1986); Mason et al. (1986)
UDP-glucuronosyl-transferase:		
p-nitrophenol	SD	Thunberg et al. (1980, 1984); Ahlborg et al. (1987)
	CD	Lucier et al. (1973, 1975a, 1986); Hook et al. (1975a)
	Wistar	Aitio et al. (1979); Thunberg & Hîkansson (1983)
o-aminophenol	Wistar	Aitio et al. (1979)
4-methylumbelliferone	Wistar	Aitio & Parkki (1978)

increased, while glutathione peroxidase, both total and Se-dependent, and the content of reduced glutathione were reduced by TCDD treatment (Hassan et al., 1983, 1985a,b,c).

The following hepatic enzyme activities involved in drug metabolism have been reported to be unaffected by TCDD treatment in the rat: N-and O-demethylation (Lucier et al., 1973; Poland & Glover, 1973a; Hook et al., 1975a; Beatty et al., 1978; Kitchin & Woods, 1979; Madhukar & Matsumura, 1981), epoxide hydratase (EH) (Aitio & Parkki, 1978), β-glucuronidase (Lucier et al., 1973, 1975) and NADPH cytochrome c reductase (Poland & Glover, 1974; Aitio & Parkki, 1978; Kitchin & Woods, 1979; Madhukar & Matsumura, 1981). The glucuronide conjugation of bilirubin (Aitio et al., 1979), estrone, and testosterone (Lucier et al., 1975a) by liver microsomes from TCDD-treated rats was not different when compared to control rats.

Some hepatic enzyme activities not belonging to the MFO system, which are affected by TCDD treatment include aldehyde dehydrogenase (Deitrich et al., 1978; Lindahl et al., 1978), δ-aminolevulinic acid synthetase (see section 7.4.3), DT-diaphorase (Beatty & Neal, 1977), transglutaminase (see section 7.4.4), ornithine decarboxylase (Nebert et al., 1980; Potter et al., 1982; Farrell & Safe, 1986), plasma membrane ATPases (see section 7.4.2.2), porphyrinogen carboxylase (see section 8.4.3), prostaglandin synthetase (see section 7.4.9), enzymes involved in testosterone metabolism (see section 7.4.9), and RNA polymerase (Kurl et al., 1982).

Prenatal and postnatal exposure via milk to TCDD, at doses of 3 μg/kg body weight to pregnant rats on days 5, 10 and 16 of gestation, induced hepatic AHH and UDPGT activities in the offspring. The effect was seen 8 days post-partum and persisted for at least 2 weeks. The inductive effect was due both to exposure to TCDD via milk and to the activation of an inducing mechanism after birth. Fetal liver AHH was slightly increased during late gestation, although the UDPGT activity and the cytochrome P-450 content were not (Lucier et al., 1975b).

Administration of 2.5 μg TCDD/kg body weight to pregnant rats on day 17 of gestation increased the AHH- and N-hydroxylation activities and cytochrome P-450 content in the fetal liver on day 20 of gestation (Berry et al., 1976).

AHH induction due to TCDD has been reported to occur also in the brain (Hook et al., 1975a), kidney (Poland & Glover, 1973a; Hook et al., 1975a; Aitio & Parkki, 1978; Potter et al., 1982; Nagayama et al., 1983), lung (Poland & Glover, 1973a; Hook et al., 1975a; Aitio & Parkki, 1978; Nagayama et al., 1983), prostate (Lee & Suzuki, 1980; Haaparanta et al., 1983; Nagayama et al., 1983), thymus (Nagayama et al., 1983), and intestine (Poland & Glover,

1973a; Hook et al., 1975a), but intestinal AHH activity was found to be unaffected by 17 and 20 µg TCDD/kg body weight (Aitio & Parkki, 1978; Manis & Apap, 1979). Testicular (Poland & Glover, 1973a; Hook et al., 1975a; Aitio & Parkki, 1978) and adrenal (Guenthner et al., 1979) AHH activities were not induced by sublethal doses of TCDD. The O-deethylation activity in kidney, lung, and prostate was increased, but no effect was seen on the activity in testes or intestine (Aitio & Parkki, 1978; Haaparanta et al., 1983). UDPGT activities in kidney, lung, intestine, and brain were increased, while no effect was seen on testicular UDPGT (Hook et al., 1975a). Similar results were reported by Aitio & Parkki (1978), though in their study intestinal UDPGT was not affected.

Renal biphenyl hydroxylation activity has been found to increase after TCDD treatment, but no effect on this enzyme activity was seen in lung, intestine, brain, or testes (Hook et al., 1975a). Elevated levels of cytochrome P-450 were found in prostate (Lee & Suzuki, 1980) and mammary gland (Rikans et al., 1979), but not in adrenals (Guenthner et al., 1979). Less testicular cytochrome P-450 was found after a single dose of 25 µg TCDD/kg body weight (Tofilon & Piper, 1982). The GSH tranferase activity was increased in the lung but not in kidney, intestine, testes (Aitio & Parkki, 1978), or prostate (Lee & Suzuki, 1980).

Neither EH nor NADPH cytochrome c reductase were inducible by TCDD in kidney, lung, intestine, testes (Aitio & Parkki, 1978), mammary gland (Rikans et al, 1979), or prostate (Lee & Suzuki, 1980). The ED_{50} values for hepatic AHH and EROD induction were determined in immature male Wistar rats 13 days after a single ip dose of 2,3,7-triCDD, TCDD, 1,3,7,8-tetraCDD, 1,2,3,7,8-pentaCDD, 1,2,4,7,8-pentaCDD or 1,2,3,4,7,8-hexaCDD (Mason et al., 1986). The order of enzyme-inducing capacity was TCDD > 1,2,3,7,8-pentaCDD > 1,2,3,4,7,8-hexaCDD > 1,2,4,7,8-pentaCDD > 2,3,7-triCDD > 1,3,7,8-tetraCDD (Table 56).

7.4.8.2 Studies on mice

Enzyme induction studies in mice have been performed mainly with two strains genetically separated at the Ah locus, thus making them responsive (C57Bl/6 (B6)) or non-responsive (DBA/2 (D2)) to induction of hepatic cytochrome P-450-related enzyme activities by aromatic hydrocarbons, e.g., 3-methylcholanthrene (3-MC). However, the extraordinary potency of TCDD for enzyme induction revealed increased hepatic cytochrome P-450 content as well as AHH and O-deethylase activities both in B6 and D2 mice after sublethal exposure to TCDD (Poland & Glover, 1974a,b,c; Jones & Sweeney, 1977; Greenlee & Poland, 1978). Studies of MFO induction in five responsive and

Table 56. Structure activity relationships for some PCDDs

PCDD Congener	*In vitro* EC_{50} values (M)[a]			*In vivo* ED_{50} values (µmol/kg)[b]				LD_{50} [c]
	Receptor binding	AHH	EROD	AHH	EROD	Body weight	Thymic atrophy	Guinea-pig µg/kg body weight
1-	> 1.0×10^{-4}	> 1.0×10^{-4}	> 1.0×10^{-4}					
2, 8-	3.2×10^{-6}	> 1.0×10^{-4}	> 1.0×10^{-4}					> 300 000
1, 2, 4-	1.3×10^{-5}	4.8×10^{-5}	2.2×10^{-6}					
2, 3, 6-	2.2×10^{-7}							
2, 3, 7-	7.1×10^{-8}	3.6×10^{-7}	1.4×10^{-7}	19.6	19.6		98.1	29 400
1, 2, 3, 4-	1.3×10^{-6}	3.7×10^{-6}	2.4×10^{-6}					
1, 2, 3, 8-		6.1×10^{-7}						
1, 3, 7, 8-	7.9×10^{-7}	5.9×10^{-7}	3.2×10^{-7}	31.2	77.6	132	100	
2, 3, 6, 7-	1.6×10^{-7}	6.1×10^{-8}	1.1×10^{-8}					
2, 3, 7, 8-	1.0×10^{-8}	7.2×10^{-11}	1.9×10^{-10}	0.004	0.003	0.05	0.09	2
1, 2, 3, 4, 7-	6.4×10^{-6}	6.6×10^{-7}	8.2×10^{-7}					
1, 2, 3, 7, 8-	7.9×10^{-8}	1.1×10^{-8}	1.7×10^{-8}	0.031	0.056	0.62	0.17	3.1
1, 2, 4, 7, 8-	1.1×10^{-6}	2.1×10^{-8}	1.1×10^{-8}	2.82	0.56	34	11.2	1125
1, 2, 3, 4, 7, 8-	2.8×10^{-7}	2.1×10^{-9}	4.1×10^{-9}	0.03	0.130	1.63	1.07	72.5
1, 2, 3, 6, 7, 8-[c]	5.7×10^{-10}	3.1×10^{-8}						70-100
1, 2, 3, 7, 8, 9-[c]	1.4×10^{-9}	4.6×10^{-8}						60-100
1, 2, 3, 4, 6, 7, 8[c]		1.3×10^{-7}						> 600
1, 2, 3, 4, 6, 7, 9-[c]		3.7×10^{-6}						
1, 2, 3, 4, 6, 7, 8, 9-	> 1.0×10^{-5}	> 1.0×10^{-4}	> 1.0×10^{-4}					

[a] Estimated concentrations needed to displace 50% of ^{3}H-TCDD bound to liver cytosol receptor from Wistar rats and to produce 50% maximum enzyme induction in the rat hepatoma 11-4-II E cell line (Bradlaw & Casterline, 1979; Mason et al., 1986).

[b] Studies in immature male Wistar rats (Mason et al., 1986).

[c] McConnell et al., 1978b.

five non-responsive strains of mice by Poland & Glover (1974a,b,c) revealed that there were no consistent differences between the strains when considering the extent to which TCDD induced AHH, O-deethylase, N-demethylase and O-demethylase activities in the liver, kidney, lung, skin, or bowel. The ED_{50} for hepatic AHH induction was determined to be 10^{-9} mol/kg body weight in the responsive strain and $\geq 10^{-8}$ mol/kg body weight in the non-responsive strain (Poland & Glover, 1975). Fully induced hepatic AHH activity was obtained both in responsive (C57Bl/6 and AKR/Qdj) and non-responsive (DBA/2 and DDD) strains of mice 3 days after an ip dose of 30 µg TCDD/kg body weight (Nagayama et al., 1985a). Both AHH and EROD were induced in C57Bl/6 mice 7 days after an ip dose of 0.32 µg/kg body weight (Bannister et al., 1986). Both hepatic AHH and ornithine decarboxylase activities were similarly induced in C57Bl/6 and DBA/2 mice after a single ip dose of 100 µg TCDD/kg body weight, but at 2 µg TCDD/kg body weight these enzymes were induced only in the C57Bl/6 strain (Nebert et al., 1980). Two daily doses of 0.1 µg TCDD, topically applied, increased the epidermal AHH activity in two strains of hairless mice (Puhvel et al., 1982). Contrary to observations in rats, TCDD induces testicular AHH activity both in B6 and D2 mice 40h after an ip dose of 50 µg/kg body weight (Mattison & Thorgeirsson, 1978).

7.4.8.3 Studies on guinea-pigs

The guinea-pig, the species most sensitive to the toxic effects of TCDD, does not respond with liver toxicity or with extensive enzyme induction.

Hook et al. (1975a) investigated the effect of a single oral dose of 0.175 µg TCDD/kg body weight on Hartley guinea-pig MFO and UDPGT activities in liver, kidney, and lung. AHH induction was found only in the kidney. In none of the tissues was there an effect on UDPGT activity. The biphenyl 4-hydroxylase activity was increased in all tissues, whereas hepatic biphenyl 2-hydroxylase was decreased. With three daily doses of 1 µg TCDD/kg body weight, Hassan et al. (1983) found an increase in hepatic AHH 6 days post-treatment. They also found slightly increased *in vitro* lipid peroxidation but no effect on glutathione content or on the enzyme activities facilitating peroxidation, reduction, or transfer of glutathione. The DT-diaphorase activity was not affected by a single oral dose of 0.6, 3.0, or 6.0 µg TCDD/kg body weight (Beatty & Neal, 1977). The maximal increases were 4.4 and 22 times for AHH and EROD activities, respectively. The testicular cytochrome P-450 content in Hartley guinea-pigs was decreased by 50% one day after a single dose of 1 µg TCDD/kg body weight. The effect persisted for at least 9 days

(Tofilon, 1980). No effect was seen on microsomal haeme content or on the activities of NADPH-cytochrome C reductase and sorbitol dehydrogenase, the marker enzyme for testicular protein synthesis. Thus, the decrease in cytochrome P-450 induced by TCDD does not seem to be a nonspecific inhibition of protein synthesis.

7.4.8.4 Studies on rabbits

Studies on enzymes in rabbits have been performed in the New Zealand albino strain exposed to single doses of 10 to 30 µg TCDD/kg body weight for 1 to 5 days. Both in adults (Johnson & Muller-Eberhard, 1977a,b) and in neonates exposed in utero (Norman et al., 1978; Kohli & Goldstein, 1981), TCDD increased the content of cytochrome P-450. It also induced the formation of immunologically distinct cytochromes P-450 in adult and neonatal liver (Norman et al., 1978). Increased cytochrome P-450 was observed in the kidney but not in the lung (Liem et al., 1980; Kohli & Goldstein, 1981). Renal and pulmonary cytochrome P-450 reductase, investigated by Liem et al. (1980), were not affected by TCDD treatment. Data on MFO induction and suppression are conflicting. Liem et al. (1980) reported increased AHH and O-deethylase activities in lung and kidney, whereas Hook et al. (1975a) saw no effect on the AHH activity in the lung and reported a decrease in hepatic AHH activity after a single oral dose of 0.5 µg TCDD/kg body weight. Biphenyl 4-hydroxylase induction was seen in the liver by Johnson et al. (1979). Hook et al. (1975a) detected such induction in lung, but no effect in the liver and kidney (Hook et al 1975a). Furthermore, Hook et al. (1975a) reported no effects on biphenyl-2-hydroxylation and UDPGT activities in liver, kidney, or lung. A decrease in hepatic, but not in renal or pulmonary N-demethylation, was found by these authors.

7.4.8.5 Studies on hamsters

Golden Syrian hamsters are among the animals most resistant to acute lethal effects induced by TCDD. Although the liver is a target tissue, hepatic enzyme induction has barely been studied in this species. When given an oral dose of 200 µg/TCDD/kg body weight for a period of 3 days, increased hepatic glutathione-S-transferase and glutathione reductase activities were found, but no effects were seen on AHH or glutathione peroxidase activities. Neither the hepatic level of glutathione nor the in vitro lipid peroxidation were affected (Hassan et al., 1983). The ED_{50} values for induction of hepatic ECOD and reduced NAD(P), menadione oxidoreductase activities, and cytochrome P-450 content in male Golden Syrian hamsters were 1.0, 2.0, and 0.5 µg TCDD/kg body weight, i.e. extremely low doses as compared to doses that produce tissue damage and lethality in this species (Gasiewicz et al., 1986).

7.4.8.6 Studies on cows

Three dairy Holstein cows (500-600 kg) received a single oral dose of 0.05 (two cows) or 7.5 μg TCDD/kg body weight (Jones et al., 1986). The cow receiving the high dose was killed on day 7 and those receiving the low dose on day 14. AHH and EROD activities were markedly induced in the high-dose but not in the low-dose animals.

7.4.8.7 Studies on chick embryos

AHH and δ-aminolevulinic acid synthetase in the chick embryo have been reported to be extremely sensitive to the inductive effects of TCDD (Poland & Glover, 1973b,c). Maximal induction occurred with 155 pmol TCDD/egg. The induction was relatively long lasting, with 70% of the maximum induced activity present 5 days following a single dose of TCDD. Structure-activity studies demonstrated a good correspondence between the toxicity and induction potency of a series of dibenzo-*p*-dioxin congeners (Poland & Glover, 1973c).

ED_{50} values for the induction of hepatic microsomal EROD, AHH, and 4-dimethylaminoantipyrine-*N*-demethylase in 2-week-old white Leghorn cockerels on day 5 after TCDD exposure were 778, 302, and 561 ng/kg body weight, respectively, and aldrin epoxidase was inhibited by TCDD treatment (Sawyer et al., 1986). Hepatic and cardiac EROD activities were increased in white Leghorn chicken embryos exposed to TCDD *in ovo* at doses between 1000 and 10 000 pmol/egg (Quilley & Rifkind, 1986).

7.4.8.8 Studies on cell cultures

TCDD has a very low toxicity in cell cultures, yet it is a very potent inducer of AHH activity in these systems, including lymphocytes and primary hepatocytes, as well as established and transformed cell lines.

The inducibility of lymphocyte AHH has been investigated in mitogen-stimulated human lymphocytes from the venous blood of healthy volunteers. Kouri et al. (1974) found a dose-dependent increase in AHH activity (0, 0.1, 1.0, 10, or 100 ng TCDD/ml medium for 24 h). The optimal dose was about 10 ng/ml, and the maximal induction was by a factor of 2 to 3. On the contrary, Gurtoo et al. (1979) found no dose-response correlation, in the dose range 1.7 to 20 ng TCDD/ml, when measuring lymphocyte AHH induction. To circumvent the limitation of prior mitogen activation when studying AHH induction in lymphocytes, Freedman et al. (1979) used the human B-lymphocyte RPMI-1788 cell line, which does not require prior activation for the induction of AHH activity. The optimal concentration to stimulate AHH activity was determined to be 10 ng/ml medium. Highly variable induction of AHH (between 3- and 28-fold) was obtained by Nagayama et al. (1985b) in human lymphoblastoid cell lines derived from the peripheral blood of healthy volunteers of both sexes and of variable ages. The cells were exposed to 7.5 ng TCDD/ml medium for 48 h.

In a study by Niwa et al. (1975), the estimated ED_{50} values for AHH induction by TCDD in 11 established cell lines, in fetal primary cultures from five animal species and cultured human lymphocytes, ranged from 0.04 ng/ml medium in C57Bl/6 mouse cultures and 0.08 ng/ml in the rat hepatoma H-4-IIE cell line to more than 66 ng/ml in the HTC rat hepatoma cell line. TCDD was demonstrated to be the most potent AHH inducer out of 24 chlorinated dibenzo-_p_-dioxin analogues (Bradlaw et al., 1980) tested in a rat hepatoma cell culture extremely sensitive to AHH induction, the ED_{50} being about 0.5 pg/10^6 cells. A 165-fold increase in AHH-activity and a 54-fold increase in EROD activity were obtained in rat hepatoma H-4-IIE cells when exposed to 2 x 10^{-10} mol TCDD/litre for 3 days (Keys et al., 1986). In this system co-exposure of TCDD with 1,3,6,8-tetraCDF and 2,4,6,8-tetraCDF reduced the TCDD-induced enzyme induction, whereas co-exposure of TCDD and TCDF resulted in an additive effect on enzyme induction (Keys et al., 1986). The EC_{50} values for AHH and EROD induction in the same cell system varied over 7 orders of magnitude for 14 different PCDDs (Table 56), the most potent being TCDD and the least potent being 2,3,6-triCDD (Mason et al., 1986). A 2- to 650-fold AHH induction was observable in 8 of 22 different cell cultures exposed to 10^{-9} mol TCDD/litre for 24 h (Knutson & Poland, 1980a). The cells were derived from tissues and/or species susceptible to TCDD toxicity _in vivo_. Nanomolar concentrations of TCDD induced AHH activity in keratinocyte cultures of human (Willey et al., 1984) and animal origin (Knutson & Poland, 1980a).

Five human squamous carcinoma cell lines derived from tumours of the epidermis and tongue responded to TCDD with increased _O_-deethylase activity, the EC_{50} being 10^{-10} to 10^{-9} mol/litre (Hudson et al., 1983a).

Steward & Byard (1981) treated primary hepatocytes isolated from Sprague Dawley rats, for 48 h with various concentrations of TCDD. They found a 2-fold induction of the AHH activity with 3 pg TCDD/10^6 cells. Maximal induction occurred with 2.4 ng TCDD/10^6 cells. Primary hepatocytes, isolated from adult male Wistar rats, exhibited a linear increase (from 2- to 4-fold) in AHH activity when exposed to TCDD in the range 10^{-11} to 10^{-8} mol/litre for 72 h (Jansing & Shain, 1985). Primary hepatocytes from TCDD-treated (5, 10, or 25 µg TCDD/kg body weight) rats, isolated 2 to 30 days post-treatment, showed decreased ouabain and α-aminoisobutyric acid uptake as well as tyrosine aminotransferase activity (Yang et al., 1983a). Treatment of rats with 25 µg 1,3,6,8-tetraCDD/kg body weight did not affect these parameters. Neither could these effects be demonstrated in primary hepatocytes from control rats that were treated with TCDD (50, 100, or 200 nmol/litre medium) in vitro for 48 h.

The induction of AHH and EROD activities of a complex PCDD/PCDF mixture from a fly ash extract has been reported (Safe et al., 1987).

7.4.9 Endocrine effects

Human exposure to TCDD has resulted in hirsutism and chloracne (Table 64), symptoms that suggest an alteration in endocrine regulation. Furthermore, chronic exposure to TCDD impaired reproduction in experimental animals, possibly by interfering with the estrous cycle (Kociba et al., 1976; Allen et al., 1977; Barsotti et al., 1979; Murray et al., 1979). The ability of TCDD to mimic natural steroids with steroid-like actions has prompted studies on the binding of TCDD to steroid hormone receptors.

Over-production of glucocorticoids mimics some of the symptoms of TCDD toxicity, e.g., involution of lymphoid tissues, oedema, and mobilization of fatty acids from adipose tissues. Thus TCDD might increase glucocorticoid activity by binding to glucocorticoid receptors. However, TCDD was unable to displace ^{3}H-dexamethasone, a potent synthetic glucocorticoid, from the normal rat cytosol glucocorticoid receptor even when present in 200-fold molar excess (Neal et al., 1979). Poland et al. (1976) demonstrated that cortisol and synthetic glucocorticoids did not bind to the TCDD receptor. An increase in the plasma level of corticosterone was found in male Sprague Dawley rats 7 and 14 days after a single oral dose of 50 µg TCDD/kg body weight (Neal et al., 1979). With the method used, a variety of fluorescent adrenocortical steroid hormone derivatives was measured. In contrast, Balk & Piper (1984), using a competitive binding radioassay for corticosterone, reported decreased blood levels (29 and 26% of controls) of corticosterone in male Sprague Dawley rats on days 14 and 21, respectively, after a single oral dose of 25 µg TCDD/kg body weight. Accumulation of 11-β-hydroxy-progesterone in the blood of TCDD-treated rats was noticed on day 14 (Balk & Piper, 1984). Neal et al. (1979) reported 100% mortality within 6 days in adrenalectomized rats given 10, 20, 40, or 80 µg TCDD/kg body weight. Adrenalectomy and hypophysectomy could not prevent liver lesions, reduced growth rate, or thymic involution in female Fisher-344 rats given a single oral dose of 10 or 20 μg TCDD/kg body weight (van Logten et al., 1980). Thymic effects of TCDD became even more severe after hypophysectomy. Daily sc injections of 0.25 mg growth hormone had a positive influence on body weight gain but did not protect against thymic involution in hypophysectomized rats.

Single oral or interperitoneal doses of TCDD between 7 and 100 μg/kg body weight decreased the serum thyroxine (T4) level in the rat (Bastomsky, 1977; Potter et al., 1983, 1986b; McKinney et al., 1985; Pazdernik & Rozman, 1985; Rozman et al., 1985b), but not in the guinea-pig, after a single oral dose of 2 μg/kg body weight (McKinney et al., 1985). The serum triiodothyronine (T3) level in TCDD-treated rats was reported to be increased (Bastomsky, 1977; Potter et al., 1986b), unaffected (Potter et al., 1983), or decreased (Pazdernik & Rozman, 1985; Rozman et al., 1985b). Increased serum thyrotropin (TSH) (Bastomsky, 1977; Potter et al., 1986b), increased thyroid ^{131}I-uptake and increased biliary excretion of T_4, but not of T_3 (Bastomsky, 1977) have been reported in TCDD-treated rats.

Rats treated with TCDD at doses up to about 30 μg TCDD/kg body weight and pair-fed controls had similar serum T_4, T_3, and TSH levels when compared to *ad libitum* fed control rats (Potter et al., 1983, 1986b). Thus, it is unlikely that hypophagia is responsible for the TCDD-induced changes in serum thyroid hormone levels. When mature TCDD-treated rats were compared to pair-fed controls, there were no functional alterations in thyroid status or thermogenesis, including increased serum levels of T_3, T_4, and TSH after acute cold challenge, increased total oxygen consumption after moderate cold exposure or decreased basal metabolic rate as compared to *ad libitum* fed control rats (Potter et al., 1986b). A significant hypothermia was, however, observed in young TCDD-exposed rats receiving 45 μg/kg body weight as a single ip dose (Potter et al., 1983).

Available data on serum T_4, T_3, and TSH levels are not sufficient to state whether TCDD-treated rats are functionally hypothyroid, euthyroid, or hyperthyroid.

In ovo exposure of white Leghorn chicken embryos to TCDD in the dose range 1 to 10 000 pmol/egg increased the cardiac release of prostaglandins (Quilley & Rifkind, 1986). Potter et al. (1983) reported decreased levels of insulin in serum and pancreas and of somatostatin in the gastric antrum of Sprague Dawley rats 7 days after a single ip dose of 45 μg TCDD/kg body weight, when compared to pair-fed control rats. The somatostatin levels in serum, liver, and pancreas were not affected, neither was the serum glucagon level.

The finding that steroids are an endogenous substrate for the hepatic MFO system (Kuntzman et al., 1965) suggests that compounds, such as TCDD, that influence the activity of this enzyme system may alter steroid metabolism _in vivo_, and consequently also the magnitude of steroid-mediated functions. As demonstrated by Gustafsson & Ingelman-Sundberg (1979), the metabolic profiles of 4-androstene-3,17-dione, 5α-androstane-3α,17β-diol and 4-pregnene-3,20-dione in hepatic microsomes from SD rats, treated with 20 μg TCDD/kg body weight for 4 consecutive days, were changed when compared to control rats 1 day post-treatment. The changes were most pronounced in female rats. When five daily doses of 1 μg TCDD/kg body weight were given to pregnant rats for 12 or 13 days during gestation, hepatic microsomes showed decreased ability to form catechol estrogens and to hydroxylate testosterone. However, this decrease did not relate to altered circulating estradiol levels (Shiverick & Muther, 1983). TCDD treatment did not affect the glucuronidation of testosterone and estrogen (Lucier et al., 1975a) or prostaglandin synthesis (Kohli & Goldstein, 1981). TCDD decreased the hepatic and uterine estrogen receptor levels in 25-day-old Long-Evans rats 2 to 10 days after treatment with single ip doses of 20 or 80 μg/kg body weight (Romkes et al., 1987). Decreased estrogen receptor levels in the liver and uterus also occurred 2 days after treatment with 1,2,7,8-tetraCDD, 1,2,3,7,8-pentaCDD, and 1,2,4,7,8-pentaCDD, but dose-response relationships were present only for TCDD and 1,2,3,7,8-pentaCDD. The estradiol-induced increases in hepatic and uterine estrogen receptor levels were counteracted by simultaneous TCDD treatment, although the effect of TCDD was not dose dependent. Hepatic hydroxylation of testosterone in 2β- and 16α-positions was not affected in male Sprague Dawley rats (190-200 g) 3 days prior to a single oral dose of 15 μg TCDD/kg body weight (Hook et al., 1975b). Somewhat younger male Wistar rats (100 g) treated with a single dose of 0.06 μmol TCDD/kg body weight exhibited increased levels of 7α-hydroxytestosterone and decreased levels of 3α-, 16α- and 16β-hydroxylated testosterone, as well as of androstenedione, in hepatic microsomes when compared to control rats (Keys et al., 1985). Decreased cytochrome P-450 content was found in guinea-pig (Tofilon, 1980) and rat (Tofilon & Piper, 1982) testes for at least one week after oral TCDD treatment of 1 μg/kg and 25 μg/kg body weight, respectively. Testicular AHH activity was induced by TCDD in mice (Mattison & Thorgeirsson, 1978), but not in rats after a single oral dose of 20 μg TCDD/kg body weight (Aitio & Parkki, 1978). Mittler et al. (1984) studied the effect of single ip doses of 0.2, 1, or 5 μg TCDD/kg body weight on testicular 16-α-testosterone hydroxylase (16-TH), 6-β-hydroxytestosterone (6-HT), and

7-α-hydroxy testosterone (7-HT) activities in young Sprague Dawley rats 90 h after exposure. Seminiferus 16-TH activity was increased from a non-detectable level to 0.07-0.14 pg/mg protein and interstitial 6-HT activity was increased 4-fold in TCDD-treated animals. The 7-HT activity was not affected by TCDD, neither in the seminiferous tubules nor in the interstitial fraction. Serum testosterone and dihydrotestosterone were depressed dose-dependently by TCDD treatment, the ED_{50}s being about 15 µg/kg body weight in male Sprague Dawley rats, when compared to pair-fed and _ad libitum_ fed controls (Moore et al., 1985). The plasma clearance and biliary excretion of ^{3}H-testosterone was not affected in Sprague Dawley rats treated with 100 µg TCDD/kg body weight before an i.v. injection of ^{3}H-testosterone, neither did castrated rats with implanted testosterone-leaking capsules respond to a dose of 15 or 100 µg TCDD/kg body weight with decreased accessory sex organ weights (Moore & Peterson, 1985). Increased AHH and _O_-deethylase activities and cytochrome P-450 content have been reported in rat prostate after single ip and oral doses, respectively, of 10 µg/TCDD/kg body weight (Haaparanta et al., 1983; Lee & Suzuki, 1980).

7.4.10 Vitamin A storage

Decreased hepatic vitamin A storage has been reported in animals exposed to various chlorinated aromatic compounds (Table 57). Compared to other chlorinated hydrocarbons for which this effect has been evaluated, TCDD is more potent in its ability to reduce the vitamin A content of the liver.

A single oral dose of 10 µg TCDD/kg body weight decreased both the total amount and the concentration of vitamin A in the liver of adult male Sprague Dawley rats (Thunberg et al., 1979). The decrease was evident 4 days after dosing and progressed with time. After 8 weeks the treated animals had a total liver vitamin A content corresponding to 33% of that of controls. Decreased dietary intake of vitamin A could not account for this difference. In a four-week study TCDD was given as a single oral dose of 0, 0.1, 1.0, or 10 µg per kg body weight to adult male Sprague Dawley rats fed _ad libitum_ with pelleted diets containing 1.2 (low), 3.0 (normal), or 6.0 (high) mg vitamin A/kg diet (Thunberg et al, 1980). Both the concentration and the total amount of vitamin A were decreased in a dose-dependent manner in the animals receiving the high vitamin A diet. In the animals on the normal and low vitamin A diets, significant differences were seen only at doses of 1.0 and 10 µg TCDD/kg body weight. A significant increase in the UDPGT activity was observed in all dietary groups treated with 1.0 and 10 µg TCDD per kg body weight, suggestive of an increased excretion

Table 57. The potency of various chlorinated cyclic hydrocarbons to reduce hepatic vitamin A content in the rat

Compound (Reference)	Strain/sex/age	Dose and route of administration	Duration of the study	% Reduction of hepatic vitamin A
Arochlor 1242 (Cecil et al., 1973)	*Rattus norvegicus*/M,F[f]/21 days	100 mg/kg in diet[a]	2 months	49
p,*p*-DDT (Cecil et al., 1973)	*Rattus norvegicus*/M,F/21 days	100 mg/kg in diet[a]	2 months	38
Methoxychlor (Davison & Cox, 1976)	Sprague Dawley/NR[f]/23 days	10 mg/kg in diet[b]	16 weeks	7
		100 mg/kg in diet		12
		1000 mg/kg in diet		37
		10 000 mg/kg in diet		68
PCB (Innami et al., 1976)	Sprague Dawley/M/21 days	100 mg/kg in diet[c]	8 weeks	82
TCDD (Thunberg et al., 1979)	Sprague Dawley/M/NR (single oral dose)	10 μg/kg bw[f]	7 days	29
			14 days	39
			28 days	59
			56 days	67

Table 57 (contd).

Compound (Reference)	Strain/sex/age	Dose and route of administration	Duration of the study	% Reduction of hepatic vitamin A
TCDD (Thunberg et al., 1980)	Sprague Dawley/M/NR	0.1 µg/kg bw[g]	28 days	2
		1.0 µg/kg bw[g]		27
		10.0 µg/kg bw[g]		65
TCDD (Hakansson, 1988)	Sprague Dawley/M/2 months	15 µg/kg bw[g]	44 days	59[d] 88[e]
		30 µg/kg bw[g]		78[d] 98[e]
		60 µg/kg bw[g]		81[d] 97[e]
		120 µg/kg bw[g]		90[d] 99[e]
Toxaphene (Thunberg et al., 1984)	Sprague Dawley/M/NR	20 mg/kg bw[h]	4 weeks	0

a 9-12 mg vitamin A/kg diet *ad libitum*.
b 33 000 IU vitamin A/kg diet *ad libitum*.
c 3000 IU vitamin A/kg diet *ad libitum*.
d 21 000 IU vitamin A/kg diet *ad libitum*.
e 8000 IU vitamin A/kg diet *ad libitum*.
f M = male; F = female; NR = not reported; bw = body weight.
g Single oral doses.
h Orally twice weekly.

of vitamin A conjugated with glucuronic acid (Thunberg & Hakansson, 1983). However, no correlation between the UDPGT activity and the reduction of hepatic vitamin A levels was seen when homozygous Gunn rats lacking inducible UDPGT were treated with a single oral dose of 20 µg/kg body weight (Aitio et al., 1979) nor in heterozygous Gunn rats with inducible UDPGT after a single oral dose of 10 µg/kg body weight (Thunberg & Hakansson, 1983).

Male Sprague Dawley rats received a single oral dose of 10 µg TCDD/kg body weight 4 days prior to the oral administration of a single physiological dose of labelled vitamin A, (11,12-^{3}H)retinylacetate (RA) (Hakansson & Ahlborg, 1985a). The distribution and elimination of the radiolabel, and the vitamin A content in various tissues were determined 1, 6, 12, 24, 72, and 192 h after the administration of ^{3}H-vitamin A. The body burden of radioactivity remained around 40% of the administered dose in control rats throughout the study, whereas in TCDD-pretreated rats the body burden decreased continuously from 21% at 12 h after administration to 11% at the end of the study. More of the radiolabel was recovered in the kidney, testes, epididymis, and serum of TCDD-treated animals than in controls, when calculated as percentage of body burden, whereas less was recovered in the liver. Forty percent of the dose was eliminated via faeces and urine in TCDD-treated rats, compared to 23% in controls. More radioactivity was eliminated in faeces than in urine both in control and TCDD-pretreated animals, although urinary elimination was more pronounced in TCDD-pretreated than in control rats. It was concluded that TCDD-treated rats handled the newly administered dose of vitamin A in a similar way to rats deficient in Vitamin A (Huque, 1981; Blomhoff et al., 1982). This finding is remarkable since the TCDD-treated animals in this study still had considerable stores of hepatic vitamin A, and did not show decreased levels of serum vitamin A, i.e., they were not deficient in vitamin A. In a similarly designed study the effect of a single oral dose of 10 µg TCDD/kg body weight on the endogenous pool of vitamin A (radiolabelled 15-^{3}H-retinol given 5 to 7 days prior to TCDD treatment) was studied in Sprague Dawley rats with stores of low liver vitamin A (Hakansson et al., 1986). It was demonstrated that endogenously stored vitamin A was rapidly depleted from the liver of TCDD-treated rats and was eliminated both in faeces and in urine. An increased distribution of the vitamin A stored in the liver to extrahepatic tissues was also seen in the treated rats.

To elucidate whether dietary vitamin A would reduce TCDD toxicity, Hakansson (1988) fed male Sprague Dawley rats _ad libitum_ from weaning throughout the experiment with diets containing 2000 (I), 5000 (II), 8000 (III), or 21 000 (IV) IU of vitamin A/kg. A single oral dose of TCDD (15, 30, 60, or 120 µg TCDD/kg body weight) was given when the rats were 8 weeks old and the animals were killed 44 days post-treatment. With diet IV, TCDD reduced in a dose-dependent manner hepatic vitamin A by 59 to 90%. With diets II and III, reduction of hepatic vitamin A was more than 95% after dosing with 15 and 30 µg TCDD/kg, respectively. In control animals fed diet I, total hepatic vitamin A was less than 1 µg and TCDD had no further effect at any dose. Serum vitamin A was dose-dependently decreased by TCDD treatment in dietary groups I, II, and III, whereas in dietary group IV TCDD increased serum vitamin A. Only with the highest TCDD dose was there a counteraction by dietary vitamin A on all of the above parameters.

A single dose of 10 µg TCDD/kg body weight to female Sprague Dawley rats on the day of delivery affected the vitamin A content in the liver and kidney of the offspring (Hakansson et al., 1987). The effect became clearly visible after weaning, i.e., when the dietary intake of vitamin A was high enough to allow for storage. At the end of the study (postnatal day 32), the vitamin A content in the liver was 225 µg in control pups and 102 µg in TCDD-exposed pups. The corresponding values for the kidney vitamin A content were 1.4 and 8.4 µg, respectively. The TCDD-induced effects on vitamin A levels in the liver and kidneys followed a similar time-course as the growth reduction, i.e., a minor effect throughout the lactation period, which became more pronounced post-weaning. This was in contrast to the liver enlargement and thymus involution in TCDD-exposed pups, which were most pronounced throughout lactation and tended to diminish post-weaning.

Single oral doses of 0, 1, 5 and 10 µg TCDD/kg body weight or a mixture of PCDDs and PCDFs, reconstituting the levels found in human milk, were given to male Sprague Dawley rats (80 g) in corn oil (Ahlborg et al., 1987). The mixture was given at three dose levels resulting in 1, 5, or 10 µg TCDD/kg body weight. Four weeks after dosing there was a dose-dependent decrease in hepatic vitamin A in TCDD-treated rats; no further effect was seen in the animals treated with PCDD/PCDF mixtures. In contrast, mixture treatment had an additive effect, as compared to TCDD alone, on the increases in renal vitamin A and hepatic cytochrome P-450 contents, AHH activity, and UDPGT activity.

Taken together these data indicate that TCDD interferes with the storage mechanism for vitamin A. In the liver this mechanism has been thoroughly investigated (Hirosawa & Yamada, 1973; Blomhoff et al., 1982; Olson & Gunning, 1983). As dietary vitamin A seems unable to counteract all toxic effects, this would imply either that the effect on vitamin A storage is secondary to TCDD toxicity or that the cellular utilization of vitamin A is affected by TCDD.

7.5 Embryotoxicity and Reproductive Effects

The teratogenic potential of TCDD was first demonstrated in rats and mice by Courtney & Moore (1971). This followed the finding that 2,4,5-trichlorophenoxyacetic acid contaminated with 30 mg TCDD/kg was teratogenic in two strains of mice and one strain of rat (Courtney et al., 1970), leading to an increased incidence of cleft palate and cystic kidney in both strains of mice and cystic kidney in rats. Further studies have revealed that TCDD is fetotoxic rather than teratogenic in the rat, producing subcutaneous oedema, haemorrhages, and slight kidney anomalies (see section 7.5.1). In contrast, TCDD produces a specific teratogenic response, consisting of cleft palate and kidney malformations, in several strains of mice (see section 7.5.2 and Table 58). Extra ribs, minor abnormalities in the palate, and cardiovascular malformations have been demonstrated in rabbits, monkeys, and chickens, respectively, after exposure to TCDD in utero (see sections 8.5.3-8.5.6). Impaired reproductive performance due to TCDD exposure has been demonstrated in rats and monkeys (see sections 8.5.1 and 8.5.4).

7.5.1 Studies on rats

The initial studies on the embryotoxic effects of TCDD in the rat were performed with Charles River CD (Courtney & Moore, 1971), Sprague Dawley (Sparschu et al., 1971), and Wistar rats (Khera & Ruddick, 1973). In these studies maternal toxicity was noted at doses > 0.5 (Sparschu et al., 1971) or 1 µg/kg body weight per day (Khera & Ruddick, 1973). Decreases in gestational survival, fetal weight, and post-natal survival were reported at dose levels in the range 0.125-0.5 µg TCDD/kg body weight per day on gestation days 6-15 or 5-14. Haemorrhages, mainly intestinal, and subcutaneous oedema were common findings at similar doses. The teratogenic findings were limited to kidney anomalies, described as unilocular cystinephrotic kidney or as hydronephrosis, in the CD rat at or above 0.5 µg TCDD/kg per day (Courtney & Moore, 1971). Slightly dilated renal pelvis was reported in the F_1 generation at the 0.01 µg/kg per day dose level in a three-generation reproductive study of TCDD in Sprague Dawley rats (Murray et al., 1979). Giavini et al. (1983) found an increased incidence of renal anomalies in Charles River CD offspring exposed to 2 µg TCDD/kg body weight on gestation days 0 to 2, but not in Sprague Dawley offspring when the dam was given daily oral doses of 0, 0.125,

0.5, and 2 μg TCDD/kg body weight for 2 weeks before mating (Giavini et al., 1982a).

Sparschu et al. (1971) found an increased number of resorption sites in Sprague Dawley rats at doses $\geq$ 0.5 μg TCDD/kg per day, but no effect on ovulation rate and preimplantation loss was reported even at 2 μg/kg per day. TCDD exposure (0.1, 0.5, or 2.0 μg/kg per day) on gestation days 0 to 2 had no effect on the reproductive performance of Sprague Dawley rats (Giavini et al., 1983). In contrast, impaired reproductive performance was found in Charles River CD rats after receiving TCDD for two weeks before mating (Giavini et al., 1982a). The number of resorption sites was elevated at doses of 0.5 μg TCDD/kg per day or more, whereas the ovulation rate and preimplantation loss was affected only at 2 μg/kg per day.

The male reproductive ability was affected by TCDD treatment only at toxic doses, as judged by studies of Khera & Ruddick (1973) and Murray et al. (1979). Nevertheless, decreased mating frequency was noted in the groups, of the F_0 generation that received 0.1 μg TCDD/kg per day in the diet (Murray et al., 1979). No effect on the mating frequency was found by Giavini et al. (1982a, 1983).

In a three-generation reproduction study, Murray et al. (1979) maintained Sprague Dawley rats on diets providing doses of 0, 0.001, 0.01, or 0.1 μg TCDD/kg body weight per day. The F_0 generation received the diet for 90 days before mating. No toxic effects were observed in the F_0 generation but decreased body weight and reduced food consumption were noted in the F_1 and F_2 generations at 0.01 μg/kg per day. Fertility was greatly reduced at 0.1 μg/kg per day in the F_0 generation. This group was discontinued because of the low number of offspring. In the F_1 and F_2 generations fertility was significantly reduced at 0.001 and 0.01 μg/kg per day, respectively. At 0.01 μg/kg per day, litter sizes were reduced, and fetal and neonatal survival were decreased as well as postnatal growth. Murray et al. (1979) concluded that doses of 0.1 and 0.01 μg/kg per day impaired reproduction in rats. A dose of 0.001 μg/kg per day had no effect on fertility, litter size, postnatal body weight, or neonatal survival and was therefore suggested to be a no-effect dose for reproductive lesions.

Reevaluation of these data by Murray et al. (1979) using another statistical model, including pooling of the data from the four generations, led to the conclusion that the 0.001 μg/kg per day dose level did affect reproduction and thus was not a no-effect level, but a low-effect level (Nisbet & Paxton, 1982). Kimbrough et al. (1984) considered that the data by Murray et al. (1979) could not be used for risk assessment calculations due to the great variation in fertility index both in controls and exposed rats.

No embryotoxic and/or reproductive effects were found when female Wistar rats were exposed to 1,2,3,4-tetraCDD (50, 100, 200, 400, or 800 µg/kg body weight per day), 2,7-diCDD (250, 500, 1000 or 2000 µg/kg body weight per day); 2,3-diCDD (1000 or 2000 µg/kg body weight per day), or 2-monoCDD (1000 or 2000 µg/kg body weight per day) on gestation days 6-15 (Khera & Ruddick, 1973). The maturation process of the lung was not affected in Sherman rats exposed to 2,7-diCDD (40 µg/kg per day on gestation days 7-15) (Kimbrough et al., 1974).

7.5.2 Studies on mice

TCDD induced embryo mortality in NMRI mice was significantly increased at doses of 4.5 and 9 µg TCDD/kg body weight per day when given on gestation days 6-15, but no embryotoxic effect was observed when daily doses of 9 µg/kg body weight were given on gestation days 9-13 (Neubert & Dillman, 1982). The number of resorptions on day 13 of gestation in NMRI mice was increased, as compared to controls, when 25 µg TCDD/kg body weight was given, divided into five daily doses on days 7-11 of gestation, but no effect was observed when the same dose was given as single ip injections on days 7 or 10 of gestation (Nau & Bass, 1981). A single ip dose of 30 µg TCDD/kg body weight on gestation day 11 had no effect on the fetal mortality in C57Bl/6 mice on days 12, 13, or 14 of gestation (Weber & Birnbaum, 1985). Decreased pre- and postnatal survival rates and retarded postnatal development were observed in NMRI mice given four oral doses of 12.5 µg TCDD/kg body weight on gestation days 14-17 (Nau et al., 1986). The cumulative mortality was 45%, 68.5%, and 75% in exposed offspring on postnatal days 1, 14, and 22, respectively, as compared to 6% in controls on day 22.

Table 58 summarizes the early studies on the teratogenic effects of TCDD in various strains of mice. These studies (Courtney & Moore, 1971; Neubert & Dillman, 1972; Courtney, 1976; Smith et al., 1976), revealed that TCDD is a specific teratogen in mice causing increased frequencies of kidney anomalies and cleft palate at doses well below those which result in fetal mortality and maternal toxicity.

The TCDD-induced kidney anomaly is morphologically described as a progressive hydronephrosis, preferentially occurring in the right kidney, and never accompanied by hydroureter or abnormal nephron development (Courtney & Moore, 1971; Moore et al., 1973; Birnbaum et al., 1985; Weber et al., 1985).

The fetal kidney seems to be more susceptible to TCDD exposure than the developing palate (Courtney & Moore, 1971; Moore et al., 1973; Birnbaum et al., 1986; Weber et al.,

Table 58. Early studies on embryotoxic effects of TCDD in mice

Strain/sex[b] (reference)	Route/vehicle/dose (µg/kg body weight day)	Treatment/ observation (days)[a]	Parental toxicity	Embryotoxic effects
CD-1/F (Courtney & Moore, 1971)	subcutaneous/ DMSO/1.0, 3.0	6-15 / 18	No effect	Increased incidence of kidney anomalies at doses ≥ 1 µg/kg per day.
BDA/2J (Courtney & Moore, 1971)	subcutaneous/ DMSO/3.0	6-15 / 17	Increased relative liver weight	Increased incidence of cleft palate and kidney anomalies.
C56BL/6J (Courtney & Moore, 1971)	subcutaneous/ DMSO/3.0	6-15 / 17	Increased relative liver weight	Increased incidence of cleft palate and kidney anomalies.
NMRI/F (Neubert & Dillman, 1972)	oral/rape seed oil/0.3, 3.0, 4.5, 9.0	6-15 / 18	None reported	Increased number of resorptions at 9 µg/kg per day. Increased incidence of cleft palate at doses ≥ 3 µg/kg per day.
C56BL/6J (Neubert & Dillman, 1972)	oral/corn oil:acetone (9:1)/1.0, 3.0	10-13 / 18	None reported	Increased incidence of cleft palate at doses ≥ 3 µg/kg per day increased incidence of kidney anomalies at doses ≥ 1 µg/kg per day.

Table 58 (contd).

CD-1/F (Courtney, 1976)	oral/corn oil:anisole (95:5)/25, 50, 100, 200, 400	7-16 / 18	Increased maternal relative liver weight at 25 and 50 µg/kg per day. Marked oedema and vaginal bleeding at doses > 200 µg/kg per day.	Increased fetal mortality at all doses. Increased incidence of kidney anomalies and cleft palate at doses ≥ 25 µg/kg per day and 50 µg/kg per day, respectively. Increased incidence of club foot was found in the high-dose group. Hydrocephalus and open eyes were seen occasionally.
CF-1 (Smith et al., 1976)	oral/corn oil:acetone (98:2)/0.001, 0.01, 0.1, 1.0, 3.0	6-15 / 18	Increased maternal relative liver weight at 3 µg/kg per day.	Increased number of resorptions at 1 µg/kg per day. Increased incidence of cleft palate at doses ≥ 1 µg/kg per day. Dilated renal pelvis occurred at 3 µg/kg per day.

[a] First day of gestation designated day zero.
[b] F = female.

1984). The incidence of kidney anomalies after a single dose of 1 μg TCDD/kg body weight on gestation day 10 in C57Bl/6 mice was 34.3%. If the same dose was divided and given on gestation days 10-13, the incidence of kidney anomalies was 58.9%. The incidences of cleft palate in the same studies were 0 and 1.9%, respectively (Moore et al., 1973). In contrast, in the CF-1 strain of mice, cleft palate was a more sensitive parameter than hydronephrosis, occurring at 1 and 3 μg TCDD/kg body weight per day on gestation days 6 to 15, respectively (Smith et al., 1976). It would appear that 3 μg TCDD/kg per day on gestation days 10-13 is close to a threshold dose for cleft palate induction in C57Bl/6 mice (Moore et al., 1973; Birnbaum et al., 1986). The maximum increase in cleft palate incidence is produced if TCDD is administered on any individual day from gestation day 8-10 in C57Bl/6 mice (Pratt et al., 1984) or on gestation day 10-11 in NMRI mice (Nau & Bass, 1981; Neubert & Dillman, 1982; Krowke, 1986). The cleft palate incidence in C57Bl/6 mice was more pronounced (36%) when TCDD was given as a single oral dose of 12 μg/kg body weight on gestation day 11 than if 3 μg/kg body weight per day was given on gestation days 10-13 (Birnbaum et al., 1985). No difference was seen in the incidence of kidney anomalies with the same treatment. TCDD is not a potent inducer of cleft palate when given on day 13 of gestation or later (Neubert & Dillman, 1982; Pratt et al., 1984). Examination of cryostat sections taken from C57Bl/6 embryos during the time of palatal elevation and fusion demonstrated that TCDD does not interfere with growth, elevation, or initial contact of the palatal shelves but does interfere with the firm adhesion and/or degeneration of the medial epithelial cells, i.e., programmed epithelial cell death does not appear to occur in the medial epithelium in embryos exposed to TCDD (Pratt et al., 1984). The cleft palates that were observed were complete clefts of the entire hard and soft palate and no clefts of the primary palate were observed (Pratt et al., 1984).

Poland & Glover (1980) reported that in nine out of ten inbred strains of mice, the susceptibility to cleft palate formation produced by TCDD (30 μg TCDD/kg body weight sc on day 10 of pregnancy) followed the distribution of the Ah locus within that strain. The five strains with a low affinity TCDD receptor in the liver (DBA/2, RI, AKR, SWR, and 129) developed cleft palate at an incidence of 0 to 3% while four of the five strains with a high affinity TCDD receptor in the liver (C57Bl/6, A, BALB/cBy, and SEC) developed cleft palate at an incidence of 54 to 95%. The only strain with a high affinity hepatic TCDD receptor that did not develop cleft palate was CBA. Mid-gestational mice embryos from C57Bl/6 exhibit high levels of the TCDD receptor in the maxillary processes and secondary palatal shelves whereas no specific binding of TCDD could be demonstrated in the AKR strain (Dencker & Pratt, 1981). Evidence that TCDD interferes in embryonic development by directly interacting with embryonic cells rather than being secondary to maternal effects was presented by D'Argy et al., (1984) in a study where mouse blastocysts were transplanted between NMRI (sensitive) and DBA (non-sensitive) dams on gestation day 3. TCDD treatment (30 µg/kg body weight) on gestation day 10 resulted in 75 to 100% incidence of cleft palate among NMRI fetuses whether they remained in their own dams or as aliens in DBA dams. Also, none of the DBA fetuses developed cleft palate whether or not they remained in their own dams or as aliens in NMRI dams.

Attempts to modify and further characterize the TCDD-induced cleft palate formation have been performed with several interacting substances. The non-teratogenic β-naphthoflavone (βN) enhanced the TCDD-induced fetal mortality and the increase in the incidence of cleft palate in C57Bl/6 and NMRI mice when βN was administered simultaneously or 8 h before TCDD, but not 24 h before or after (Hassoun & Dencker, 1982). TCDD was given as a single ip dose of 25 or 16 µg/kg body weight to C57Bl/6 and NMRI mice, respectively, on gestation days 10, 11, 12, or 13. TCDD-induced cleft palate incidence was enhanced by 2,3,4,5,3',4'-hexachlorobiphenyl, but not 2,4,5,2',4',5'-hexachlorobiphenyl, in C57Bl/6 mice, although none of the isomers alone were teratogenic at the doses used (Birnbaum et al., 1985). Neither of the hexachlorobiphenyls used affected the incidence of renal anomalies, as compared to TCDD alone.

A dose-related enhancement of the TCDD-induced incidence of cleft palate was found in C57Bl/6 mice exposed to either triiodothyronine or thyroxine, as compared to TCDD alone (Lamb et al., 1986). The hydrocortisone-induced cleft palate response was enhanced by simultaneous administration of TCDD in C57Bl/6 mice (Birnbaum et al., 1986). Co-administration of TCDD and TCDF to C57Bl/6 mice on gestation day 10 resulted in a cleft palate incidence compatible with an additive toxicity model in which TCDF contributes to the toxicity of TCDD in a weight ratio of 1:30 (Weber et al., 1985). Also 1,2,3,7,8-pentaCDD and 1,2,3,4,7,8-hexaCDD had additive effects on the TCDD-induced cleft palate incidence in NMRI mice (Krowke, 1986). No clearly dose-related teratogenic effects were observed in C57Bl/6 mice exposed to oral doses of 1,2,3,4-tetraCDD (100, 250, 500, or 1000 µg/kg per day), octaCDD (5 or 20 mg/kg per day) or to a mixture of 40% 2,7-diCDD and 60% 2,3,7-triCDD (100 or 200 µg/kg per day) on gestation days 7-16 (Courtney, 1976).

7.5.3 Studies on rabbits

New Zealand rabbits were administered TCDD by gavage in doses of 0, 0.1, 0.25, 0.5, and 1 μg/kg per day on days 6-15 of gestation and the fetuses were examined on day 28 of gestation (Giavani et al., 1982b). Above 0.25 μg/kg per day, decreased maternal weight gain and unspecified signs of maternal toxicity were reported. At doses of 0.5 and 1 μg/kg per day, there were 2/15 and 4/10 maternal deaths, respectively. An increase in abortion and resorption rates occurred at doses above 0.25 μg/kg per day, with no live fetuses detected in the 1 μg per kg per day dose group. There was a significant increase in extra ribs, compared to a level of 33.3% in the controls to 82, 66.6, and 82%. In the 0.1, 0.25, and 0.5 μg/kg per day dose groups, 82, 66.6, and 82% extra ribs were noted. There were no increases in specific soft tissue anomalies.

7.5.4 Studies on monkeys

The effect of exposure to TCDD in the diet, before mating and throughout gestation, on the reproductive performance and production of progeny of healthy, fertile rhesus monkeys (*Macaca mulatta*) was studied by Allen and co-workers (Allen et al., 1979a,b; Barsotti et al., 1979; Schantz et al., 1979). At a level of 500 ng TCDD/kg diet (11 ng/kg body weight per day), there were no effects on the length, intensity, or duration of the menstrual cycle, but decreases in serum estradiol and progesterone levels were observed (Barsotti et al., 1979). Mating with control males at the end of the sixth month resulted in three pregnancies, out of which two resulted in abortion, and three animals failed to conceive. The remaining TCDD-treated female was not bred due to toxic symptoms. The two females that survived the study were returned to a control diet and later gave birth to well developed infants. After 7 months on the 50 ng TCDD/kg diet (1.5 ng/kg body weight per day), the reproductive outcome was: four abortions, one stillbirth, two failures to conceive and two normal births (Schantz et al., 1979).

All controls conceived and gave birth to normal infants (Barsotti et al., 1979; Schantz et al., 1979).

McNulty (1984) demonstrated that rhesus monkeys (*Macaca mulatta*) receiving 1 μg TCDD/kg body weight either as a single dose on gestation days 25, 30, 35, or 40, or divided into nine doses between gestation days 20-40, failed to give birth normally. Of 16 pregnancies 13 resulted in abortions. Two of the three live fetuses, obtained by Caesarean section on day 145 of gestation, showed minor abnormalities in the palate. Maternal toxicity, manifest in 8 out of 16 females, appeared only after a period of 44-111 days after abortion. From the results obtained it was not possible to conclude whether fetal death was a direct effect of TCDD on the fetus or placenta or an indirect effect through maternal toxicity.

7.5.5 Studies on chickens

Treatment of fertile White Leghorn chicken eggs, on day 0 of development, with single doses of TCDD, ranging from 0.009 to 77.5 pmol/egg, resulted in a dose-related increase in the following types of cardiovascular malformations: ventricular septal defects, aortic arch anomalies, aortic arch anomaly plus ventricular septal defect, and conotruncal malformation (Cheung et al., 1981). The dose producing cardiovascular malformations in 50% of the embryos was about 1 pmole TCDD/egg.

A dose-dependent decrease in hatchability and increased incidences of beak, brain, and leg malformations were found in the embryos when fertile White Leghorn eggs were injected with toxic fat material containing 0.9, 1.8, or 4.5 ng of a mixture of dioxins (14% diCDDs, 1% triCDDs, 38 to 45% tetraCDDs, 13% pentaCDDs, 14% hexaCDDs, 12% heptaCDDs, 8% octaCDD) (Flick et al., 1973).

7.6 Mutagenicity and Related End-Points

7.6.1 Mutagenicity

7.6.1.1 Studies on bacteria

Results from bacterial mutagenicity tests with TCDD are conflicting.

In studies by Hussain et al. (1972) and Seiler (1973), a positive response was reported in the *Salmonella typhimurium* strain TA 1532 without metabolic activation in a plate test after preincubation of bacteria in medium containing TCDD and also in a spot test. A mutagenic response was also obtained with *Escherichia coli* Sd-4, measuring reversion to streptomycin independence (Hussain et al., 1972). OctaCDD was not mutagenic to various strains of *Salmonella typhimurium* (Seiler, 1973) without metabolic activation. More recent publications, however, do not report any mutagenic effect of TCDD in the Ames' *Salmonella* plate incorporation assay using strains TA 1530, TA 1532, TA 1535, TA 1537, TA 1538, TA 98, or TA 100 in the presence or absence of metabolic activation systems from rat and Syrian hamster liver (Gilbert et al., 1980; Geiger & Neal, 1981; Mortelmans, 1984). In these studies the earlier reported positive tester strain TA 1532 was either replaced by strain TA 1537 (Geiger & Neal, 1981; Mortelmans, 1984) or was tested in addition to TA 1537 (Gilbert et al.,

1980). Strain TA 1537 has been derived from TA 1532 and is more sensitive, due to its improved uptake of large molecules. TCDD was tested in the dose range 0.2-2000 μg/plate. Due to the limited solubility of TCDD, a maximal dose in the Salmonella system was reported to be 20 μg TCDD/plate (Geiger & Neal, 1981).

7.6.1.2 Studies on eukaryotic cells

Bronzetti et al. (1983) reported a mutagenic response of TCDD in yeast in an in vitro suspension test and a host-mediated assay. In both assays Saccharomyces cerevisiae strain D7 was used. Positive responses were obtained in vitro in the presence of metabolic activation at doses of TCDD up to 10 μg TCDD/ml, and in the host-mediated assay after treatment of mice with a single dose of TCDD (25 μg/kg body weight).

In L5178Y mouse lymphoma cells, TCDD induced mutations in a dose-dependent manner at doses of 0.05-0.5 μg TCDD/ml; survival of cells at the highest concentration was at least 75% (Rogers et al., 1982).

7.6.1.3 In vivo studies

A dominant lethal test on male Wistar rats has been reported by Khera & Ruddick (1973). The rats were given 4, 8, or 12 μg TCDD/kg body weight per day orally for seven consecutive days, after which seven sequential mating trials, 5 days at a time, were conducted in the surviving males. Nine days after separation of females from the males, the females were killed. The highest dose was lethal for all males exposed (20/20); 8 μg/kg per day killed 11/20 males, and 4 μg/kg per day was lethal for 2/20. All animals in the control group survived.

The results did not indicate a dominant lethal effect during the 35 days post-treatment period, corresponding to the postmeiotic stages of spermatogenesis.

7.6.2 Interaction with nucleic acids

Poland & Glover (1979) found that very little TCDD bound to rat liver nucleic acids after treatment with ^{3}H-TCDD in vivo; the maximum covalently bound TCDD was calculated to be 6 and 12 pmol per mol of nucleotide residues from DNA and RNA, respectively. After iv injection of ^{3}H-TCDD in rats, the radioactivity taken up by the liver cytosol decreased at the same rate as the radioactivity in the nuclear fraction increased. The radioactivity in the nuclei was at a maximum 2 h after injection (Carlstedt-Duke et al., 1982). Guenthner et al. (1979) demonstrated *in vitro* metabolism of TCDD to reactive intermediates that bound covalently to cellular macromolecules, principally to proteins. However, no isomer-specific methods were used for analysis of metabolites in this study.

Liver slices from Sprague Dawley rats treated with 5 µg TCDD incorporated twice the level of thymidine into nuclear DNA 10 days post-treatment than did controls (Conaway & Matsumura, 1975). Christian & Peterson (1983a) found no effect on the *in vivo* incorporation of thymidine into liver DNA 35 to 36 h after the administration of 10 µg TCDD/kg body weight to Sprague Dawley rats. DNA synthesis in Porton rats, stimulated by 70% hepatectomy and measured as the 1 h *in vivo* incorporation of thymidine, was not affected by treatment with 10 or 200 µg TCDD/kg body weight 0, 24, or 72 h before the hepatectomy was performed (Greig et al., 1974). In contrast, Dickins et al. (1981) found an 8- to 10-fold increase in DNA synthesis in response to the proliferation caused by a 1/3 hepatectomy in Sprague Dawley rats given 5 µg TCDD/kg body weight 5 days prior to the hepatectomy. In this study thymidine incorporation into DNA was measured *in vitro* at various times after hepatectomy. The TCDD-induced increase was most pronounced 24 to 32 h after the hepatectomy. The somewhat conflicting results may be due to differences in the *in vivo* and *in vitro* incorporation of thymidine, as well as to differences in the time points studied. According to Dickins et al. (1981), the discrepancy in proliferative DNA synthesis could be due to the degree of hepatectomy. Thus 70% hepatectomy would by itself enhance DNA synthesis to near maximum level, making it difficult to measure any effect of TCDD under the experimental conditions. This suggestion was confirmed by Christian & Peterson (1983a), who compared the effect of TCDD on proliferative DNA synthesis after 1/3 and 2/3 hepatectomy. This study also revealed that the effect could be seen only when a certain amount of time, namely 5 to 10 days, elapsed between TCDD administration and hepatectomy.

The transfectivity of bacteriophage Qβ/RNA was evaluated after treatment *in vitro* with TCDD. No effect was noticed in the tested dose range (0.2-4 µg TCDD/ml) (Kondorosi et al., 1973).

The effect of TCDD on the repair of DNA damage induced by 2-aminofluorene (AF) and 2-acetylaminofluorene (AAF) in primary hepatocytes from B6 and D2 mice has been investigated (Moller et al., 1984). Pretreatment *in vivo* with TCDD (50 µmol/litre) resulted in a slight increase in DNA damage (measured by the alkaline elution technique) following incubation with either AF or AAF for 60 min, suggesting induction of aromatic amine activating enzymes.

7.6.3 Cytogenetic effects

Green & Mooreland (1975) and Loprieno et al. (1982a) did not observe any induction of chromosomal aberrations in rats administered TCDD intraperitoneally or by gavage (5 to 20 μg/kg body weight). Later Green et al. (1977) showed a significant increase in the induction of chromosomal abnormalities in bone marrow cells of male rats at doses of 2 and 4 μg TCDD/kg body weight and in females at 4 μg/kg body weight. In a study by Meyne et al. (1985) C57Bl/6 or DBA/2 mice (with high- and low-affinity TCDD receptors, respectively) were ip injected at doses 0, 50, 100, and 150 μg/kg body weight. There was no increase in the frequency of chromosomal aberrations in bone marrow cells of the TCDD-treated mice of either strain 8, 16, or 24 h after treatment. All doses were high enough to induce hepatotoxic damage in C57Bl/6 mice. In male and female CD-1 mice, however, a weak but significant increase in chromosomal aberrations was obtained 96 h post-treatment (ip 10 μg TCDD/kg body weight) (Loprieno et al., 1982b).

Lamb et al. (1981) evaluated the frequency of sister chromatid exchange (SCE) in bone marrow cells of C57Bl/6 mice given single ip injections of mixtures of chlorinated phenoxy acids that contained 0.16, 1.2, or 2.4 μg TCDD/kg body weight. The mean SCE frequency in treated and in control mice did not differ significantly. Mice fed diets containing the same daily doses as above for 4 to 8 weeks did not show any increase in SCE frequencies.

At doses (50, 100, and 150 μg per kg body weight) hepatotoxic to C57Bl/6 mice, there was no significant increase of SCEs in C57Bl/6 or DBA/2 mice 18 h after ip injection of TCDD (Meyne et al., 1985). Meyne et al. (1985) also performed a micronucleus test under the same conditions as above. Mice, killed 24 or 48 h after treatment, did not show any increase of micronuclei in polychromatic erythrocytes of bone marrow in either strain.

7.6.4 Cell transformation

Single treatments (11 concentrations in the range 0 to 5 μmol/litre) of mouse embryo fibroblast (C3H/10T1/2) tissue cultures with TCDD did not transform or initiate the process of transformation in cultures subsequently exposed to 12-*O*-tetradecanoylphorbol-13-acetate (Abernethy et al., 1985). Continued treatment of these cells with low concentrations (≥ 4 pmol/litre) of TCDD enhanced the production of foci in cultures pretreated with *N*-methyl-*N*'-nitro-*N*-nitrosoguanidine. Maximal enhancement occurred at 40 pmol/litre. Higher doses, 120 to 4000 pmol/litre, did not further increase the incidence of foci production. Promotion of transformation is thus the predominant effect of TCDD in the C3H/10T1/2 cell-transformation system.

7.7 Carcinogenicity

7.7.1 Long-term animal studies on single compounds

Several studies on the carcinogenicity of TCDD and related compounds have been performed.

The data from studies using oral exposure are summarized in Table 59. Van Miller et al. (1977) exposed male Sprague Dawley rats to various dietary levels of TCDD ranging from 0.001 μg/kg and 1 μg/kg to 1 mg/kg for 78 weeks. Pronounced mortality was observed at higher doses. Neoplastic changes in different organs were noted in a number of rats that died. At 95 weeks, the small number of surviving animals were killed. At dietary levels of 5, 50, and 500 ppt TCDD (ng/kg feed), a variety of tumours were noted, but no particular trend emerged. However, at a level of 5 μg/kg feed, four squamous cell tumours of the lung, four neoplastic nodules (hyperplastic nodules), and two cholangiocarcinomas of the liver were found in seven rats.

Kociba et al. (1978) fed groups of 50 male and female Sprague Dawley rats 0.1, 0.01, and 0.001 μg TCDD/kg body weight for 2 years. 86 male and 86 female control rats received the vehicle only. The doses corresponded to 2193, 208, and 22 ng TCDD/kg diet. A variety of tumours were found in the control and experimental groups. Tumours caused by the ingestion of TCDD were confined to the liver, lungs, hard palate/nasal turbinates, and tongue. In the female rats that had received doses of 0.1 and 0.01 μg/kg body weight, a statistically significant increase of neoplastic nodules (hyperplastic nodules, hepatomas) of the liver was noted, and in the rats that had received 0.1 μg TCDD/kg body weight there was a statistically significant increase of hepatocellular carcinomas. Epithelial tumours along the respiratory tract, tongue, and hard palate consisted of well differentiated squamous cell carcinomas. There was an increased incidence, compared with the controls, of squamous cell carcinomas of the hard palate and nasal turbinate in both male and female rats receiving 0.1 μg TCDD/kg body weight, while the incidence of squamous cell carcinoma of the lungs at this dose showed an increase only in the females. The authors also noted a decreased incidence of tumours of the pituitary gland, uterus, mammary glands, pancreas, and adrenal glands in the treated groups, possibly secondary to an effect on the hormonal functions of different glands. This decrease was in some instances statistically significant.

Table 59. Carcinogenicity bioassays of PCDDs after oral administration

Compound (Reference)	Exposure: route, dose, frequency and duration-treatment/test	Species/strain/sex	Tumour type and incidence
2,3,7,8-TCDD (Van Miller et al., 1977)	Oral (diet), 0.0, 0.001, 0.005, 0.05, 0.5, 1.0, 5.0 µg/kg. 78/95 weeks	Rat/Sprague Dawley/M	all tumours: 0/10 at 0.0, 0/10 at 0.001, 5/10 at 0.005, 3/10 at 0.05, 4/10 at 0.5, 4/10 at 1.0, and 7/10 at 5.0 µg/kg
2,3,7,8-TCDD (Kociba et al., 1978)	Oral (diet), 0.0, 0.001, 0.01, 0.1 µg/kg body weight per day. 105/105 weeks	Rat/Sprague Dawley/M	squamous cell carcinoma hard palate: 4/50 at 0.1 µg/kg per day; squamous cell carcinoma tongue: 1/50 at 0.001 and 0.01, 3/50 at 0.1 µg/kg per day; adenoma of adrenal cortex: 2/5 at 0.01 and 5/50 at 0.1 µg/kg per day
		Rat/Sprague Dawley/F	hepatocellular carcinoma: 0/86 at 0.0, 0/50 at 0.001, 2/50 at 0.01, and 11/49 at 0.1 µg/kg per day; squamous cell carcinoma of tongue: 1/50 at 0.01 and 4/49 at 0.1 µg/kg per day, squamous cell carcinoma of lung: 7/49 at 0.1 µg/kg per day.
2,3,7,8-TCDD (NIH, 1982a)	Oral (gavage corn oil:acetone, 9:1), 0.0, 0.1, 0.05, 0.5 µg/kg body weight per week. 104/105-107 weeks	Rats/Osborne-Mendel/M	follicular cell adenomas or carcinoma of thyroid: 1/69 at 0.0, 5/48 at 0.10, 8/50 at 0.05, and 11/50 at 0.5 µg/kg per week

Table 59 (contd - 2).

		Rats/Osborne-Mendel/F	follicular cell adenomas or carcinoma of thyroid: 3/73 at 0.0, 2/45 at 0.1, 1/49 at 0.05, and 6/47 at 0.5 µg/kg per week; neoplastic nodules or hepatocellular carcinoma: 5/75 at 0.0, 1/49 at 0.1, 3/50 at 0.05, and 14/49 at 0.5 µg/kg per week
2,3,7,8-TCDD (NIH, 1982a)	Oral (gavage corn oil:acetone, 9:1), Males 0.0, 0.01, 0.05, 0.5 µg/kg body weight per week. Females 0.0, 0.04, 0.2, 2.0 µg/kg body weight per week, 104/105 weeks	Mice/B6C3F$_1$8/M	hepatocellular carcinoma: 8/73 at 0.0, 9/49 at 0.01, 8/49 at 0.05, and 17/50 at 0.5 µg/kg per week
		Mice/B6C3F$_1$8/F	hepatocellular carcinoma: 1/73 at 0.0, 2/50 at 0.04, 2/48 at 0.2, and 6/47 at 2.0 µg/kg per week; follicular cell adenomas of thyroid: 0/69 at 0.0, 3/50 at 0.04, 1/47 at 0.2, and 5/46 at 2.0 µg/kg per week
1,2,3,6,7,8/ 1,2,3,7,8,9-hexaCDD (1:2) (NIH, 1980b)	Oral (gavage corn oil:acetone, 9:1), 0.0, 1.25, 2.5, 5.0 µg/kg body weight per week, 104/105 weeks	Rats/Osborne-Mendel/M	liver neoplastic nodules or hepatocellular carcinoma: 0/74 at 0.0, 0/49 at 1.25, 1/50 at 2.5, and 4/48 at 5.0 µg/kg per week
		Rats/Osborne-Mendel/F	liver neoplastic nodules or hepatocellular carcinoma: 5/75 at 0.0, 10/50 at 1.25, 12/50 at 2.5, and 30/50 at 5.0 µg/kg per week
1,2,3,6,7,8-/ 1,2,3,7,8,9-hexaCDD (1.2) (NIH, 1980b)	Oral (gavage corn oil:acetone, 9:1), Males 0.0, 1.25, 2.5, 5.0 µg/kg body weight per week Females 0.0, 2.5, 5.0, 10.0 µg/kg body weight per week, 104/105-108 weeks	Mice(B6C3F$_1$)/M	hepatocellular adenomas or carcinomas: 15/73 at 0.0, 14/50 at 1.25, 14.49 at 2.5, and 24/48 at 5.0 µg/kg per week
		Mice(B6C3F$_1$)/F	hepatocellular adenomas or carcinomas: 3/73 at 0.0, 4/48 at 2.5, 6.47 at 5.0, and 10/47 at 10.0 µg/kg per week

Table 59 (contd - 3).

Compound (Reference)	Exposure: route, dose, frequency and duration-treatment/test	Species/strain/sex	Tumour type and incidence
Dibenzo-*p*-dioxin (NCI, 1977)	Oral (diet), 0, 5000, 10 000 mg/kg diet, 87-90/91-97 weeks	Mice/B6C3F_1/M	hepatocellular carcinoma: 4/49 at 0, 7/50 at 5000, and 3/48 at 10 000 mg/kg diet; hepatocellular adenomas: 4/49 at 0, 1/50 at 5000, and 2/48 at 10,000 mg/kg diet; malignant tumours: 5/49 at 0, 11/50 at 5000, and 8/50 at 10 000 mg/kg diet
		Mice/B6C3F_1/F	malignant tumours: 8/50 at 0, 9/49 at 5000, and 3/39 at 10,000 mg/kg diet; hepatocellular carcinoma: 1/47 at 5000 mg/kg diet
2,7-diCDD (NCI, 1979)	Oral (diet), 0, 5000, 10 000 mg/kg diet, 110/110-117 weeks.	Rats/Osborne-Mendel/M	malignant tumours: 5/33 at 0, 7/34 at 5000, and 4/33 at 10 000 mg/kg diet; hepatocellular adenoma: 1/33 at 0; hepatocellular carcinoma: 1/33 at 10,000 mg/kg diet
		Rats/Osborne-Mendel/F	malignant tumours: 5/31 at 0; 4/33 at 5000, and 5/30 at 10 000 mg/kg diet

Two further studies on the carcinogenicity of TCDD are available (NIH, 1982a; NIH, 1982b). The TCDD used in these studies was reported to be 99.4% pure, based on gas chromatographic analysis.

In two gavage studies both Osborne-Mendel rats and B6C3F1 mice were used (NIH, 1982a). All animals were about 6 weeks old. Dosages, duration, and outcome are summarized in Table 59. The statistical analysis performed was similar to that in the dermal study (NIH, 1982b). Mean body weights of the high-dose groups of rats were lower than those of the corresponding controls after week 55 and 45 for males and females, respectively, but no other clinical signs were observed. No such dose-related depression in mean body weight gain was observed in mice when compared to the vehicle-control groups.

In the male rats, increased incidences of follicular cell adenomas or carcinomas in the thyroid were dose related and were significantly higher ($P < 0.001$) in the high-dose group than in the vehicle controls (1%, 10%, 16%, and 22%). In the female rats, an increase (though not statistically significant) was seen only in the high-dose group (4%, 4%, 2%, and 13%). The incidence of neoplastic nodules of the liver in the high-dose group of female rats was significantly ($P < 0.006$) higher than that in the vehicle-control group (7%, 2%, 6%, and 28%).

In male and female mice, incidences of hepatocellular carcinomas were dose related and, in the high-dose groups, were significantly ($P < 0.002$ and 0.014, respectively) higher than those in the corresponding vehicle-control groups (males: 11%, 18%, 16%, and 34%; females: 1%, 4%, 4%, and 13%).

Follicular cell adenomas in the thyroid occurred at dose-related incidences in female mice, and were significantly ($P < 0.009$) higher in the high-dose groups than those in the vehicle controls (0%, 6%, 2%, and 11%). In conclusion, under the conditions of this bioassay, TCDD was carcinogenic for Osborne-Mendel rats, inducing follicular cell thyroid adenomas in males and neoplastic nodules of the liver in females. TCDD was also carcinogenic for B6C3F1 mice, inducing hepatocellular carcinomas in males and females and follicular cell thyroid adenomas in females.

Toth et al. (1979) administered TCDD orally by gavage to groups of 45 male Swiss/H/Riop mice at doses of 0, 0.007, 0.7, and 7 µg/kg body weight once a week for one year, and the animals were followed for their lifetime. Liver tumours were found at 18%, 29%, 48%, and 30%, respectively. The tumour incidence at 0.7 µg/kg was significantly higher when compared to controls ($P < 0.01$), while the increase at the highest dose level (7 µg/kg) was not statistically significant ($P = 0.11$). The latter finding may be due to a much reduced average survival in comparison with the control group (average life span 424 and 588 days, respectively).

In a study using dermal application of TCDD (NIH, 1982b), male and female Swiss-Webster mice were about 6 weeks old at the beginning of the bioassay. The one-tailed Fisher exact test was used to compare the tumour incidence of a control group with that of a group of dosed animals. Mean body weights of dosed animals were essentially the same as those of the corresponding vehicle-control groups, but less than those of the untreated controls, for males throughout the study and for females during the first 80 weeks. The incidence of fibrosarcoma in the integumentary system of female mice treated with TCDD or TCDD and dimethylbenzathraline (DMBA) was significantly higher than that of the controls ($P < 0.007$ and $P < 0.010$, respectively). An increase in the same tumour type, although not statistically significant ($P = 0.084$), was also observed in the male mice (7% and 21% for the control and TCDD-treated groups, respectively). In conclusion, under the conditions of this bioassay, TCDD was carcinogenic for female Swiss-Webster mice, causing fibrosarcomas in the integumentary system. However, the study has been criticized in several areas, namely, a maximal tolerated dose (MTD) was not achieved, especially in male mice, only one dose per sex was used, and the number of mice (30) in the TCDD-exposed groups was considered less than optimal.

7.7.2 Long-term animal studies with mixed compounds

Toth et al. (1979) studied groups of 100 male and 100 female, 10-week-old random-bred Swiss H/Riop mice that were given weekly oral doses of 2,4,5-trichlorophenoxyethanol (TCPE) at 67-70 mg/kg body weight, together with 0.112 µg TCDD/kg body weight or 0.007 µg TCDD/kg body weight in 0.5% carboxymethyl cellulose by gastric intubation for 12 months. The incidences of liver tumours in males after 2 years were reported to be 48% and 58% in the two treated groups, compared with 26-33% in the untreated male mice of the colony that survived up to 3 years. Three additional groups of mice were given 7 mg TCPE/kg body weight with 0.0007 µg TCDD/kg body weight, 0.7 mg TCPE/kg body weight with 0.00007 µg TCDD/kg body weight, or 7 mg TCPE/kg body weight with 0.7 µg TCDD/kg body weight. There was no increased incidence of liver tumours in any of the treatment groups.

A 1:2 mixture of 1,2,3,6,7,8- and 1,2,3,7,8,9-hexachlorodibenzo-p-dioxins (HxCDDs) has been tested for carcinogenicity by dermal application to mice and by gavage in rats and mice (NIH, 1980a,). The following impurities were detected in the mixture: pentaCDD 0.04%, TCDD 0.09%, triCDD 0.004%, and bromopentaCDD < 0.004%. The specific isomers of these impurities were not identified. The doses used and duration of the gavage studies (NIH, 1980b) are given in Table 59. In both species and either sex, only tumours of the liver occurred at a significantly greater incidence than controls. In male rats and male and female mice, the liver tumour incidence was significantly increased over control values only in the high dose groups (5 µg/kg per week), while in female rats the incidence was significantly greater at both medium- and high-dose levels (2.5-5 µg/kg per week). In the dermal study, no treatment-related tumours were recorded in either the carcinogenicity bioassay or the tumour promotion assay using DMBA as an initiator (NIH, 1980a). It was concluded that the mixture of hexaCDDs tested was carcinogenic to rats and mice following administration by gavage. However, there was no tumorigenic activity when hexaCDD was applied to mouse skin.

When added to the diet in concentrations up to 10 000 mg/kg, 2,7 dichlorodibenzo-*p*-dioxin and dibenzo-*p*-dioxin were found to be non-carcinogenic in chronic feeding studies in mice and rats of either sex (NCI, 1977; NCI, 1979).

7.7.3 Short-term and interaction studies

Poland & Glover (1979) estimated the maximum covalent binding of TCDD *in vivo* to rat liver protein, ribosomal RNA (rRNA), and DNA after ^{3}H-TCDD (39 Ci/mmol) was administered to immature male and female Sprague Dawley rats (105-135 g) as a single ip injection of 7.5 µg/kg. The rats were killed 12 h, 24 h, 48 h, or 7 days after dosing with TCDD. The level of radioactivity in the liver varied from 18 to 64% of the administered dose, and only a small fraction was associated with the purified macromolecular fractions. The radioactivity associated with rRNA and DNA was very low and essentially all the unextracted radioactivity was associated with protein (0.03 to 0.1% of the total radioactivity in the liver). The maximum amount of ^{3}H-TCDD that could have been covalently bound to DNA was estimated as 1.8×10^{-17} mol TCDD per mg DNA, or 6.2 nmol TCDD per mol DNA nucleotide, which means binding of about 1 molecule TCDD to the DNA in 35 cells. Phenobarbital treatment, or prior administration of TCDD did not significantly alter the amount of unextractable ^{3}H-TCDD associated with any macromolecular fraction. Similarly, there were no differences in the levels of ^{3}H-TCDD associated with protein, rRNA, or DNA in male or female rats pretreated with TCDD.

TCDD was found to be a carcinogen in chronic feeding studies in rats and mice. Most carcinogens bind covalently, either directly or after a conversion to electrophilic intermediates, to protein, rRNA, and DNA to the extent of 10^{-4} to 10^{-6} mol of carcinogen per mol of amino acid or nucleotide residue. The maximum binding of TCDD is 4-6 orders of magnitude lower than that of most chemical carcinogens and is of questionable biological significance. The results obtained in the study of Poland & Glover (1979) thus indicate that it is unlikely that the mechanism of TCDD-induced carcinogenesis would include the covalent binding of TCDD.

In female Charles River CD-1 mice, TCDD was found to be a weak initiator when given alone in a single dose of 2 μg/mouse by dermal application (Di Giovanni et al., 1977). In these studies 12-O-tetradecanoylphorbol-13-acetate (TPA) was used as a promoter. When TCDD and 7,12-dimethylbenzanthracene were given together, a slight additive effect was found. As mentioned earlier, in a study on a hexaCDD mixture, no treatment-related tumours were found in a tumour promotion test on mice using DMBA as an initiator (NIH, 1980a).

The possible role of TCDD as a promoter in diethylnitrosamine-induced hepatocarcinogenesis was studied by Pitot et al. (1980) in female Charles River rats (200-250 g). A single oral dose (10 mg/kg) of diethylnitrosamine (DEN) was given 24 h after a 70% hepatectomy, and treatment with TCDD (0.14 or 1.4 μg/kg sc once every 2 weeks for 7 months) was started one week after the hepatectomy. The promoting effect of TCDD in this 2-stage model of liver cancer was also compared with the effect of a known promoting agent, phenobarbital (0.05% in the diet for 7 months). Enzyme-altered foci, which are thought to be precursors of hepatocellular carcinomas, were greatly increased in number, total volume, and phenotypic heterogeneity by the administration of TCDD. A significant incidence of hepatocellular carcinomas (5 out of 7) was observed in the DEN-treated rats that were given the high dose of TCDD, but no carcinomas were seen in the rats treated with DEN only (0 out of 4). The results indicated that TCDD was a potent promoting agent for hepatocarcinogenesis, and the authors suggested that all the tumours associated with the chronic administration of TCDD arise from its promoting activity of cells previously initiated by exposure to carcinogens in the environment.

Studies utilizing a two-stage system of mouse skin tumorigenesis (Berry et al., 1979), which allows separate evaluation of the initiation and promotion phases of carcinogenesis, have demonstrated that TCDD does not promote the development of skin tumours at a dose of 0.1 μg given twice weekly, whereas in the animals pretreated with 1.0 μg TCDD for 1, 3, or 5 days prior to initiation with DMBA, TCDD was shown to act as a potent inhibitor of PAH-induced skin tumour initiation. Almost complete inhibition (96%) was achieved with a single non-toxic topical dose of 0.1 μg, and 3 days pretreatment with 0.01 μg TCDD gave over 80% inhibition. The authors suggested that this potent anticarcinogenic effect of TCDD may be related to its ability to induce epidermal enzyme pathways involved in detoxifying PAH carcinogens in the skin. According to Kimbrough (1979), TCDD and other compounds of this type, which are potent enzyme inducers, may prevent or enhance the tumour-inducing ability of other chemicals by enhancing the metabolism of these xenobiotics.

Poland et al. (1982) studied the promoting effects of TCDD in the mouse skin two-stage tumorigenesis model. The effects of TCDD and TPA were compared in DMBA-initiated HRS/S mice that were either heterozygous or homozygous for the recessive "hairless" trait. TCDD was found to have a tumour-promoting effect only in the homozygous mice. The data suggested to the authors that TCDD might act as a promoter by a mechanism different from that of TPA.

The interaction of TCDD with 3-methylcholanthrene (3-MC) was studied by Kouri et al. (1978), who found that TCDD was a co-carcinogen with 3-MC when administered by subcutaneous injection. Both sexes of two inbred strains of mice (C57B1/6C and DBA/2), responsive and non-responsive to the induction of AHH by 3-MC, respectively, were used. TCDD at a concentration of 1 or 100 μg/kg body weight was administered as a single dose alone or in combination with 3-MC (150 μg/kg). The duration of the study was 36 weeks. The number of animals in each group at the start of the experiment was not stated, but seems to have been between 30 and 100. No subcutaneous tumours were observed in controls or in mice treated with TCDD alone. In responsive mice no enhancement occurred, while in non-responsive mice the simultaneous administration of TCDD and 3-MC enhanced the carcinogenic response of TCDD at 100 μg/kg. At 1 μg TCDD/kg, a reduction in latency time to tumour was noted.

An anticarcinogenic effect of TCDD has been reported by Cohen et al. (1979) and by Di Giovanni et al. (1979a). When TCDD was topically applied to Sencar or CD-1 mice 72 h prior to the administration of either DMBA (10 nmol) or benzo(a)-pyrene (BP) (100 nmol), it markedly decreased the skin tumour initiation by both DMBA and BP. This inhibition of tumorigenesis correlated with the decreased <u>in vivo</u> binding of DMBA to DNA after TCDD administration, but not with the total binding of BP to DNA. However, the hydrocarbon-deoxyribonucleoside adducts from the DNA of TCDD-pretreated mice showed a striking absence of BP-7,8-dihyrodiol-9,10-epoxide adduct bound to guanine. It is suggested, accordingly, that the formation of this adduct may be a critical step in BP-induced skin carcinogenesis in mice. In further studies of the tumour-inhibitory effect of TCDD (Di Giovanni et al. 1980), it was demonstrated that exposure of CD-1 mice to TCDD 3 days before initiation with BP or 3-MC resulted in a decreased tumour yield, compared to acetone-pretreated animals, while treatment with TCDD 5 min before and 1 day after initiation failed to affect the tumour yield. However, when TCDD was administered 3 days or 5 min before or 1 day after initiation with BP-diol epoxide, there was a decreased tumour yield in all cases. The authors concluded that the ability of TCDD to inhibit tumour yield when administered after the BP-diol epoxide, indicated the possible existence of more than one mechanism involved in the anticarcinogenic effect of TCDD.

7.8 Mechanisms of Action

The toxicity of TCDD apparently depends on the fact that the four lateral positions of the molecule are occupied by chlorine (see section 7.8.1) Toxicity decreases with decreasing lateral substitution and increasing total chlorine substitution. As has been outlined in sections 7.1-7.7, TCDD toxicity involves many different types of symptoms and these symptoms vary from species to species and from tissue to tissue, both quantitatively and qualitatively. Furthermore, age- and sex-related differences in sensitivity to TCDD have been reported. Characteristic for TCDD toxicity is also the delay in expression of toxicity, from 2 weeks to 2 months, seen in all species. It has been suggested that the initial event in TCDD-induced toxicity is the binding of TCDD to the so-called Ah receptor. This complex, whether of cytosolic or nuclear origin, exerts its action in the nucleus by triggering a pleiotropic response including the induction of mixed function oxidases. Present knowledge, however, rules out enzyme induction *per se* as being the cause of toxicity and death (see section 7.8.1). Although the toxicokinetics of TCDD vary between species, these differences are not sufficient to explain the variabilities in sensitivity to TCDD toxicity (see section 7.8.2). Available data indicate an involvement of TCDD in processes regulating cellular differentiation and/or division. Alterations in the regulation of such processes, which are not equally active in all cells throughout the organism, would be expected to result in effects that vary among tissues as well as among species (see section 7.8.3).

7.8.1 Receptor-mediated effects

The binding of TCDD to the Ah receptor has been postulated to be the necessary first step in the induction of cytochrome P-450 synthesis and of related enzyme activities, as well as in the mechanism of toxicity (Poland et al., 1976; Okey et al., 1979; Poland & Glover, 1979; Poland & Knutson, 1982). So far, no conclusive data exist for the direct involvement of the Ah receptor in the TCDD-induced toxicity.

Knowledge of the mechanism involved in the Ah locus enzyme-induction response has grown rapidly since the initial findings that binding of TCDD to the receptor resulted in increased levels of cytochrome P-450 mRNA in genetic variants of mice (Tukey et al., 1982) and mouse hepatoma cell lines (Israel & Whitlock, 1983). These findings have been confirmed and further expanded in studies using mice genetics and recombinant DNA techniques (Tukey et al., 1982; Miller et al., 1983; Gonzales et al., 1984; Israel & Whitlock, 1984; Jones et al., 1984, 1985, 1986; Okino et al., 1985; Tuteja et al., 1985; Kimura et al., 1986), thus providing more data to the understanding of the mechanism for the Ah locus enzyme induction.

In early experiments (Poland et al., 1976; Carlstedt-Duke, 1979; Okey et al., 1979), Ah receptors appeared to be localized in the cytosol when in its unoccupied state and was translocated into nuclei only when occupied by a ligand (Greenlee & Poland, 1979; Okey et al, 1980; Poellinger et al., 1982; Gasiewicz & Rucci, 1984). However, Whitlock & Galeazzi (1984) concluded that unoccupied Ah receptor in the intact cell was primarily located in the nucleus and that apparent cytosolic Ah receptor was a redistribution artifact. Following the distribution of Ah receptor and three cytosolic marker enzymes between the nuclear and cytosolic fractions during fractionation (Denison et al., 1986a,c), it was again concluded that unoccupied Ah receptor is primarily cytosolic or that this receptor protein is in equilibrium between the cytoplasm and nucleus.

However, it is generally agreed that the ultimate biological regulation by the Ah receptor is due to specific interaction of ligand-receptor complexes with chromatin sites (Greenlee & Poland, 1979; Okey et al., 1979, 1980; Mason and Okey, 1982; Poellinger et al., 1982; Poland and Knutson, 1982; Tukey et al., 1982a; Gonzales et al., 1984; Israel & Whitlock, 1984).

Several investigators have estimated the molecular size and other physicochemical properties for the cytosolic hepatic Ah receptor (Okey et al., 1979, 1980, 1982; Tukey et al., 1982b; Poellinger et al., 1983; Gasiewicz et al., 1983a,b; Denison et al., 1986a; Hannah et al., 1986). To obtain reliable results in the isolation and characterization of the Ah receptor, it is necessary to use perfused liver, in order to reduce the contribution from blood proteins, and to use a radioactive ligand of high purity and specific activity quality (Poellinger et al., 1983; Denison et al., 1986a). Furthermore, the ionic strength of the medium during isolation has a marked effect upon the apparent molecular weight of the receptor (Denison et al., 1986a). The physicochemical data for the Ah receptor presented in Table 60 were obtained from two studies (Denison et al., 1986a,c; Poellinger et al., 1983) in which the receptor was isolated from perfused liver of Sprague Dawley rats under conditions of high ionic strength.

Table 60. Physicochemical data for the hepatic Ah receptor in Sprague Dawley rats

Physicochemical data	Denison et al. (1986a)	Poellinger et al. (1983)
Stokes radius (nm)	5.2 ± 0.2	6.1 ± 0.2
Sedimentation coefficient (S)	5.6 ± 0.6	4.4
Relative molecular mass	121 000	111 000

The receptor protein has been found also in extrahepatic tissues (Carlstedt-Duke, 1979; Carlstedt-Duke et al., 1979, 1981; Johansson et al., 1982; Mason & Okey, 1982; Gasiewicz & Rucci, 1984; Gasiewicz et al., 1984; Furuhashi et al., 1986; Kurl et al., 1985; Söderkvist et al., 1986). Different mammalian species possess Ah receptors with similar, though not identical, properties (Gasiewicz & Rucci, 1984; Denison et al., 1986a, b; Kurl et al., 1985). Jaiswal et al. (1985a, b) have shown species differences in the TCDD-inducible P-450 gene subfamily. Humans appear to only have the P_1-450. The function of human P_1-450 may be equivalent to a combination of P_1-450 and P_3-450 in the mouse. A complete lack of measurable cytosolic and almost total absence of inducer-receptor complexes in the nucleus of human MCF-1 cells (cells derived from an adenocarcinoma of the breast) were reported. This absence was out of proportion to the ability of TCDD to induce AHH and acetamide-4-hydroxylase activities in these cells. Further studies in different cell lines are thus needed to characterize the level of receptor in humans. The only non-mammalian species demonstrated to have significant Ah receptor is the chick embryo (Denison et al., 1986b). However, no detectable level of the receptor was found in 2-week-old White Leghorn chickens (Sawyer et al., 1986). Based on certain similarities in the biochemical behaviour between the Ah receptor and steroid hormone receptors, it has been proposed that there is a natural ligand for the Ah receptor (Neal et al., 1979; Poland et al., 1976). So far such a ligand has not been identified, either among steroid hormones (Poland et al., 1976; Carlstedt-Duke et al., 1979; Romkes et al., 1987) or among certain dietary factors (Johansson et al., 1982), although lumichrome, a metabolite of riboflavin, was suggested as an endogenous ligand for the receptor (Kurl & Villee, 1985). TCDD does not bind to the glucocorticoid, estrogen or progesterone receptors (Neal et al., 1979; Romkes et al., 1987). Monoclonal anti-glucocorticoid receptor-IgG antibodies did not react with the TCDD receptor (Poellinger et al., 1983) and the hydrophobic properties of the Ah receptor were more pronounced than those of the steroid hormone receptors (Poellinger & Gullberg, 1985).

Convincing data for the importance of the receptor in TCDD-induced toxicity could be based on structure activity relationships, i.e., that the binding affinities of TCDD and other PCDDs or PCDFs to the receptor correlate with their biological potencies. The binding affinities of PCDDs and PCDFs have been demonstrated to correlate with their biological potencies, particularly the induction of enzyme activities as well as the production of acute toxic effects (Tables 56 and 61) (Poland & Kende, 1976; Poland et al., 1976; Knutson & Poland, 1982).

Furthermore, the structure-activity relationships observed for enzyme induction, thymic atrophy, body weight loss, and LD_{50} values were comparable to the structure-activity relationships observed for receptor binding (Tables 56, 61) (Bandiera et al., 1984a,b; Mason et al., 1985, 1986; Sawyer & Safe, 1985; Safe et al., 1986). Interactive studies, i.e., studies where PCDD and PCDF congeners have been given both separately and as mixtures, have also been used to investigate the role of the Ah receptor in the mechanism of action of TCDD. Depending on the mechanism of action the biological responses may be synergistic potentiated, additive, unaffected, or antagonistic. Such studies have been performed for enzyme induction (Sawyer & Safe, 1985; Keys et al., 1986; Ahlborg et al., 1987), vitamin A reduction (Hakansson et al., 1987), teratogenicity (Birnbaum et al., 1985; Weber et al., 1985), thymic atrophy (Bannister & Safe, 1987), and immune suppression (Rizzardini et al., 1983). So far this kind of data is scattered and difficult to interpret.

Polymorphism in the Ah locus, which is suggested to be structural gene for the cytosolic receptor, seems to determine the sensitivity of genetically different strains of mice to TCDD and congeners. Ah responsive strains of mice, e.g., C57Bl/6, are characterized by (a) high hepatic levels of the TCDD receptor protein, (b) highly elevated levels of hepatic cytochrome P-448 and associated enzyme activities in response to treatment with 3-MC, and (c) sensitivity to the ulcerative action of DMBA on the skin. Ah-non-responsive mice, e.g., DBA/2, lack these attributes (Nebert et al., 1975). Based on these findings several genetic studies have been performed to elucidate the role of the receptor in TCDD toxicity. Contrary to 3-MC, TCDD induces AHH activity and several toxic effects

Table 61. Structure-activity relationships for some PCDFs

	In vitro EC_{50} values (mol/litre)[a,b]			*In vivo* ED_{50} values (µmol/kg)			LD_{50} [c]
PCDF congener	Receptor binding	AHH	EROD	AHH	Body weight loss	Thymic atrophy	Guinea-pig µg/kg body weight
Dibenzofuran	$< 10^{-3}$	ND	ND				
2-	2.8×10^{-4}	ND	ND				
3-	4.2×10^{-5}	ND	ND				
4-	$< 10^{-3}$	1.0×10^{-5}	1.71×10^{-5}				
2,3-	4.72×10^{-6}	2.19×10^{-6}	4.84×10^{-6}				
2,6-	2.46×10^{-4}	6.17×10^{-5}	6.31×10^{-5}				
2,8-	2.57×10^{-4}	3.95×10^{-5}	4.0×10^{-5}				
1,3,6-	4.40×10^{-6}	2.53×10^{-6}	3.37×10^{-6}				
1,3,8-	8.50×10^{-5}	1.94×10^{-5}	3.02×10^{-5}				
2,3,4-	1.9×10^{-5}	1.51×10^{-7}	2.48×10^{-7}				
2,3,8-	1.0×10^{-6}	2.49×10^{-6}	1.56×10^{-6}				
2,6,7-	4.5×10^{-7}	2.80×10^{-6}	3.13×10^{-6}				
2,3,4,6-	3.5×10^{-7}	1.32×10^{-6}	1.13×10^{-6}				
2,3,4,7-	2.51×10^{-8}	1.79×10^{-8}	1.48×10^{-8}	46	34	7.8	
2,3,4,8-	2.0×10^{-7}	4.14×10^{-8}	3.76×10^{-8}	ND	130	> 150	
2,3,6,8-	2.2×10^{-7}	1.04×10^{-6}	7.79×10^{-7}				
2,3,7,8-	4.1×10^{-8}	3.91×10^{-9}	2.02×10^{-9}	0.65	3.2	3.6	5-10
1,2,3,6-	3.54×10^{-7}	$> 10^{-4}$	$> 10^{-4}$	> 160	> 250	> 250	
1,2,3,7-	1.12×10^{-7}	2.7×10^{-5}	6.3×10^{-5}	110	87	110	
1,2,4,8-	$> 10^{-5}$	1.20×10^{-5}	9.26×10^{-5}				
1,2,4,6,7-	6.77×10^{-8}	3.25×10^{-7}	3.48×10^{-7}				
1,2,4,7,9-	2.0×10^{-5}	3.77×10^{-8}	3.84×10^{-8}				
1,2,3,4,8-	1.2×10^{-7}	2.09×10^{-7}	1.63×10^{-7}				
1,2,3,7,8-	7.45×10^{-8}	2.54×10^{-9}	3.06×10^{-9}	1.5	2.6	1.8	
1,2,3,7,9-	3.98×10^{-7}	8.6×10^{-8}	8.6×10^{-8}	15	49	23	
1,2,4,6,8-	3.09×10^{-6}	1.0×10^{-5}	1.2×10^{-5}	> 150	7150	> 150	
1,2,4,7,8-	1.3×10^{-6}	1.06×10^{-7}	1.48×10^{-7}	7.8	49	46	
1,3,4,7,8-	2.0×10^{-7}	1.60×10^{-9}	1.40×10^{-9}	3.5	26	0.70	

Table 61 (contd).

2,3,4,7,8-	1.5×10^{-8}	2.56×10^{-10}	1.34×10^{-10}	0.037	1.0	0.26
2,3,4,7,9-	2.0×10^{-7}	7.9×10^{-9}	5.8×10^{-9}	7.0	22	5.5
1,2,3,4,7,8-	2.3×10^{-7}	3.56×10^{-10}	3.79×10^{-10}	0.29	1.3	0.56
1,2,3,6,7,8-	2.7×10^{-7}	1.47×10^{-9}	1.24×10^{-9}	0.35	3.2	0.90
1,2,4,6,7,8-	8.3×10^{-6}	4.24×10^{-8}	2.93×10^{-8}			
2,3,4,6,7,8-	4.7×10^{-8}	6.87×10^{-10}	5.75×10^{-10}	0.27	2.8	0.90

a Estimated concentration needed to displace 50% of ^{3}H-TCDD bound to liver cytosol receptor from Wistar rats and to produce 50% maximum enzyme induction in the rat hepatoma H-4-IIE cell line (Bandiera et al., 1984b).

b Studies in immature male Wistar rats (Mason et al., 1985).

c Moore et al. (1979).

both in Ah-responsive and Ah-non-responsive strains of mice. However, the dose required to produce the effect in an Ah-non-responsive strain is approximately 10-fold greater than that needed for a responsive strain, thus demonstrating that the Ah-non-responsive strain also contains the TCDD-receptor but that this receptor is defective (Okey & Vella, 1982).

Crosses and backcrosses of C57BL/6 and DBA/2 mice have shown that sensitivity to TCDD-induced thymic atrophy immune system disturbances (section 7.4.5) and teratogenic effects (section 7.5.2) segregate with the Ah locus. Furthermore, data from studies of DBA/2 mice given either single or multiple doses of TCDD (Jones & Sweeney, 1980; Smith et al., 1981) suggest that the LD_{50} in this strain of mice is at least 5-fold greater than the values recorded for the C57Bl/6 and C57Bl/10 strains (Vos et al., 1974; Jones & Greig, 1975; Smith et al., 1981). TCDD-induced hepatic porphyria has also been shown to segregate with the Ah locus in mice (Jones & Sweeney, 1980). However, Greig et al. (1984) found that additional genetic loci must be involved in this lesion. The correlative differences between the C57Bl/6 and DBA/2 strains of mice, in terms of altered specific binding of TCDD and sensitivity to this compound, may be unique and may not be applicable to other species (Gasiewicz & Rucci, 1984).

Less convincing data for the model of receptor-mediated toxicity of TCDD arise from studies of toxicity, receptor levels, and/or enzyme induction of TCDD in various species, tissues, and cell cultures. Despite enormous variability in recorded LD_{50} values for guinea-pig, rat, mouse, rabbit, and hamster (Table 47), the amounts and physical properties of the hepatic as well as the extrahepatic receptors, do not vary extensively in these species (Poland & Knutson, 1982; Gasiewicz & Rucci, 1984). Furthermore, although recorded LD_{50} values for TCDD vary more than 100 times in chick embryos, C3H/HeN mice, and Sprague Dawley rats, the ED_{50} doses for AHH induction in these species are comparable (Poland & Glover, 1974b). In the guinea-pig, the most TCDD-susceptible species, enzyme induction is several times lower even at lethal doses. A number of cell types, including primary cultures and established and transformed cell lines from several species and tissues, are inducible for AHH activity, indicating the presence of the receptor, yet toxicity is not expressed in these systems (Knutson & Poland, 1980a).

Available data thus suggest that the receptor for TCDD may be a prerequisite, but is not sufficient in itself for the expression of TCDD toxicity.

7.8.2 Toxicokinetics

The interspecies variation in sensitivity to TCDD may be attributable, at least in part, to different rates at which various species distribute, metabolize, and excrete the compound. Table 62 summarizes some of the data on the elimination, toxicity, and metabolism of TCDD in different species, some previously discussed in section 6. Distribution data (section 6.1) has been obtained mainly from animals exposed to toxic doses of TCDD. Interspecies comparisons based on these data are difficult to perform, since studies in different species have been performed with non-comparable relative toxic doses and collection of data has occurred at variable time-points. However, the available data suggest that tissue levels alone cannot explain the interspecies differences in pathology and acute toxicity of TCDD. For example, the molar concentration of TCDD in the hamster may be orders of magnitude greater than in the rat and mice, without development of hepatotoxicity, yet definite liver damage occurs both in rats and mice.

Based on the findings that the toxicity of TCDD is lower in rats after the stimulation of hepatic mixed function oxidases (Beatty et al., 1978), and that the metabolites of TCDD are less toxic than the parent compound (Weber et al., 1982a; Mason & Safe, 1986) (see section 7.1.5), the metabolism of TCDD has been considered as a detoxification mechanism.

Following the administration of TCDD, most of it appears to be eliminated through a first-order process in most species (see section 7.1). In all species investigated TCDD is largely eliminated in the faeces (Table 48). Only in hamsters and certain strains of mice is urinary elimination a major route of excretion (Table 41). Available data demonstrate that TCDD is converted to more polar metabolites prior to elimination in the urine and bile (Table 62). Unchanged TCDD does not appear in the bile or urine of any species, but it is the major excretory product in the faeces of mice, guinea-pigs, and hamsters (Table 62). As the urine and bile appear to be free of unmetabolized TCDD, the existence of unchanged TCDD in faeces indicates that a significant amount of unchanged TCDD may be excreted into the intestinal lumen by some route other than bile.

The metabolic profiles of TCDD in excreta differs between species, but generally urinary metabolites are more polar than biliary or faecal metabolites. Furthermore, several metabolites, both in urine and bile, are glucuronide conjugates.

The apparent absence of TCDD metabolites in the tissues of all species, except for the guinea-pig (Table 62), suggests that, once formed, the metabolites of TCDD are readily excreted. Another factor, besides metabolism, that may influence the total rate of elimination of TCDD is the amount of adipose tissue stores, which may vary between species.

Table 62. Rates of elimination, toxicity, and metabolic transformation of TCDD in different species

Species/strain	Elimination half-life (days)	LD_{50} value (µg/kg body weight)	TCDD-derived radioactivity occurring in: Urine	Bile	Faeces	Tissues
Rats[a, b, c, d]						
Sprague Dawley	17-31	25-60	5 polar metabolites	4-8 polar metabolites; little, if any, unchanged TCDD.		unchanged TCDD
Mice[e, f, g]						
C57BL/6, DBA/2, B6D2F$_1$	10-24	114-2570	4-7 polar metabolites	4-6 polar metabolites	3-4 polar metabolites, unchanged TCDD.	unchanged TCDD
Guinea-pig[h]						
Hartley	22-94	0.6-2.5	4 polar metabolites	5 polar metabolites	mainly unchanged TCDD	unchanged TCDD, polar metabolites
Hamsters[a, i]						
Golden Syrian	12-15	1157-5051	4 polar metabolites	5-6 polar metabolites	metabolites, unchanged TCDD	unchanged TCDD
Dogs[j]						
Beagle	not reported	not reported		metabolites		

[a] Gasiewicz et al., 1983a. [b] Poiger & Schlatter, 1979. [c] Ramsey et al., 1982. [d] Rose et al., 1976.
[e] Gasiewicz et al., 1983b. [f] Koshakji et al., 1984. [g] Vinopal & Cassida, 1973. [h] Olson, 1986.
[i] Olson et al, 1980a. [j] Poiger et al., 1982.

At present there is no clear relationship between the ability of a given species to excrete TCDD and/or its metabolites and the acute toxicity of TCDD in that species. However, the somewhat greater rate of elimination of TCDD in the hamster and the lower rate of elimination in the guinea-pig (Table 62) may contribute to their relative resistance and sensitivity, respectively, to the acute toxic effects of TCDD.

The rate of metabolism and excretion of PCDDs and PCDFs varies with molecular structure. In most species PCDFs are much more readily eliminated than their PCDD counterparts. Less halogenated congeners are usually metabolised and excreted more rapidly than the more halogenated ones, especially the 2,3,7,8-substituted congeners (see sections 6 and 9).

7.8.3 Impairment of normal cellular regulatory systems

When considered together, the diverse pattern of toxic effects, the species- and tissue-specific responses, and the time-course for effects, as well as the non-toxic action of TCDD on most cell cultures *in vitro*, seem to indicate that TCDD-induced toxicity occurs as a result of an impairment of a normal cellular regulatory system. Such a system might be present in all cells throughout the organism, though the activity may vary with cell type, tissue, age, sex, and strain, and/or species.

7.8.3.1 Endocrine imbalance

In many aspects, TCDD toxicity mimics endocrine imbalance, although no evidence exists to indicate a direct involvement of hormones in the toxic action of TCDD (section 7.4.9).

7.8.3.2 Body weight regulation

The most reliable and consistent symptom of TCDD toxicity among all experimental animals is weight loss. The cause of the body weight loss seems to be reduced food intake, apparently occurring secondarily to a physiological adjustment that reduces the body weight to a maintenance level lower than normal. The physiological trigger for controlling this body weight set-point might be a target for TCDD action (section 7.4.1).

7.8.3.3 Plasma membrane function

The changes in the surface characteristics of the plasma membranes induced by TCDD *in vivo* (7.4.2.2) resemble changes occurring in precancerous and transformed cells (Pitot &

Sirica, 1980). Such changes, including reduction of gap junctions and surface glyco-proteins, would be expected to curtail cell-cell communication and to reduce intercellular recognition and attachment events implicated in the process of tumour promotion.

It has been shown by Pitot et al. (1980) that TCDD promotes diethylnitrosamine (DEN)-induced hepatocarcinoma in rats. In this study, canalicular ATPase was used as a marker in detecting enzyme-altered foci, whose number increased when TCDD was given to DEN-treated partially hepatectomized rats. The foci exhibited decreased ATPase activity in agreement with previous observations that TCDD _in vivo_ reduces the ATPase level in canaliculi-rich plasma membranes.

TCDD, unlike other well known promoters, requires a prolonged treatment period _in vivo_ to exert its effect. The lack of effect of TCDD _in vitro_ would imply that the promoter activity is mediated through some _in vivo_ process and not by its direct interaction with plasma membranes.

7.8.3.4 Impaired vitamin A storage

The histomorphological appearance of chloracne, the most characteristic and prominent sign of TCDD-induced toxicity in humans, resembles in some respects effects seen in the skin of patients suffering from vitamin A deficiency (Kimbrough, 1974).

Many of the effects of TCDD poisoning observed in animal studies, including failure of normal growth, keratosis, epithelial lesions, immunosuppression, and reproductive and teratological effects, are similar to the effects of dietary vitamin A deficiency (Thunberg et al., 1980). The most intriguing similarities between symptoms due to vitamin A deficiency and TCDD toxicity concern effects on epithelial tissues, particularly the process of keratinization. TCDD induces terminal differentiation of epithelial tissues both _in vivo_ and _in vitro_. However, lack of epithelial degeneration (programmed cell death) of the medial epithelial cells of palatal shelves has been reported in mice exposed to TCDD _in utero_ (Pratt et al., 1984).

Vitamin A is essential for normal differentiation. It diminishes the expression of differentiation in stratified squamous epithelia and accentuates the expression of differentiation in secretory epithelia. Vitamin A deficiency can convert secretory epithelia to squamous epithelia, while excess of the vitamin can convert stratified squamous epithelia to secretory epithelia (Wolf, 1980). With the use of cultured human keratinocytes, it has been demonstrated that vitamin A at the cellular level affects cell motility, cell-cell interaction, and epithelial morphogenesis. At the molecular level, vitamin A determines, by controlling the level of the corresponding mRNA, the nature of keratins synthesized (Fuchs & Green, 1981). Keratins constitute a cytoskeleton in epithelial cells, and the keratin pattern may be used as a marker for epithelial differentiation (Sun et al., 1979, 1983a,b). Removal of vitamin A from the medium of cultivated human keratinocytes of various origin led to increased synthesis of large keratins and reduced synthesis of lower molecular weight keratins (Fuchs & Green, 1981). This pattern was reversed by the addition of vitamin A to the medium. Each tissue and cell type controlled its synthesis of keratins differently, depending on the vitamin A concentration in the medium. The ability of TCDD to impair vitamin A storage (section 7.4.10) may be responsible for some of the toxic effects produced by TCDD.

7.8.4 Lipid peroxidation

Based on indirect lines of evidence, Sweeney & Jones (1983) proposed that increased *in vivo* lipid peroxidation, resulting in the formation of free radicals, might be a mechanism of TCDD toxicity. Firstly, lipofuscin pigments, considered to be by-products of lipid peroxidation, accumulate in the heart muscle cells of TCDD-treated rats (Albro et al., 1978). Secondly, iron deficiency inhibits *in vitro* lipid peroxidation (Bus & Gibson, 1979; Sweeney et al., 1979) and has been demonstrated to reduce hepatic TCDD toxicity *in vivo* in rats (Sweeney et al., 1979). Thirdly, 0.25% butylated hydroxyanisole (BHA) in the diet has been shown to provide protection from TCDD-induced porphyria and lipid accumulation in mice. In contrast, 0.01% vitamin E, another antioxidant, in the diet had no protective effect (Hassan et al., 1985a,b). Stohs et al. (1983) demonstrated increased *in vivo* (conjugated diene method) and *in vitro* (microsomal malondialdehyde formation) hepatic lipid peroxidation in female Sprague Dawley rats given a total of 70 µg/kg body weight in three daily oral doses of 10, 20, and 40 µg TCDD/kg body weight, or a single oral dose of 80 µg TCDD/kg body weight. Lipid peroxidation was determined at days 1, 6, and 11 after the last treatment. The maximal increase of lipid peroxidation *in vivo* was 2-fold one day post-treatment, whereas the 5- to 6-fold increase in *in vitro* lipid peroxidation reached its maximum at 6 days post-treatment. The TCDD-induced *in vitro* lipid peroxidation could be inhibited by repeated treatment with BHA, glutathione, vitamin E, and vitamin A (Hassan et al., 1985a,b). Dietary selenium had no inhibitory effect on TCDD-induced lipid peroxidation (Hassan et al., 1985c).

Robertson et al. (1985) found no evidence for TCDD-induced *in vivo* lipid peroxidation, as judged by levels of exhaled endogenous ethane, and metabolic clearance of both externally and internally applied exogenous ethane in male Sprague Dawley rats after a single ip dose of 60 µg TCDD/kg body weight. Neither was there a correlation between TCDD-induced lipid peroxidation in vitro and sensitivity towards the lethal effect of TCDD in Sprague Dawley rats, Golden Syrian hamsters or guinea-pigs (Hassan et al., 1983). Hepatic microsomes from Sprague Dawley rats and Golden Syrian hamsters exposed to TCDD in vitro responded with increased lipid peroxidation only in the presence of Fe^{3+}-ADP in the incubation mixture (Albro et al., 1986).

From all these data on TCDD and lipid peroxidation, it was concluded by Albro et al. (1986) that it was premature to attempt to define a relationship between lipid peroxidation and TCDD-induced lethality.

8. EFFECT OF PCDDs ON HUMAN BEINGS - EPIDEMIOLOGICAL AND CASE STUDIES

8.1 Occupational Studies - Historical Perspective

The illness most frequently observed in workers engaged in the manufacture of trichlorophenol, 2,4,5-T, and related products is a skin disease called chloracne. This skin disease has also been called "Pernakrankheit" (perchlorinated naphthalene illness or halogen wax acne) and was described by Herxheimer (1899). In addition to the halogenated phenols, chloracne is caused by a number of chlorinated compounds such as the chlorinated biphenyls and chlorinated naphthalenes (Muller, 1937; Braun, 1955; Crow, 1970; Kimbrough, 1974).

Although chloracne is well known to those engaged in the treatment of occupational diseases, many outbreaks that have occurred over the years, particularly in the USA, have not been reported in the scientific literature. In the Federal Republic of Germany, chloracne is now considered an occupational disease for which compensation is mandatory (Braun, 1970).

Herxheimer (1899) also described general toxic signs and symptoms in his patients, such as lack of appetite, weight loss, headache, and vertigo. After his original observations and publication, several other reports followed. The technique of obtaining chlorine gas consisted of an electrolytic procedure where a mixture of potassium, sodium, and magnesium chlorides was subjected to a current with a central carbon electrode where the chlorine was obtained and piped off. The workers who took care of the chlorine gas never developed chloracne thus refuting the original hypothesis by Herxheimer. By contrast, those who handled the electrodes and cleaned the reaction vessels were those afflicted with chloracne. Already at this time chlorinated phenolic compounds were considered as possible noxious agents (Fraenkel, 1902). This however could never be proven and even at present, when satisfactory analytical techniques are now available, no analysis of the so-called "tuffy tar" has been carried out.

Another class of chlorinated organic compounds causing skin damage appeared during the First World War (1914-1918). At this time perchlorinated naphthalenes had come into use as insulation materials, e.g., in the radio and electronic industry. The first description of Pernakrankheit was that by Wauer (1918). The use of the unspecified technical mixture of chlorinated naphthalenes spread all over the world and caused numerous intoxications notably among workers in manufacture. The perna disease has been summarized by von Wedel et al. (1943) and described in particular detailed by Braun (1955).

Apart from chloracne the systemic effects of the same compounds have been dealt with by Drinker et al. (1937) and Greenburg et al. (1939).

Both in man and experimental animals, serious liver damage occurred after exposure to chlorinated naphthalenes, consisting of liver necrosis and toxic jaundice (acute yellow liver atrophy). Among several hundred cases of chloracne due to these compounds, Braun (1955) tabulated 24 deaths due to toxic jaundice and 14 recoveries. It should be pointed out that a fulminant liver disease with jaundice of this kind is an extremely rare condition. For comparison, it has never occurred after exposure to trichlorophenol (TCP) and TCDD as described below. Note should also be taken of the fact that not only were the perchlorinated naphthalenes an ill identified mixture of chemical species, but exposure frequently occurred at the same time to mixtures of chlorinated biphenyls, the latter now known to be contaminated with chlorinated dibenzofurans. The potentiation of toxicity by these mixtures and other chlorinated compounds were discussed by Drinker et al. (1937), Greenburg et al. (1939), von Wedel et al. (1943), and Risse-Sunderman (1959).

Several accidental ingestions of chloracnegenic compounds have occurred. They are of particular importance in relation to discussions on whether chloracne is a systemic or local disease. The so-called Yusho disease is discussed in section 11.

Herzberg (1947) described several cases of chloracne, in which other toxic signs and symptoms were seen, due to consumption of "chlorinated paraffin" used as a substitute for butter during cooking in postwar Berlin. Among general signs and symptoms observed were gastrointestinal disturbances with abdominal pain, headache, pain in joints, neuropathy, depression, and lack of appetite. The dermatological symptoms were erythema, exanthema, comedones, and retention cysts in sebaceous glands. It was noted as remarkable that the skin signs had a follicular predilection, as in seborrhoea (face, head, bosom, and back). The slow development of chloracne, and particularily the fact that the sebaceous glands were affected, led the author to conclude that it was a secretory disease (Ausscheidungstoxikose). With regard to the chloracnegenic component, it is unlikely that paraffin itself was active. Herzberg speculated that something else, possibly a pyrolysis product that arose during cooking, could have caused the disease.

Accidents in chemical plants involved in the manufacture of chlorinated phenolic compounds are listed in Table 63. It should be stressed that all these intoxications are due to mixtures, e.g., TCP and TCDD and other compounds. Summaries

Table 63. Summary of accidents in chemical plants involving the manufacture of chlorinated phenolic compounds

Country and date	Product[a]	Cause of exposure	Personnel affected	Years from incident to last observation	References
Germany 1910	CP	Explosion + occupational	5	Same year	Teleky (1913), Wahle (1914), Dohmeier & Janson (1983)
United States 1949	TCP	Explosion + Occupational	228	30	Ashe & Suskind (1949, 1950), Suskind et al. (1953), Suskind (1978), Huff et al. (1980), Zack & Suskind (1980) Zack & Gaffey (1983), Moses et al. (1984), Suskind & Hertzberg (1984)
Federal Republic of Germany 1949	TCP (PCP)	Occupational	17	1	Baader et al. (1951)
Federal Republic of Germany 1952	TCP	Occupational	60		Bauer et al. (1961)
Federal Republic of Germany 1952-1953	TCP	Occupational	37		Hay (1977)
Federal Republic of Germany 1953	TCP	Explosion + Occupational	75	29	Hoffman (1957), Goldmann (1972, 1973), Huff et al. (1980), Thiess et al. (1982)
France 1953	TCP	Explosion + Occupational	17	2	Dugois & Colomb (1956, 1957), Dugois et al. (1958)
Federal Republic of Germany 1954	TCP, 2,4,5-T	Occupational	31	24	Schultz (1957a,b), Bauer et al. (1961), Kimmig & Schultz (1957a,b) Kleu & Göltz (1971), von Krause & Brassow (1978)

Table 63 (contd - 2).

Country and date	Product[a]	Cause of exposure	Personnel affected	Years from incident to last observation	References
Federal Republic of Germany 1954	TCP 2,4,5-T	Occupational	24	4	Risse-Sundermann (1959)
United States 1956	2,4,5-T 2,4,5-T	Occupational	48	6	Bleiberg et al. (1964), Poland et al. (1971)
United States 1956	TCP	Occupational	Many		Hay (1977)
Italy 1959	TCP	Explosion + Occupational	5	2	Hofman et al. (1962)
United States 1959	TCP	Occupational			Hay (1977)
United States 1960	TCP	Occupational	Many		Hay (1977)
Netherlands 1963	TCP 2,4,5-T	Explosion	106	11	Dalderup, (1974a,b), Berlin et al. (1976), Huff et al. (1980)
USSR 1964	2,4,5-T	Occupational	128		Telegina et al. (1970), IARC (1977)
United States 1964	TCP	Occupational	61	6	Vahrenholt (1977), Cook et al. (1980), Ott et al. (1980)
Czechoslovakia 1964-1969	TCP	Occupational	80	6	Jirásek et al. (1973, 1976), Pazderova et al. (1974, 1980, 1981)
United Kingdom 1968	TCP	Explosion	90	14	May (1973, 1982), Huff et al. (1980)
Japan 1970	2,4,5-T	Occupational	25	3	Mivra et al. (1974)

Table 63 (contd - 3).

USSR 1972	TCP	Occupational	1	1	Zelikov & Danilov (1974)
Austria 1972-1973	2,4,5-T	Occupational	50		Forth (1977), Hay (1977)
Federal Republic of Germany 1974	2,4,5-T	Occupational	5		Forth (1977), Hay (1977)
Italy 1976	TCP	Explosion	193	8	Reggiani (1977, 1978, 1983a), Vahrenholt (1977), Filippini et al. (1981), Abate et al. (1982), Ideo et al. (1982)

[a] Products: TCP = trichlorophenols; CP = chlorophenols; PCP = pentachlorophenol; 2,4,5-T = 2,4,5-trichlorophenoxyacetic acid.

of the industrial accidents are to be found in Holmstedt (1980) and only some of them will be dealt with here.

The first reported intoxication with a mixture probably containing TCDD, although the chemical structure was not given, occurred in February 1910. Five people were said to have been contaminated after a reactor explosion and two of these were described in some detail in a dermatological thesis (Teleky, 1913; Wahle 1914). Wahle (1914), however, in his thesis emphazised that this intoxication was not due to any of the chlorinated naphthalene derivatives that were well known by then.

An industrial poisoning was reported in 1949, due to the formation of TCDD in uncontrolled exothermic reactions occurring during the manufacture of TCP at a 2,4,5-T-producing factory in Nitro, West Virginia, USA. The temperature in one of the reactors containing tetrachlorobenzene, methanol, and sodium hydroxide increased, a relief valve opened, and the contents of the vessel were discharged into the interior of the building and over a wide area outside of the building. A total of 228 people were affected.

Symptoms included chloracne, nausea, vomiting, headaches, severe muscular aches and pains, fatigue, emotional instability, and intolerance to cold. Laboratory findings showed an increase in total serum lipids and an initially prolonged prothrombin time. Among those affected were not only workmen, but also laboratory personnel, medical personnel, and even the Safety Director who visited the area of exposure. Several wives who had never visited the plant also developed acne, usually at the same time as their husbands working at the plant. A man from the nearby town who purchased a truck that was parked in the vicinity of the accident at the time it occurred, and his child, also developed chloracne. The disabling symptoms, which kept men from their jobs for as long as 2 years, were severe aches and pains and fatigability, the manifestations of peripheral neuropathy. Liver tests 4 years later were normal, but mild cases of acne were common. TCDD was still an unknown chemical. The follow-up to this accident will be discussed in section 8.4.

In 1953, at the Badische Anilin and Soda Fabrik, during the alkaline hydrolysis of 1,2,4,5-tetrachlorobenzene to 2,4,5-trichlorophenol, the temperature and pressure in an autoclave increased rapidly and resulted in an exothermic reaction releasing a great deal of steam through a safety valve of the reaction vessel. This steam covered the walls, windows, doors, and machinery in the rooms of four floors, and finally precipitated in solid form on everything in these rooms. Forty-two workers involved in the clean-up operations developed chloracne, and even after the extensive clean-up operations occasional workers still developed chloracne.

Thereafter the autoclaves were used for 2 years without incident but in 1958 a mechanic who conducted repair work on an autoclave subsequently developed chloracne (Hofmann, 1957; Goldmann, 1972). In 1968 and 1969 the building containing the autoclaves was dismantled. Goldmann (1972, 1973) conducted a study of the 42 workers exposed in this accident. In 21 cases, the chloracne was preceded by a non-specific dermatitis and in two cases very persistent chronic conjunctivitis and blepharitis were observed; 14 cases also showed involvement of other organs. In four instances the liver was affected, and microscopic examination of the liver again showed a very characteristic grey pigment that did not stain positive for iron. A transient involvement of the myocardium was also noted. In five instances the upper respiratory tract was involved with tracheitis and bronchitis. There was one instance of haemorrhagic pleuritis and one instance of afebrile gingivitis and stomatitis. In a number of cases a high susceptibility to infection was noted, sometimes accompanied by a decrease in gamma-globulin. One worker died of pancreatitis, in seven cases the central nervous system was affected, three instances of toxic polyneuritis were recorded, and in two instances hearing, sense of smell, and taste were impaired. The child of one of these workers also developed chloracne, and in most of the workers active chloracne persisted for many years - in one instance for 18 years. Follow-up studies are described in section 9.4.

Of particular interest is a study by Risse-Sundermann (1959). According to oral reports by the treating physician, all 24 members of a team working in a trichlorophenol operation became ill after the production process was switched to the pressurized phenol process in the spring and summer of 1954. Slightly different acneiform skin conditions appeared as symptoms of the toxic exposure. In addition, the patients suffered from dizziness, nausea, vomiting, lacrimation, burning of the eyes, difficulty in hearing, gastrointestinal spasms, intolerance to fatty foods, diarrhoea, jaundice, hepatitis (which was fatal in one case), and paresthesias and hyperesthesias, as well as extreme irritability. One patient became psychotic and committed suicide. In addition, some of the patients complained of impotence.

Ten workers at this chemical factory were followed for five years by Risse-Sundermann (1959). In addition to the signs and symptoms mentioned above, she noticed swollen lymph glands and a considerable decrease in body weight. The patients underwent neurological examination, with no objective signs being observable. Of particular interest in this well documented study is the fact that in three patients the general symptoms (e.g., tiredness, depression, lack of appetite, stomach pains, sexual dysfunction) preceded that of the skin manifestations .

Bauer et al. (1961) reported a study of workers affected by three different outbreaks of chloracne. In this study more than 100 workers were examined. Of these, 31 Hamburg workers had been exposed 5 years ealier. Nine were examined in detail and their symptoms tabulated. Initially, there was dermatitis and irritation of the face, sometimes accompanied by conjunctivitis, and followed by the gradual development of chloracne and patchy pigmentation of the skin. In some cases irritations of the mucous membranes of the face and upper respiratory tract, together with a persistent blepharoconjunctivitis, were also noted. In the follow-up study, a number of cases of liver injury were observed and, at liver biopsy, a typical grey pigment was observed in liver sections, which did not stain positive for iron. Viral hepatitis was suspected. In a few cases, chronic bronchitis and occasional myocardial damage were also observed. In all cases, fatigue was the main complaint and muscle weakness and muscle pain were described by the workers, particularly in the proximal muscles of the lower extremities. All nine also reported decreased libido. In a few instances, paresthesia and hyperesthesia or pronounced sensory neuropathy were observed, and minor circumscribed pareses were found. A psychovegetative syndrome occurred in most of the workers. Other signs recorded were: inability to concentrate, memory deficits, sleep disturbances, particularly increased somnolence, decreased drive, and alcohol intolerance. Psychological tests also showed abnormalities.

Following the malfunction of a reaction vessel in northern Italy, in which 2,4,5-trichlorophenol was produced, the temperature in the vessel increased rapidly and an intense black vapour filled the work-room covering everything with a black deposit. Five workers engaged in clean-up operations developed chloracne (Hofmann & Meneghini, 1962). None of those involved in the clean-up exhibited any involvement of general systemic toxicity (even after 16 months) that could be related to exposure to the tar and soot. However, one 15-year-old worker developed folliculitis and superficial nodular elements on the face a few days after initial exposure. A slow but progressive generalization of the dermatosis developed on the trunk, scalp, and lower extremities. An examination several months later revealed no damage to the renal or liver parenchyma. However, this worker was found to still suffer from outbursts of chloracne in 1980 (Holmstedt, 1980).

Duverne et al. (1964) reported a case that occurred at a plant at Lyon, France, where products that used 2,4,5 trichlorophenol as a starting material were manufactured. This worker developed chloracne as well as serofibrinous pleuritis.

Ten workers also developed chloracne at a plant near Grenoble, France, which produced 2,4,5-trichlorophenol that served as the starting material for phenoxy pesticides and germicides for cosmetics. These workers showed symptoms of systemic poisoning similar to those reported by Goldmann (1972), and hepatic insufficiency with lipaemia and elevated serum cholesterol levels (Dugois & Colomb, 1956). Another accident resulting in TCDD exposure of workers occurred in the same factory in 1966 (Dugois et al., 1967).

An exothermic reaction resulted in an explosion at a plant in Chesterfield, England, in 1968. The company made 2,4,5-trichlorophenol from tetrachlorobenzene and the explosion occurred during the process involving ethylene glycol and caustic soda under atmospheric pressure (Milnes, 1971). In this incident, 79 workers developed chloracne but there was no evidence of systemic illness (May, 1973). In 1971, 3 years after the explosion, two workers who had not been involved in the explosion or its aftermath were employed as pipe-fitters at a new installation, away from the site of the explosion, to refit one of the cleaned tanks. They both developed severe chloracne, and the son of one of these workers and the wife of the other also developed this condition (Jensen & Walker, 1972). May (1973) cited two incidents involving explosions in a similar process. In the first incident, fatal injuries were recorded; in the second incident, all 50 exposed persons fell ill after 10 days and had liver injury.

In the USA, an outbreak of chloracne occurred among workers manufacturing 2,4-dichlorophenoxyacetic acid and 2,4,5-trichlorophenoxyacetic acid (Bleiberg et al., 1964); 29 workers developed chloracne and 11 of these had elevated urinary uroporphyrins and exhibited varying degrees of acquired porphyria cutanea tarda. At least one of these workers had abnormal liver-function tests and microscopic examination of a liver biopsy specimen showed parenchymal cell regeneration and haemofuscin pigment. Many of the workers with chloracne showed hyperpigmentation of the skin. A second study of the workers at this plant was conducted in 1969 by Poland et al. (1971). A total of 73 male employees were examined, and moderate to severe chloracne was found in 13 workers (18%), mild chloracne in 35 (48%), hyperpigmentation in 30, and uroporphyrinuria in 1. No definite systemic illness could be documented in these workers. Of those studied, 33 had been employed at the plant for 0-4 years, 10 for 4-8 years, and 30 for more than 9 years. The mean duration of employment was 8.3 ± 7.6 years (mean $\pm$ 1 SD). The trichlorophenol manufactured in this plant contained 10-25 mg TCDD/kg. Twenty-six of the workers seen by Bleiberg et al. (1964) were also seen in a follow-up study. Six months prior to the second survey (Poland et al., 1971), the manufacturing process was altered so that the 2,4,5-T produced contained less than 1 mg TCDD/kg.

In 1964, in the USSR, many workers developed chloracne while engaged in producing 2,4,5-T. Production was then discontinued (Telegina & Bikbulatova, 1970).

On 10 July 1976, an explosion occurred at the ICMESA plant at Meda, near Seveso, Italy, when 12 workers were present. All 176 workers of the plant were examined 3 or 4 weeks after the accident. Chloracne was suspected in 1 of them; the others showed minor symptoms that could not be correlated with exposure. Alkaline phosphatase and δ-glutamyltransferase seemed slightly increased in 32 and 37 cases, respectively, while five workers showed a reduction in their δ-aminolevulinic acid dehydratase blood levels, and three showed moderately increased urinary gamma-aminolevulinic acid (Zedda et al., 1976). Similar findings were reported by Fara et al. (1976) and Reggiani (1978). The follow-up of the general population is described in section 8.2.

8.2 General Population Studies

8.2.1 Missouri, USA

Environmental exposures have occurred in a small area of Missouri, USA (Carter et al., 1975; Kimbrough et al., 1977; Kimbrough, 1984). In the summer of 1971 many birds, rodents, cats, dogs, insects, and horses died after exposure in a horse arena in eastern Missouri. The incident followed the spraying of "waste oil" on the horse arena for dust control. Within 3 weeks of the spraying of this arena, two other arenas were sprayed. In all, 57 adult horses died, 26 abortions occurred among the horses at the most heavily exposed farm and many foals died soon after birth. At the time, the nature of the chemical that had caused the problem was unknown. The arenas were excavated and the contaminated dirt dumped at other sites. After many fruitless attempts to identify the cause of this outbreak, it was discovered in 1973-1974 that the original soil from one of the arenas contained 5600-6500 mg trichlorophenol/kg, 31.8-33.0 mg TCDD/kg, and 1350-1590 mg polychlorinated biphenyls/kg. Because of this finding, the episode was reinvestigated. It was found that the salvage oil company that sprayed the three arenas routinely collected discarded motor oil and lubricants from over 2000 service stations in eastern Missouri and southwestern Illinois. It also collected, from various sources, a limited amount of used organic solvents such as transformer oils and other compounds. A company in southwestern Missouri was finally identified as a source of TCDD. This company had manufactured trichlorophenol as an intermediate for hexachlorophene. The production of 2,4,5-trichlorophenol had generated a distillate residue which was emptied once a week into a residue storage tank. Initially this chemical waste was collected and incinerated but, in 1971 when the trichlorophenol producer experienced a financial crisis, he arranged for the chemical wastes to be disposed of by a chemical supplier. The chemical supplier subcontracted the chemical waste disposal to the salvage oil dealer. The salvage oil dealer added the toxic chemical waste to his salvage oil storage tank, having collected a total of 18 000 gallons. This material, mixed with salvage oil and other chemicals, was sprayed on the riding arenas and some of it was taken to re-refining companies. Soil samples from arenas where contaminated dirt had been dumped in 1974 contained trichlorophenol levels that ranged from 1.5-32.6 mg/kg, TCDD levels that ranged from 0.22-0.85 mg/kg, and polychlorinated biphenyl levels that ranged from 10-25 mg/kg.

A 6-year old girl, who had used one of the arenas for sandbox-like play in 1971, developed epistaxis, headache, diarrhoea and lethargy, haemorrhagic cystitis, and signs of pyelonephritis. She had an uneventful recovery. Three other females exposed to the same arena had recurring headaches, skin lesions, and polyarthralgias. Two 3-year-old boys in another arena developed chloracne on the exposed skin surfaces which lasted for more than a year. Evaluation of the three female patients 5.4 years after exposure to TCDD-containing oil showed them to be in good health (Beale et al., 1977).

A comprehensive medical examination of 154 residents exposed to TCDD, and 155 unexposed residents in similar type housing in eastern Missouri, revealed no consistent differences between the two groups. The examination included a medical history, physical examination, serum and urinary chemistries, and immunological and neurological tests. The findings may suggest that long-term TCDD exposure is associated with depressed cell-mediated immunity (decreased delayed-type hypersensitivity skin reactions to standard antigens) (Hoffman et al., 1986; Stehr et al., 1986). Urinary concentrations of glucaric acid were not significantly different between persons identified as being at high or low risk (Steinberg et al., 1985).

8.2.2 Seveso, Italy

The scientific follow-up on the population of Seveso, N. Italy, which had been accidentally exposed to TCDD in 1976 (see sections 4.1.1 and 8.1), was guided by an international steering group headed by Professor M.A. Klingberg. The group completed its work in February 1984 and concluded that "it is obvious that no clear-cut adverse health effects attributable to TCDD, besides chloracne, have been observed" (Regione

Lombardia, 1984). A total of 193 people had displayed symptoms of chloracne, but at the beginning of 1984 only 20 presented active symptoms. After 15-20 days exposure to TCDD soil levels of 270-1200 μg/m^2, there was a marked incidence of chloracne. No disturbance of biochemical functions were seen when the exposure had been limited to soil with TCDD levels at or below 30-70 μg/m^2. Later evaluations failed to confirm earlier findings of a decrease in motor nerve conduction velocity in some individuals. A significant increase in urinary glucaric acid levels, indicating increased microsomal enzyme activity, was found 3 years after exposure in 67 exposed children, as compared to 86 non-exposed children (Ideo et al., 1982, 1985). The steering group found the data difficult to evaluate as analytical and individual biological variabilities were not explained (Regione Lombardia, 1984).

Studies performed on the rate of spontaneous abortions and birth defects in the Seveso area do not allow any conclusions to be drawn (Tognoni & Bonaccorsi, 1982). The hypothesis that low exposure might cause pre-pregnancy or pregnancy effects that adversely affect the outcome was tested using several exposure models. The only finding was a slightly higher rate of haemangioma among newborns in the exposed group. However, this showed up only with one of the exposure models. It was considered doubtful that this was due to TCDD exposure (Regione Lombardia, 1984).

Lymphocytes from inhabitants of Seveso were examined for chromosomal aberrations by Regianni (1980a,b) and Mottura et al. (1981). In 17 TCDD-exposed individuals examined within two weeks of the accident, no increase in chromosomal aberrations was observed (Regianni, 1980). In the abstract by Mottura et al. (1981), chromosomal aberration analysis was performed on subjects distributed into three classes: acute exposure, chronic exposure, and a control group of non-exposed subjects. No significant difference in the frequency of chromosomal aberrations in the three exposure categories was reported. Data on number of subjects, chromosomal aberrations, and exposure level and time were not given.

Tenchini et al. (1983) published a comparative cytogenetic study on induced abortions from women exposed to TCDD after the Seveso accident, and in non-exposed subjects. Chromosome analysis was performed on maternal peripheral blood, placental and umbilical cord tissues, and fetal tissues. No significant differences were found in the level of chromosomal aberrations in the blood of placenta and umbilical cord from TCDD-exposed and non-exposed women. The exception was fetal samples from non-exposed women, in which a significant increase in chromosomal aberrations was obtained, possibly an artefact due to experimental techniques. The effect of TCDD on fetal chromosomes is therefore still unclear.

Several epidemiological follow-up studies are continuing in and around Seveso.

8.2.3 Viet Nam

From 1960 to 1969 a mixture of 2,4-dichlorophenoxyacetic acid and 2,4,5-trichlorophenoxyacetic acid (Agent Orange), which was contaminated with TCDD (concentrations ranging from 0.5 to 47 mg/kg) (Kearny et al., 1972), was sprayed over areas of Viet Nam as a defoliant. The spraying from 1960 to 1965 was minimal; in 1966 it covered slightly more than 800 000 acres, in 1967 almost 1.7 million acres, in 1968 over 1.3 million acres, and in 1969 1.2 million acres. Studies have been carried out since the early 1970s to ascertain whether the exposure of the general population in Viet Nam to this herbicide could have resulted in an increased incidence of birth defects. However, the results of such investigations have not been published in readily available peer-reviewed journals, making it difficult to assess the scientific significance of the findings. Such studies have been reviewed by Westing (1984) and Constable & Hatch (1985). Those studies reviewed indicate a range of effects including spontaneous abortions, infertility, and birth defects. However, there are marked deficiencies in experimental design in most, if not all, studies, including potential bias in the selection of populations, poor record-keeping of populations and biological effects, such as congenital malformations, and a lack of control over possible confounding factors. These deficiencies make it difficult, if not impossible, to use this body of data in assessing the human health risks from exposure to phenoxy-herbicides contaminated with TCDD and other PCDDs.

Tung (1973) reported an increased incidence of liver tumours in Viet Nam. From 1955 to 1961 there were 159 cases of liver cancer out of a total of 5492 cancer cases, and from 1962 to 1968, 791 out of a total of 7911 cancer cases. Van (1984) continued Tung's investigation. Previous exposure to herbicides of 21 male cases of primary liver cancer and 42 controls was ascertained. Six of the 21 cases and three of the controls had lived or worked in areas sprayed with herbicides or had moved there shortly after spraying ceased. Residence time varied from 8 to 77 months. There is a lack of information on confounding factors and there was a chance for bias in these studies. In general, the possibility of exposure to multiple chemicals and the short latency period noted make the study by Van (1984) of little value for assessing risk (IARC, 1986).

In 1979, the United States Air Force (USAF) initiated an epidemiological study into the possible health effects from chemical exposure of Air Force personnel who conducted aerial dissemination of herbicide in Viet Nam (Operation Ranch Hand) (Lathrop et al., 1984). The purpose of this investigation was to determine whether long-term health effects exist and can be attributed to occupational exposure to herbicides. This study used a matched cohort design in a non-concurrent prospective setting, incorporating mortality, morbidity, and follow-up studies. The report presented the results of health information on 2706 Ranch Handers and comparison individuals obtained by questionnaire and 2269 Ranch Handers and comparison individuals undergoing an extensive physical examination. It was concluded that there was insufficient evidence to support a cause and effect relationship between herbicide exposure and adverse health in the Ranch Hand group at this time. The study disclosed numerous medical findings, mostly of a minor or undetermined nature, that require detailed follow-up.

In a study of 15 soldiers in Australia exposed to Agent Orange, no increases in structural chromosomal aberrations or sister chromatid exchanges were noticed, compared to a control group of 8 subjects (Mulcahy, 1980). In 1980 the Australian Commonwealth Institute of Health agreed to conduct a series of scientific investigations into the health of Viet Nam veterans and their families. After considerating the most appropriate study programme, it was decided in 1981 to conduct, as part of that programme, a case-control study of congenital anomalies and Viet Nam service (Donovan et al., 1984). The report is largely negative, as is that of Erickson et al. (1984) which reported a similar study of American veterans.

8.3 Signs and Symptoms in Humans Associated With TCDD Exposure

Many signs and symptoms have been reported in studies of human exposures to PCDDs, both occupationally and from the general environment. These have been compiled from the various studies and are shown in Table 64.

8.3.1 Skin manifestations

Chloracne is a sign of exposure to several chlorinated cyclic organic compounds, the most potent being TCDD. Chloracne thus may serve as a marker of such exposure. The most distinctive lesion in chloracne is the so-called cyst, a skin-coloured elevation that may measure from 1 mm to 1 cm in diameter, with a central opening that may be difficult to detect. Comedones that contain black or black-appearing material in their openings are also present. There may be a secondary inflammatory reaction, melanosis, and hyperkeratosis, and these skin changes may be preceded by a "cable

Table 64. Signs and symptoms reported in association with human exposure to TCDD or mixtures containing TCDD

A. Skin Manifestations

1. Chloracne
2. Hyperkeratosis
3. Hyperpigmentation
4. Hirsutism
5. Elastosis

B. Systemic Effects

1. Mild fibrosis of liver
2. Raised transaminase values in blood
3. Hypercholesterolaemia
4. Hypertriglyceridaemia
5. Loss of appetite and weight loss
6. Digestive disorders (intolerance to alcohol or fatty food, flatulence, nausea, vomiting, diarrhoea)
7. Muscular aches and pains, joint pain, lower extremity weakness
8. Swollen lymph glands
9. Cardiovascular, urinary tract, respiratory, and pancreatic disorders

C. Neurological Effects

1. Sexual dysfunction
2. Headache
3. Neuropathy
4. Sight disturbance
5. Loss of hearing, taste, and smell

D. Psychiatric Effects

1. Sleep disturbance
2. Depression
3. Loss of energy and drive
4. Uncharacteristic bouts of anger

rash" or "cable itch". These skin lesions resemble photosensitivity reactions and the bearers may suffer severe pruritus. Microscopic examination of the skin lesions shows marked dilatation of the hair follicles which are filled with keratinous material, the sebaceous glands may be partly or completely atrophied and, occasionally, hyperplasia of these glands has also been reported. Hyperkeratosis and acanthosis of the surrounding epidermis usually accompany these lesions. Atrophy of the epithelium and thinning of the epithelial walls surrounding these keratinous cysts are observed at a later stage of the disease. If the follicular cysts rupture, foreign body granulomata may also be observed. Healing of these skin lesions usually results in deeply pitted scars. The distribution of chloracne is predominantly facial, affecting in particular the malar areas, the jaws, and the regions behind the ears. At times it may involve the ear canal and, with increasing severity, also the rest of the face and neck. In more extensive cases, the outer upper arms, neck, back, abdomen, outer thighs, and genitalia may also be involved (Crow, 1970).

While the absence of chloracne does not absolutely rule out exposure to TCDD, it usually indicates that there has been no exposure to a toxic dose of the substance. "Toxic" is used here to indicate both systemic and local effects. Where there has been exposure to TCDD and chloracne has resulted, it is the only known clinical sign that persists for a long period of time, even for the remainder of the exposed person's lifetime. In a large group of people exposed to mixtures containing TCDD, the absence of chloracne usually indicates that exposure to a toxic dose was unlikely and also makes it unlikely that severe, persistent systemic disorders will result.

Hyperkeratosis is a fairly common phenomenon whereas hyperpigmentation and hirsutism are rare. It should be noted that hyperkeratosis is prominent in the exposed Seveso children who have no affected sebaceous glands. These glands develop only at puberty.

Elastosis of the skin has been noted as a long-term effect of TCDD exposure.

8.3.2 Systemic effects

Liver effects following exposure to PCDDs have been diagnosed even by histological examination, and account for temporarily raised transaminases in blood, hypercholesteraemia, and hypertriglyceridaemia. Bauer et al. (1961) and Risse-Sundermann (1959) do not however exclude viral hepatitis as a cause of such findings in their patients exposed to TCDD. Loss of appetite, weight loss, and digestive disorders are common complaints from humans exposed to either TCDD itself, or to technical mixtures containing TCDD. Muscular aches and pain and weakness in extremities have been reported, particularly after exposure to technical mixtures containing TCDD. Swollen lymph nodes have also been reported, both after exposure to "pure" TCDD and to mixtures. The cardiovascular, urinary tract, respiratory, and pancreatic disorders reported are of doubtful significance with regard to a causal relationship to TCDD exposure.

Porphyria cutanea tarda has been reported in two cases of occupational exposure where chlorinated organic compounds were manufactured in addition to trichlorophenol. These were the incidents at the factory of Diamond Alkali, Newark, New Jersey, USA, in 1956 (Poland et al., 1971) and at Spolana, Czechoslovakia, between 1964 and 1969 (Pazerova-Vejlupkova et al., 1981). The porphyria cutanea tarda observed in these cases was very unlikely to have been induced by exposure to TCDD but rather by exposure to other chlorinated organic compounds manufactured in these plants (Jones & Chelsky, 1986).

8.3.3 Neurological effects

Sexual dysfunction (lack of libido and impotence) has been reported after acute exposure to both "pure" TCDD and technical mixtures (Schulz, 1968). The frequency of its occurrence may have been underestimated to date. Headache is a frequent symptom after exposures to technical mixtures containing TCDD.

Sensory neuropathy has been noted in many instances. Usually workers in the initial stages of exposure will complain of pains in their joints after they have very acute severe chloracne; however, there are usually no abnormal physical findings in the joints, but the complaints may continue. In early studies of workers affected by TCDD, no attempts were made to objectively measure the effects on the sensory nervous system. Tests have now been developed that evaluate sensory nerves and that can be used in future field studies. The nerve conduction tests, which primarily have been used so far, are actually not very useful to measure neuropathy. Differences in nerve conduction were shown among residents from Seveso, Italy, who had chloracne and those who did not (Richert, von, 1962; Fillipini et al., 1981).

Sight disturbance may be related to alkaline exposure or to conjunctivitis related to effects on the glands of Meibom. Loss of hearing, taste, and smell have been reported in a few cases, but a causal relationship to TCDD exposure is doubtful.

8.3.4 Psychiatric effects

The symptoms have been listed in Table 64 in what is believed to be their order of frequency and degree of severity.

8.4 Epidemiological Studies

Signs and symptoms related to accidental exposure to TCDD are given in Table 64. However, it should be observed that all the accidents and occupational contamination concern exposure to a mixture of compounds where TCDD was only one component. In all cases, its concentration in the mixtures was unknown. Only two cases of intoxication with "pure" TCDD have been reported.

The story of the discovery of TCDD is by now well documented (Holmstedt, 1980; Sandermann, 1984a, b). TCDD was synthetized in 1955. Four people were intoxicated, one co-worker severely so while drying crystals. In all cases, decreased libido was the first symptom, followed by other symptoms such as moderate to severe chloracne, sleeping difficulties, inability to concentrate, depression, and, in at least one case, swelling of the lymph nodes. In all cases, the signs and symptoms disappeared within a couple of years, with the exception of the chloracne in the most heavily exposed man.

The second occasion of exposure to what one must assume to be pure TCDD is the one reported by Oliver (1975). The toxic effects on three young scientists who suffered "transient minimal exposure to TCDD" were described. Two of them suffered from typical chloracne. Delayed symptoms about two years after initial exposure occurred in two of the scientists. These symptoms were said to have included personality changes, other neurological disturbances, and hirsutism. All three scientists were found to have raised serum cholesterol levels, but no other biochemical disturbances and no porphyrinuria or liver damage were demonstrated. Whether the unusually delayed physiological effects were in fact due to the initial dioxin exposure is a question that was discussed by the author. Although conclusive evidence is lacking, it seems likely that these delayed effects were in fact due to dioxin intoxication. The conditions of exposure remain unexplained.

Of the many cases of exposure reported in Table 63, only two (at Monsanto in 1949 and at BASF in 1953) have been adequately followed up epidemiologically with matched control groups.

The workers of Monsanto, USA, have been investigated several times between 1949 and 1984. Immediately after the accident, Ashe & Suskind (1949) hospitalized and studied four cases of severe poisoning among the workers. These four workers were diagnosed as having chloracne, but by the time of examination these men had recovered from earlier symptoms of peripheral neuropathy. In 1950, a further examination of these four workers and two additional men revealed continued irritability, nervousness, and insomnia (Ashe & Suskind, 1950). A consistent loss of libido and some impotence was reported. Further clinical examination revealed hepatomegaly, altered prothrombin times, and disturbed lipid metabolism.

A further study of 36 workers from this plant was undertaken in 1953 (Suskind et al., 1953). It was noted that even those who developed, to a moderate or severe degree, the skin eruptions, pains in back, dyspnoea, fatigue, nervousness, and decreased libido generally improved. Even those suffering the most severe cutaneous eruptions initially had only a few or no lesions in 1953.

More recent studies on these workers are those of Zack & Suskind (1980) and Zack & Gaffey (1983). Zack and Gaffey reported on a 121-member study cohort, with a presumptive high-peak exposure to TCDD base on chloracne occurrence, which was followed for mortality until 1978. The entire cohort was traced; there were 32 deaths; 89 people were still alive. There was no excess in total mortality or in deaths from malignant neoplasms. The proportional mortality analysis of decedents according to exposure by 2,4,5-trichlorophenoxyacetic acid (2,4,5-T) indicated no unusual patterns of mortality. The proportional mortality ratio (PMR) for malignant neoplasms was low (PMR = 82) in the exposed group. Lung cancer was the only site among the malignant neoplasms for which the value was somewhat higher in the exposed group.

The Monsanto workers were again examined in 1984 (Suskind & Herzberg, 1984). A clinical epidemiological study was conducted to determine the long-term health effects of workplace exposures during the process of manufacturing the herbicide 2,4,5-T, including contaminants such as TCDD. The population consisted of two cohorts, 204 clearly exposed and 163 not exposed (controls). Among the exposed workers, clinical evidence of chloracne persisted in 55.7%. None of the controls experienced chloracne development. An association was found between the persistence of chloracne and the presence and severity of actinic elastosis of the skin. There was an association between exposure and the history of ulcers of the gastrointestinal tract. Pulmonary function values among those who were exposed and who currently smoked were lower than those who were not exposed and who currently smoked. No disturbances of sexual functions were found at this time after age adjustment. The data assembled in the study indicated no evidence of increased risk for cardiovascular disease, hepatic disease, renal damage, or central or peripheral nervous system problems.

Another selection of the population from the same plant has been examined by another group of epidemiologists (Moses et al., 1984). Since the degree of exposure was unknown to these investigators and since chloracne is generally considered a quite reliable indicator of heavy dioxin exposure, it was decided to use chloracne as a "surrogate" for exposure and to classify the study population by its presence or absence. It was recognized that those without chloracne, but with appropriate work-exposure history, might also have had TCDD exposure and were not therefore used as "unexposed controls". Chloracne was found in 52% of 226 workers in a 1979 cross-sectional survey at the plant where 2,4,5-T had been manufactured from 1948 to 1969. Mean duration of residual chloracne was 26 years, and in 29 subjects it had been present for 30 years. A significantly increased prevalence of abnormal gamma-glutamyl transpeptidase (GGT) and higher mean GGT were found in those with chloracne compared to those without. Although mean triglyceride values were higher in those with chloracne, the difference was not statistically significant. Neurological examination showed a statistically significant higher prevalence of abnormal sensory findings in those with chloracne. Increased prevalence of angina and reported myocardial infarction in those with chloracne was not significant when age-adjusted. Increased prevalence of reported sexual dysfunction and decreased libido in those with chloracne, compared to those without, was statistically significant after age adjustment. No differences were found between those with and without chloracne in serum cholesterol, total urinary porphyrins, or in reproductive outcomes. Exposure to TCDD in 2,4,5-T production may thus result in apparently permanent changes in the skin. Sensory changes in peripheral nerves and possible changes in liver metabolism in those with current or past chloracne are also suggested by these data. Based on worker histories, even severe acute toxicological effects of TCDD are reversible, or improve markedly over time. While the cross-sectional nature of this study, the low participation rate, and the highly select nature of the population limit the conclusions that can be drawn, it is unlikely that permanent, severe, and debilitating toxicological sequelae are inevitable after exposure to TCDD sufficient to produce chloracne. It must be noted, however, that individual susceptibility may make certain workers with heavy exposures more vulnerable.

The exposure of workers at BASF in 1953 has been the subject of several reviews, the latest one being that of Thiess et al. (1982). Twenty-seven years after the accident that occurred in the BASF Ludwigshafen plant, a mortality study was undertaken of people exposed in the uncontrolled reaction which occurred during the trichlorophenol process. The follow-up was 100% successful and involved 74 people. Overall mortality (21 deaths) did not differ in this group from the rate expected in three external reference populations, or from that observed in two internal comparison groups, where 18-20 deaths were observed. Of the 21 deceased people, 7 had had cancer, compared with 4.1 expected. In addition, two other cases of cancer (one bronchial carcinoma and one carcinoma of the prostate) were still alive at the time of writing. Three deaths due to stomach cancer at ages 64, 66, and 69 years, were found, compared with 0.6 expected from regional mortality data. One stomach cancer occurred among 148 individuals in the two comparison cohorts. The incidence of cancer in these workers was considerably greater than expected and cannot be explained only as a chance event. Of 74 people, 66 had severe chloracne or severe dermatitis. There is a possibility that some members of the BASF cohort were exposed to other unknown occupational hazards before or after the accident. However, the use of two internal comparison groups composed of matched controls from the same factory was designed to control for, as far as possible, other occupational exposures that could be important etiological or confounding factors. Because of the small size of the cohort and the small absolute number of deaths from any particular cause, the results of this study do not permit any definite conclusions concerning the carcinogenic effect of exposure.

In comparison with the above-mentioned, well conducted long-term epidemiological studies, a host of other follow-up studies have been published, none of which used adequate controls. They are, therefore, of less value but will be briefly summarized here.

Jirasek et al. (1973, 1976) and Pazderova et al. (1974, 1980, 1981) examined 55 of a total of 80 workers who suffered intoxication during the manufacture of sodium pentachlorophenate and the sodium salt and butyl ester of 2,4,5-T. One worker died from severe acute intoxication at an early stage (Jirasek et al., 1976), and 76 workers developed chloracne. The following additional symptoms were found: porphyria cutanea tarda, disorders of the metabolism of lipids, porphyrins, and carbohydrates, and alteration of plasma proteins. Hepatic lesions were also present. Neurological and electromyographic (EMG) examinations revealed peripheral nerve changes in 17 people, first detected in 8 people during the second year of the study. A neurasthenic syndrome was also observed. The patients with porphyria cutanea tarda showed hyperpigmentation, hypertrichosis, and bullosis actinica mechanica. Porphyrin excretion in urine ranged from 172 to 2230 μg/24 h. Polyneuropathies, confirmed by EMG examination, were noted, predominantly in the lower extremities. In this outbreak, the disease was progressive during the first 2 years; subsequently the dermatological symptoms as well as the porphyric disease and the neurological disorders improved. The impaired lipid metabolism improved only very slowly.

In this plant, the toxic substances were led off through the breathing zone of the workers. The concentrations of the chlorinated hydrocarbons in the air were never measured. Due to insufficient data, the real hygienic conditions at the work place could not be accurately reconstructed. The manufacturing of 2,4,5-T was halted permanently in 1968 so that it was impossible to obtain the necessary information in an adequate manner. From 1959 to 1964, according to information from the plant, only sodium pentachlorophenate was manufactured. Not until 1965 was the manufacture of sodium 2,4,5-T commenced on a pilot scale, and later the butyl ester of 2,4,5-T was also manufactured. After each year of production, something was always changed or modified in the process and technology so that actually there was never full-scale production in the true sense of the word. Many of the herbicides manufactured could not be found from the documentation (Pazderova et al., 1974). The uncertain mixture of compounds involved in the Spolana episode makes interpretation of signs and symptoms almost impossible. In all likelihood the porphyria observed was due to the hexachlorobenzene stated to be produced at this factory.

Signs of disturbance in the porphyrin metabolism in workers manufacturing 2,4,5-T was also described by Poland et al. (1971). Chloracne was not correlated significantly with job location within the plant, duration of employment, or coproporphyrin excretion. Although 11 subjects with uroporphyria and at least three with overt porphyria cutanea tarda had been found in a study of the same plant six years earlier (Bleiberg et al., 1964), no clinical porphyria could be documented at the time of the second investigation, and only one worker had persistent uroporphyrinuria. Evidence of toxicity in other organ systems was markedly less than that reported in previous studies and in most instances there was no difference from normal populations. In all likelihood the porphyria cutanea tarda in this case, as in the study from Czechoslovakia, was due to a compound other than TCDD. This is corroborated by a recent re-evaluation of the literature (Jones & Chelsky, 1986).

A study from northern Germany was published by Bauer et al. (1961). It is not clear where the cases orginated and only nine patients were studied in depth. A summary of the findings from these patients, and another person suffering from chloracne after occupational exposure to trichlorphenol, was reported by Kleu & Göltz (1971). These patients were followed for 15 years after exposure. The severity and types of symptoms varied in a dose-related manner. Major complaints were decreased sexual activity, muscular weakness, easy fatigability, irritability, and loss of appetite and memory. The authors concluded that a permanent defect had occurred, the late form of which resembled a cerebral involutionary syndrome, combined with mental depression and neurasthenia.

A follow-up study of 11 of the 24 employees at Boehringer exhibiting skin lesions in 1955 was published by von Krause & Brassow (1978). Many continued to suffer from their earlier complaints. In seven of the eleven, nausea and intolerance to heavy fatty food was still common, and six men complained of alcohol intolerance. Although conjunctivitis had disappeared, chloracne was still clearly visible in most of the 11 subjects. Neurological problems were still severe in six of the workers.

Ten years after the incident at Coalite in 1968 when 79 workers developed chloracne due to exposure to a chlorophenol-TCDD mixture, a study was undertaken to establish the state of health of the affected employees (46) remaining in the company's employment (May, 1982). Forty-one of the 46 employees participated. The opportunity was used to examine effects on mortality, morbidity, carcinogenesis, reproduction, teratogenicity, fetotoxicity, biochemistry, immunology, and genetic changes. Concurrently, two control groups were established, one with no dioxin exposure and the other with possible dioxin exposure. These groups were selected from within the works and matched the study group with respect to sex and age, but it was not possible to match them for occupation and social status. Half the affected subjects still had minor chloracne. Other than this finding, the authors concluded that the subjects had not been had been adversely affected in any way.

Data on the mortality of workers at the Dow Chemical company have been provided in two papers (Cook et al., 1980; Ott et al., 1980). The first of these studies describes the mortality of a cohort of 61 males involved in the preparation of trichlorophenol. Forty-nine of these workers developed chloracne, presumably as a result of skin absorption of the process contaminant TCDD. Within the limitations posed by cohort size and length of follow-up, the exposure to chlorophenol-TCDD mixtures did not appear to have adversely affected mortality experience. Overall, four deaths occurred and 7.8 were expected. Of these, one death was due to cardiovascular disease (3.8 expected) and three deaths were attributed to cancer (1.6 expected). None of the findings was statistically significant. The second paper examined the mortality experience of 204 people exposed to 2,4,5-T during its manufacture from 1950 to 1971. Length of employment within the 2,4,5-T process area ranged from less than one year to a maximum of approximately ten years. Efforts to minimize TCDD contamination of the product resulted in non-detectable concentrations (less than 1 mg/kg) near the end of this period. Within the scope of this mortality survey, no adverse effects were observed with respect to occupational exposure to 2,4,5-T or to its feedstock, 2,4,5-trichlorophenol.

Hardell and his co-workers in Sweden have conducted a series of case-control studies and reported an increased risk of soft-tissue sarcomas in men who were exposed to phenoxy herbicides and/or chlorophenols (Hardell & Sandsstrom, 1979; Hardell, 1981; Hardell et al., 1981; Hardell & Ericksson, 1981). These authors also reported a case-control study that suggested that phenoxyacetic acids and chlorophenols may predispose to Hodgkin's lymphoma (Hardell et al., 1981). The relative risk was higher for a group exposed to phenoxy herbicides including 2,4,5-T and chlorophenols, i.e., pesticides that may be contaminated with PCDDs and PCDFs. However, an increased risk was still found in a group exposed mainly to phenoxy herbicides such as MCPA, 2,4-D, mecoprop and dichloroprop, i.e., pesticides with low or no contamination with PCDDs and PCDFs.

Analysis of fat levels of PCDDs and PCDFs in patients with soft tissue sarcomas and in controls failed to reveal any differences between the two groups (Nygren et al., 1986) (section 4.4.4.1).

A cohort study on Swedish farmers and gardeners has been carried out recently (Wiklund & Holm, 1986). Despite the greatly increased use of phenoxyacetic acid herbicides from 1947 to 1970, no time-related increase in the relative risk of soft-tissue sarcoma was found in the cohort or in any of the subcohorts. The same was found by Hoar et al. (1986) although the latter study points to an increase in non-Hodgkin lymphoma. It should be noted that in all these studies the majority of the herbicides used did not contain TCDD.

In follow-up studies of workers exposed to 2,4,5-T and its precursor 2,4,5-trichlorophenol (and therefore, presumably, also to TCDD), no excessive deaths due to any cause were registered (Cook et al., 1980; Ott et al., 1980; Zack & Suskind, 1980; Zack & Gaffey, 1983).

Honchar & Halperin (1981) merged the above four cohorts and found that three (2.9%) of the total 105 deaths were reported to be from soft-tissue sarcoma. Based on national statistics only 0.07% was expected to be due to this cause. Fingerhut et al. (1984) reviewed the employment records, medical and pathological reports, tissue specimens, and death certificates for these three cases and four additional cases of deaths from soft tissue sarcomas in these and related cohorts reported by Cook (1981), Moses & Selikoff (1981), and Johnson et al. (1981). Three out of the seven cases had a record of chloracne and one of dermatitis. After review of the tissue specimens, five of the seven cases were diagnosed as soft-tissue sarcoma. The remaining two (which were among the three cases in the merged cohort of Honchar & Halperin (1981)) were found to be carcinoma. For three of the cases with confirmed soft-tissue sarcoma the exposure was not well documented, although an undocumented contact with 2,4,5-T, 2,4,5-trichlorophenol, or TCDD could not be excluded.

8.5 Human Experimental Studies

Poiger & Schlatter (1986) studied a human volunteer after ingestion of a single dose of 1.14 µg ^{3}H-TCDD/kg body weight. The absorption from the intestine was > 87% and adipose tissue levels were 3.09 ($\pm$ 0.05) and 2.85 ($\pm$ 0.28) ng/kg after 13 and 69 days, respectively. The estimated half-life of TCDD was 2120 days.

Gorski et al. (1984) calculated the half-lives of 1,2,3,6,7,8-hexaCDD, 1,2,3,4,6,7,8-heptaCDD and octaCDF to be about 3.5, 3.6 and 2 years, respectively. The estimation was based on the analysis of fat tissue biopsies collected with an interval of 28 months from one 14-year-old girl who for a period of about 2-3 years had been exposed to technical pentachlorophenol. Analysis was performed by gas chromatography with electron capture detection, and the isomers were confirmed by the use of several different packed and capillary columns.

9. TOXICOKINETICS OF PCDFs

9.1 Uptake, Distribution, and Excretion

Toxicokinetic data for TCDF and other PCDFs arise from iv injections or gastrointestinal exposure. There are no studies on exposure via the respiratory tract or via dermal application.

9.1.1 Studies with 2,3,7,8-tetrachlorodibenzofuran (2,3,7,8-TCDF)

Table 65 summarizes the distribution of radioactivity to the major tissue depots at various time-points after an iv injection of ^{14}C-TCDF into rats and mice. Similar studies in guinea-pigs and monkeys are summarized in Table 66. Tables 67 and 68 give the tissue distribution of ^{14}C-TCDF in more detail for rats and mice, respectively.

TCDF has been used for kinetic studies in the rat (Birnbaum et al., 1980), mouse (Decad et al., 1981a), guinea-pig (Decad et al., 1981b), and monkey (Birnbaum et al., 1981). A single iv dose of 30.6 µg ^{14}C-TCDF/kg body weight was given to rats, mice, and monkeys, while the guinea-pigs received an iv dose of 6 µg/kg body weight. The distribution of the radio-label was followed in tissues and excreta for 3 weeks in rats and monkeys, for 10 days in mice, and for 9 days in guinea-pigs. The distribution of radioactivity in the main tissues and excreta of the different species at some of the intervals studied is presented in Tables 65 and 66 along with the respective half-lives and LD_{50} values for TCDF. Radioactivity recovered from the tissues represented the parent compound, while radioactivity in faeces and urine represented metabolites of TCDF. In the faeces of guinea-pigs only the parent substance was present. Analysis by thin-layer chromatography revealed Rf values of 0.5 and 0.1 for metabolites of TCDF in faeces and urine as compared to an Rf of 0.8 for the parent compound.

TCDF has a short half-life (2-4 days) and is quickly eliminated from the liver, both in the rat and the mouse (Birnbaum et al., 1980; Decad et al., 1981a). Elimination occurs rapidly also from the skin and muscle, whereas retention is longer in adipose tissues. The difference in the retention of TCDF in adipose tissues between C57Bl/6 and DBA/2 mice may be explained by the fact that DBA/2 mice have substantially more adipose tissues than C57Bl/6 mice.

The distribution of TCDF in the guinea-pig was different from that in the rat or mouse (Decad et al., 1981b). The maximum uptake in the liver occurred within one hour after

Table 65. LD_{50}, whole-body half-life, and distribution of radioactivity (percentage of administered dose) at various intervals after an iv dose of 30.6 µg ^{14}C-TCDF/kg to rats[a] and mice[b]

	Fisher 344 Rats			C57BL/6 Mice			DBA/2 Mice		
	3 hr	3 days	10 days	3 h	3 days	10 days	3 h	3 days	10 days
Liver	41.4±3.6	5.9±0.3	1.3	51.0±13.4	22.7±1.8	1.1±0.3	39.4±0.6	16.8±1.4	5.6±2.0
Fat	10.0±1.0	11.1±2.3	1.8	6.0±1.6	2.9±2.1	ND	9.6±3.9	22.3±2.9	7.2±0.9
Skin	6.6±0.3	1.2±0.3	0.5	3.6±0.7	3.0±1.1	ND	5.5±4.3	3.3±0.9	ND
Muscle	5.9±0.4	0.3	< 0.3	7.5±2.8	1.5±0.9	ND	10.8±3.4	5.4±1.9	1.8±0.4
Faeces		63.1±0.6	> 85		43.1	81.9±13.0		27.7	55.8±4.8
Urine		2.0±0.4	< 6		7.7	12.6±0.1		9.2	19.9±4.6
Half-life (days)		< 2[b]			2[b]			4[b]	
LD_{50} (µg/kg)		>1000[c]			> 6000[c, d]				

[a] Birnbaum et al. (1980).
[b] Decad et al. (1981b).
[c] Moore et al. (1976).
[d] Moore et al. (1979).
ND = not detectable.

Table 66. LD_{50}, whole-body half-life, and distribution of radioactivity (percentage of administered dose) at various intervals after an iv dose of ^{14}C-TCDF in guinea-pigs[a] and monkeys[b]

	Hartley guinea-pigs			Rhesus monkeys
	3 h	3 days	9 days	21 days
Liver	23.6±3.8	29.3±0.6	54.2±14.5	1.02±0.80
Fat	31.4±0.7	56.9±7.6	21.8±11.6	3.66±2.83
Skin	22.5±0.1	17.1±+0.6	15.2±3.1	2.44±1.60
Muscle		15.6±4.5	8.8±3.0	1.55±0.14
Faeces		4.7±1.3	6.6	42.9
Urine		2.3±0.4	6.6	7.9
Half-life (days)		> 20[c]		8[a]
LD_{50} (μg/kg)		> 5[c] < 10[d]		1000[d]

[a] 6 μg/kg (Decad et al., 1981a).
[b] 30.6 μg/kg (Birnbaum et al., 1981).
[c] Moore et al. (1976).
[d] Moore et al. (1979).

Table 67. Tissue distribution of TCDF-derived radioactivity in Fisher 344 rats at 15 min, 3 h, and 24 h following a single iv dose of 30.6 μg ^{14}C-TCDF/kg [b]

Tissue	Tissue content of ^{14}C (% of dose/g tissue)[a]		
	15 min	3 h	24 h
Blood	0.12±0.04	0.04±0.01	0.03±0.01
Liver	4.4 ±0.2	5.1 ±0.4	2.2 ±0.4
Fat	0.20±0.03	0.44±0.07	0.64±0.11
Muscle	0.25±0.01	0.06±0.00	0.30±0.02
Skin	0.17±0.02	0.20±0.01	0.07±0.01
Kidneys	0.67±0.04	0.17±0.03	0.08±0.01
Adrenals	7.4 ±6.9	4.7 ±1.3	0.34±0.14
Thymus	0.52±0.12	0.54±0.13	0.07±0.03
Spleen	0.37±0.07	0.08±0.02	0.02±0.00
Testes	0.09±0.01	0.09±0.01	0.06±0.02
Brain	0.25±0.01	0.15±0.03	0.02±0.00
Lungs	1.08±0.08	0.24±0.02	0.07±0.02
Heart	0.66±0.03	0.11±0.00	0.02±0.02

[a] Mean ± SD for three animals.
[b] From: Birnbaum et al. (1980).

Table 68. Tissue distribution[a] of TCDF-derived radioactivity in C57Bl/6 and DBA/2 mice at 15 min, 3 h, and 24 h after a single iv dose of 30.6 μg ^{14}C-TCDF/kg [b]

Tissue	Tissue content of ^{14}C (% of dose/g tissue)[a]					
	15 min		3 h		24 h	
	C57Bl/6	DBA/2	C57Bl/6	DBA/2	C57Bl/6	DBA/2
Blood	1.1	ND	0.6±0.3	0.22±0.04	ND	0.2±0.0
Liver	28.0±4.2	30.7±2.8	39.3±2.8	38.0 ±3.8	25.3±4.2	19.2±1.9
Adipose	2.6±0.4	2.7±1.0	3.7±1.4	4.9 ±0.1	6.1±1.2	6.1±0.4
Muscle	1.3±0.1	1.6±0.2	0.7±0.2	0.9 ±0.3	0.3±0.1	0.8±0.1
Skin	2.2±0.1	2.3±0.7	1.4±0.2	2.7 ±0.6	1.3±0.7	2.7±0.6
Kidneys	3.4±0.3	4.1±0.5	1.1±0.3	1.3 ±0.3	0.6±0.1	0.7±0.2
Adrenals	18.8±4.9	ND	6.9±5.4	9.2	6.5	ND
Thymus	3.9±2.4	3.0±1.9	2.0±0.7	4.7 ±3.2	0.3±0.2	2.5±0.6
Spleen	1.4±0.1	1.7±0.3	0.8±0.1	0.5 ±0.1	0.2±0.1	0.27
Testes	0.4±0.1	0.6±0.1	0.5±0.2	1.0 ±0.2	0.2±0.2	0.4±0.3
Brain	1.7±0.5	2.4±0.3	0.8±0.1	1.3 ±0.3	0.2±0.3	2.7±2.7
Lungs	6.7±0.5	8.2±0.7	2.4±0.9	3.1 ±1.5	0.4±0.2	0.8±0.4
Heart	2.1±1.3	3.4±2.2	0.6±0.3	0.8 ±0.4	0.2±0.1	0.3±0.1

[a] Mean ± SD for three animals.
[b] From: Decad et al. (1981b).
ND = below limit for accurate detection.

dosing; thereafter the radioactivity was distributed in the fat and skin during the succeeding hours. After one day, as a result of loss of body fat, the radioactivity in adipose tissues was redistributed to the liver. Within 3 days after dosing there was no elimination of radioactivity from the liver and adipose tissues, whereas in the skin radioactivity decreased only slightly. The estimated half-life for TCDF in the guinea-pig was more than 20 days.

Based on data from three monkeys, the half-life for TCDF was calculated to be 8 days (Birnbaum et al., 1981). At the end of the study, more radioactivity remained in adipose tissues and skin than in the liver. The retention of TCDF in the liver of monkeys 21 days after dosing was comparable to that in the liver of the rat and C57Bl/6 mouse 10 days after injection. Urinary elimination of radioactivity was a minor route when compared to faecal elimination both in the rat, mouse, and monkey, whereas in the guinea-pig these routes were of comparable importance (Birnbaum et al., 1980, 1981; Decad et al., 1981a,b). The cumulated excretion of radioactivity 3 days post-treatment amounted to approximately 64, 51, 11, and 7% in the rat, C57Bl/6-mouse, monkey, and guinea-pig, respectively.

Against this background of data on tissue distributions, half-lives, and LD_{50} values of TCDF in the rat, guinea-pig, and monkey, Birnbaum et al. (1980, 1981) concluded that TCDF, measured as excreted radioactivity, is metabolized to less toxic compounds and that animal species with a high capacity to metabolize TCDF are more resistant to its acute toxicity. This conclusion was considered applicable also to the mouse (Decad et al., 1981a). Based on the same data King et al. (1983) produced a pharmacokinetic model for TCDF in rats, mice, and monkeys. However, there are objections to this comprehensive conclusion. First, the kinetic studies on guinea-pigs (Decad et al., 1981b) were (for analytical reasons) carried out with such a high dose of TCDF that all of the animals showed marked signs of toxicity, even within 3 days. After 9 days all the animals were killed due to toxic symptoms. It is not advisable to draw any conclusions on normal kinetic behaviour from data obtained on dying animals with their abnormal metabolism and physiology. As far as the kinetic data from the monkey are concerned, the conclusions were based on a single time-point, and the number of animals in that study was also very limited (Birnbaum et al., 1981).

Ioannou et al. (1983) calculated a whole-body half-life of approximately 40 days for a non-toxic dose of TCDF in young male Hartley guinea-pigs. Their estimation was based on the distribution of TCDF-derived radioactivity in liver, adipose tissue, skin, and muscle in three animals 36 days after a single oral dose of 4 µg TCDF/kg body weight and on certain approximations obtained from a previous study (Decad et al., 1981b). Failure to demonstrate a correlation between degree of bioaccumulation and lethality of TCDF in this study may be due partly to the calculations of body burden based on the uncertain estimate of the 40 days half-life for TCDF, which may not be valid for both toxic and non-toxic doses of TCDF.

9.1.2 Studies with other PCDFs

Young male Wistar rats absorbed approximately 68% of a single oral dose of 1.0 mg 2,3,4,7,8-pentaCDF/kg body weight given in salad oil (Yoshimura et al., 1986). The daily faecal excretion was about 0.1% of the administered dose/day, whereas no 2,3,4,7,8-pentaCDF was detected in urine. Four weeks after dosing the retention of 2,3,4,7,8-pentaCDF in the liver was 48.8% of the dose. The addition of 5% of activated charcoal beads to the diet, one week after dosing and throughout the study, increased the faecal elimination of 2,3,4,7,8-penta CDF about 3-fold, but had no effect on urinary elimination. Both the liver and extrahepatic tissues, except the kidney, from rats on basal diet supplemented with activated charcoal beads had lower levels of 2,3,4,7,8-pentaCDF than rats on basal diet only.

Yoshihara et al. (1981) administered single ip injections of 13 individual PCDF congeners (at 1, 5, or 10 µg/kg) to young male Wistar rats, and retention of the respective isomers in the liver was determined 5 days later. The great variation observed in the hepatic accumulation of the various isomers seemed to depend on the position as well as the number of chlorine atoms substituted. Isomers having vicinal hydrogens were accumulated to a lesser degree, although three of the six isomers having no vicinal hydrogens (1,3,6,8-tetraCDF, TCDF, and 1,2,4,6,8-pentaCDF) also showed low accumulation. The isomer most highly accumulated was 2,3,4,7,8-pentaCDF, more than 65% of the dose being retained, whereas only 3.8% of TCDF, which is equally potent biologically, was retained. These results would imply that there is no relationship between hepatic distribution of PCDFs and their potential for acute toxicity. All animals in this study showed toxic symptoms and liver microsomal AHH activity was strongly induced, except in the cases of the following isomers: 2,8-diCDF, 1,2,7,8-tetraCDF, 1,3,6,7-tetraCDF, 1,3,6,8-tetraCDF, 1,2,4,6,8-pentaCDF. It is important to take this into consideration when judging the kinetic data. A mixture of 14% 1,2,7,8-tetraCDF, 35% TCDF, 1% 1,2,4,7,8-pentaCDF, 49% 1,2,3,7,8-pentaCDF, 1% 2,3,4,7,8-pentaCDF, and 1% hexaCDF was administered as a single ip dose of 10 mg PCDF/kg body weight to young male Wistar rats (Kuroki et al., 1980). The retention of the isomers in the liver, 5 days post-treatment, showed good agreement with the results of Yoshihara et al. (1981).

Based on the purification of three isoenzymes of cytochrome P-450 and the recovery of ^{14}C-radioactivity from the hepatic microsomes of Wistar rats treated with ^{14}C-2,3,4,7,8-pentaCDF (single ip dose of 1 mg/kg body weight, 5 days previously), Kuroki et al. (1986) suggested that one of these isoenzymes, P-448 H, functions as the storage site of 2,3,4,7,8-pentaCDF in the rat liver.

Fly ash and crude or purified toluene extracts of PCDD- and PCDF-containing fly ash from a municipal incinerator (Zaanstad, The Netherlands) were mixed with ordinary laboratory diet for rats (van den Berg et al., 1983). Small portions (2 g) of these diets were fed to male Wistar rats (300 g) every 24 h for 19 days, at which time the animals were sacrificed. The levels of tetra-. penta-, and hexa-chlorinated PCDDs and PCDFs in samples of liver and adipose tissue from these rats were determined. Rats fed the fly ash-containing diet stored PCDDs and PCDFs in their livers at concentrations which were at least 3 to 5 times lower than those of rats fed with comparable amounts of fly ash extracts. For the pentaCDD, hexaCDF, and hexaCDD isomers these concentrations were approximately 10-20 times lower. Generally PCDFs had a higher retention in the liver of rats than the corresponding PCDDs. In the adipose tissue of rats fed with fly ash extracts, retention was higher for penta- and hexaCDDs than for the corresponding PCDFs.

In a later study, male Wistar rats (275 g) were fed a diet containing the same fly ash, pretreated with 2.5% HCl (van den Berg et al., 1986a). A control group received standard diet. All congeners retained in the livers of the rats had a 2,3,7,8-chlorine substitution pattern. With the exception of 2,3,4,7,8-pentaCDF and 2,3,4,6,7,8-hexaCDF, the retention for each congener was below 10% of the dose. The retention percentages of the various congeners in the liver were almost equal at all time-points studied (34, 59, and 99 days), thus indicating a long half-life of these congeners in the liver of the rat.

A mixture of two tetraCDFs, four pentaCDFs, and four hexaCDFs, was given as a single ip injection of 500 µg to male ICR mice (Morita & Oishi, 1977). The distribution patterns of the isomers in various tissues were followed for up to 8 weeks. Analyses were performed with GC (with electron capture detection) and isomers were identified by peak number only. PCDFs were mainly located in the liver, spleen, and fat tissues, but low to minimal amounts were found also in the kidney, testes, lungs, heart, and brain. The GC patterns of liver samples changed markedly with time, in contrast to those of the other tissues, including fat, where the GC patterns remained similar throughout the study. Most isomers with shorter retention times were readily absorbed and then rapidly disappeared from the liver. Isomers with longer retention times were slowly absorbed, and thus appeared later and persisted longer in the liver. If the mixture had been administered orally, those isomers with long retention times might have passed the gastrointestinal tract with very low absorption.

The hepatic retention of PCDDs and PCDFs after dietary intake of the above-mentioned HCl-pretreated fly ash was studied in male Golden Syrian hamsters (van den Berg et al., 1986b). The livers were analyzed for tetra-, penta-, and hexaCDDs and -CDFs after feeding the diet, which contained 25% fly ash. No detectable hepatic retention was observed after 34 days. The highest retention after 95 days was 8.4% for 2,3,4,7,8-pentaCDF, but the retention was generally below 5% of the total dose. With the exception of 2,3,4,6,7-pentaCDF, only 2,3,7,8-substituted PCDDs and PCDFs were retained. Constant relative concentrations were found for the 2,3,7,8-substituted PCDDs and PCDFs at the time-points studied.

In studies by Firestone et al. (1979), three lactating Holstein cows received commercial grade pentachlorophenol orally by gelatine capsule at a dose rate of 10 mg/kg body weight twice daily for 10 days and once daily for the following 60 days. One cow served as a control and received gelatine capsules containing only ground corn. The pentachlorophenol composite used contained ten PCDD congeners (0.1-690 mg/kg) and eight PCDF congeners (0.9-130 mg/kg). Faeces collected on day 28 of the treatment period contained three hexaCDDs (0.05-0.63 μg/kg), two heptaCDDs (21.3-33.1 μg/kg), and octaCDD (290-429 μg/kg). Faeces also contained hexa-, hepta-, and octaCDF. Milk, body fat, and blood contained only three of the PCDD congeners present in the pentachlorophenol composite, namely 1,2,3,6,7,8-hexaCDD, 1,2,3,4,6,7,8-heptaCDD, and octaCDD. Milk samples also contained hexa-, hepta-, and octaCDF. The average concentrations of 1,2,3,6,7,8-hexaCDD, 1,2,3,4,6,7,8-heptaCDD, octaCDD, and octaCDF in the composite milk fat at the end of the treatment period were 20, 40, 25, and 2 mg/kg, respectively. Similar concentrations were found in body (shoulder) fat at the end of the treatment period (13, 24, and 32 mg/kg, respectively, for 1,2,3,6,7,8-hexaCDD, 1,2,3,4,6,7,8-heptaCDD, and octaCDD). Levels of dioxins in the blood were about 1000 times below the values in milk or body fat. The average daily excretion of 1,2,3,6,7,8-hexaCDD, 1,2,3,4,6,7,8-heptaCDD, and octaCDD in the milk during days 40 to 70 of treatment was about 20, 40, and 23 μg (corresponding, respectively, to 33, 3, and 0.6% of the daily intake of PCDDs). One hundred days after cessation of treatment the average levels of 1,2,3,6,7,8-hexaCDD, 1,2,3,4,6,7,8-heptaCDD, and octaCDD in shoulder fat and milk fat were 2.5, 6.6, 5.6 mg/kg and 4.3, 6.9, 3.0 mg/kg, respectively.

9.2 Metabolic Transformation

Thirteen chlorinated compounds were detected in bile collected for 48 h from female Sprague Dawley rats given a single oral dose of 678 μg TCDF (79.4% pure)/kg body weight (Poiger et al., 1984). The four major metabolites considered to originate from TCDF were trichloromethoxy-dibenzofuran, two trichlorodimethoxy-dibenzofurans, and tetrachloromethoxy-dibenzofuran. The remaining nine metabolites, detected in minute amounts, originated most likely from contaminating PCDFs (1% triCDF, 8.4% tetraCDFs, 11.2% pentaCDFs).

Metabolites of 2-monoCDF, 2,8-diCDF, 2,3,8-triCDF, and octaCDF were determined in the urine, faeces, fat, and liver of male Wistar rats given single oral doses of 250 mg/kg body weight of the respective isomers (Veerkamp et al., 1981). Analyses were performed with GC-MS. No metabolites in any samples were found in rats given octaCDF. Monohydroxy and dihydroxy derivatives were obtained with all other isomers, whereas sulfur-containing metabolites were detected only with the monoCDF and diCDF. Metabolites from 2-monoCDF and 2,3,8-triCDF were found in urine and faeces only, but with 2,8-diCDF metabolites appeared also in the tissues.

9.3 Transfer Via Placenta and/or Milk

Nagayama et al. (1980) studied the transport of a mixture of PCDFs into the placenta and milk in the mouse (Table 69). A diet containing 0.6 mg PCDFs/kg (48% tetraCDFs, 49% pentaCDFs, and 3% hexaCDFs) was given for 18 days after mating. Nine dams were killed on day 18 of pregnancy and 10 on day 14 after delivery. After giving birth, the mothers were fed a diet free of PCDFs. The placental transport, calculated from the amount of PCDFs in the neonates, was about 0.003% of the administered dose. The isomers that remained in the tissues were TCDF and 2,3,4,7,8-pentaCDF. While the levels of PCDFs in the mothers dropped from 5.2% to 1.6% of the total intake, the whole-body levels in the sucklings increased from 0.003% at the time of birth to 0.07% after one week and to 0.14% of the total intake after 2 weeks. TCDF and 2,3,4,7,8-pentaCDF were the dominant species in both the mothers and the pups. To study the transport through milk only, the same PCDF-containing diet was given to pregnant rats for 14 days from day 18 after mating, including the lactation period (Nagayama et al., 1980) (Table 70). After 14 days 5.1% of the total intake was found in the liver of the mother. The offspring contained 0.3% and 1.2% of the dam's intake after 1 and

Table 69. Levels of PCDFs in the liver of dams and in fetuses and offspring after oral administration of PCDFs to mice for 18 days during pregnancy[f]

PCDF congener	Total intake of PCDFs by dams killed on day 18 of pregnancy (μg)[d]	% of PCDF intake in:[a]		Total intake of PCDFs by dams killed 2 weeks after delivery (μg)	% of PCDF intake in:[b]		
		liver of dam	fetus		liver of dam	offspring (week) 1	2
tetraCDF[c]	1.4±0.06[d]	5.4	ND	1.6±0.10	ND	ND	ND
tetraCDF[c]	8.1±0.32	ND	ND	9.0±0.57	ND	ND	ND
2,3,7,8-tetraCDF	11.4±9.46	5.5	0.007	12.5±0.79	0.03	0.05	T[e]
pentaCDF[c]	2.9±0.12	5.7	ND	3.1±0.20	4.0	0.10	0.27
pentaCDF[c]	13.2±0.53	3.9	0.004	14.5±0.91	0.1	0.03	T[e]
2,3,4,7,8-pentaCDF	4.9±0.20	14.5	ND	5.4±0.34	10.0	0.29	0.89
hexaCDF[c]	1.4±0.06	10.7	ND	1.6±0.10	6.4	0.28	0.76
Total	43.2±1.73	5.2	0.003	47.7±3.0	1.6	0.07	0.14

[a] Nine dams in group killed on day 18 of pregnancy.
[b] Ten dams in group killed on day 14 after delivery.
[c] Specific isomer not determined.
[d] Mean ± SEM.
[e] T = 0.01-0.1 μg/kg total congener.
[f] From: Nagayama et al. (1980).
ND = not detected.

Table 70. Levels of PCDFs in the liver of mouse dams and in offspring after oral administration of PCDFs to dams for 14 days following delivery[e]

PCDF congener	Total intake of PCDF (µg)[c]	% of PCDF intake in:[a]		
		liver of dam	offspring (week) 1	2
tetraCDF[b]	2.3±0.13	6.9	ND	ND
tetraCDF[b]	12.9±0.71	ND	ND	ND
2,3,7,8-tetraCDF	17.9±3.10	5.6	0.5	1.4
pentaCDF[b]	4.4±0.24	6.7	T[d]	0.6
pentaCDF[b]	21.0±1.14	3.7	0.4	1.6
2,3,4,7,8-pentaCDF	7.7±0.42	13.8	0.4	2.2
hexaCDF[b]	2.3±0.13	7.9	T[d]	1.5
Total	68.3±3.75	5.1	0.3	1.2

[a] Ten dams in the group.
[b] Specific isomer not known.
[c] Mean ± SEM.
[d] T = 0.01-0.1 µg/kg total congener.
[e] From: Nagayama et al. (1980).
ND = not detected.

2 weeks, respectively. The dominant isomers recovered in the offspring were TCDF, 2,3,4,7,8-pentaCDF, and one unidentified pentaCDF, i.e., the same isomers found in the largest amounts in the mother's liver. The data demonstrated that the amounts of PCDFs transferred through milk were much larger than the amounts transferred across the placenta.

Weber & Birnbaum (1985) studied the distribution and placental transfer of a single oral dose of 800 µg ^{14}C-TCDF (0.0485 µCi/µg)/kg body weight to pregnant C57Bl/6 mice on gestation day 11. Embryo mortality on gestation days 12 to 14 was in the range 7.9 to 17.8%. No detectable radioactivity was found in the embryos whereas about 0.01% of the radioactive dose was contained in the placenta. The hepatic radioactivity in the dams decreased rapidly from 30.0% of the dose on gestation day 12 to 12.1% of the dose on gestation day 14. The cumulative urinary and faecal excretion from gestation day 12 to 14 were 5.4 and 80.1% of the administered dose, respectively.

10. EFFECTS OF PCDFs ON ANIMALS

10.1 Acute Toxicity

Single oral LD_{50} values for TCDF in three species are listed in Table 71.

10.1.1 Studies on rats

No histological changes associated with TCDF toxicity could be observed in rats at oral doses up to 1000 µg TCDF/kg body weight (Moore et al., 1976). These preliminary results, which also mentioned that only mild toxicological changes occurred in rats at 6000 µg TCDF/kg body weight, have not been presented in a final report.

Intravenous administration of 30.6 µg TCDF/kg body weight to male Fisher rats has been shown to cause listlessness, excessive hair loss, and decreased weight gain 2 days post-treatment. These adverse effects were reversible and 3 weeks after dosing the animals appeared healthy with normal body weight. There were no signs of thymic or splenic atrophy or of liver hypertrophy (Birnbaum et al., 1980).

Single ip injection of 1 or 10 mg/kg body weight of nine individual PCDF isomers, with at least three chlorines in the lateral positions, to male Wistar rats produced thymus atrophy and liver hypertrophy 5 days post-treatment. Five other congeners having no more than two chlorine atoms in the lateral positions did not cause any effects on the thymus or liver within the same dose range (Yoshihara et al., 1981).

The ability of 15 individual PCDFs to affect body weight gain and thymic atrophy in immature male Wistar rats was investigated 14 days after a single ip injection (Ganon et al., 1985). The ED_{50} values for both effects were estimated for each congener (Table 61).

10.1.2 Studies on mice

Moore et al. (1976) failed to establish a lethal dose for TCDF in C57Bl/6 mice after giving single oral doses of up to 6000 µg/kg body weight with an observation period of 30 days. However, there was a transient depression in body weight gain, thymic involution, and mild hepatotoxicity when 6000 µg TCDF/kg was given subcutaneously. Poland & Glover (1980) found TCDF-induced thymus atrophy in C57Bl/6 mice 5 days after a single ip dose of 3×10^{-7} mol/kg body weight.

Single doses of 100 to 1000 µg TCDF/kg body weight to pregnant C57Bl/6 mice on gestation days 10 to 13 produced no toxic effects on the dams within the time studied (Hassoun et al., 1984a; Weber et al., 1984).

Table 71. Single lethal dose values for TCDF[a]

Species/strain	Sex/No	Age or weight	Dose tested (μg/kg[c] body weight)	Duration of study (days)	LD_{50} (μg/kg body weight)	Time to death (days)
Mice (C57B1/6)	M/8	6 weeks	0 400 600 800 1200 1500 2500 4000 6000	30	> 6000	not reported
Guinea-pigs (Hartley)	M/6	3-4 weeks	0 1 5 10 15	30	5-10	9-20
Monkeys (*Macaca mulatta*)	F/2	2.0-3.7 kg	0 300 1000 1500	60	1000	14-31

[a] From: Moore et al. (1979).
[b] M = male; F = female.
[c] Doses were given orally in corn oil.

A mixture of two tetraCDFs, four pentaCDFs and four hexaCDFs given as a single ip dose of 500 µg to ICR mice produced no deaths within 8 weeks (Morita & Oishi, 1977). CF-1 mice given a PCDF mixture containing 42% tetraCDFs, 54% pentaCDFs, and 4% hexaCDFs as a single oral (10 to 1000 mg/kg body weight), sc (10 to 200 mg/kg), or ip (10 to 100 mg/kg) dose developed no toxic signs during the first week, although a modest weight loss was noted (Nishizumi, 1978). The first deaths occurred 8 days after an oral dose of 1000 mg/kg, 5 weeks after a sc dose of 200 mg/kg, and 11 days after an ip dose of 100 mg/kg. The oral LD_{50} (30 day) was 184 mg/kg for males and 414 mg/kg for females. Hepatomegaly and thymus atrophy were consistent findings in mice that died. In surviving mice on high dosages, the liver exhibited small necrotic foci accompanied by cellular infiltrates. The hepatic lesions occurred in the centrilobular area, and enlarged hepatocytes containing foamy cytoplasm, increased numbers of lipid droplets, and proliferation of smooth endoplasmatic reticulum were also seen.

10.1.3 Studies on guinea-pigs

In studies by Moore et al. (1979), the patterns of toxicity were similar for TCDF, 2,3,4,7,8-pentaCDF, and 2,3,7,8-tetrabromodibenzofuran when given to young Hartley guinea-pigs. The single oral LD_{50} was 5-10 µg/kg body weight for all three isomers, and the time to death ranged from 8 to 26 days. Overt signs at lethal doses were immediate and progressive weight loss, rough soiled hair coat, listlessness, and dehydration. Similar symptoms appeared 3 days after an iv injection of 6 µg TCDF/kg body weight (Decad et al., 1981b). At necropsy lack of body fat and reduced body mass and thymus weight were found. Histological findings were primarily associated with the depletion of lymphoid cells in the thymic cortex, but hypocellularity of bone marrow and hyperplasia in epithelial cells of the renal pelvis, ureter, and urinary bladder were also observed. Liver lesions were not observed. Surviving animals showed mild thymic lymphoid hypoplasia only. Sublethal doses resulted in decreased body weight gain.

In a study by Ioannou et al. (1983), all three adult male Hartley guinea-pigs survived a single oral dose of 6 µg TCDF/kg body weight for at least 17 days. At 10 and 15 µg TCDF/kg body weight, deaths occurred on days 15-39 (two animals were sacrificed on day 17) and 13-20, respectively. The acute oral toxicity of soot (and of benzene extracts of the soot) containing PCDDs and PCDFs from a PCB-containing transformer fire (Binghamton, New York, USA) were studied in female Hartley guinea-pigs (Silkworth et al., 1982). As discussed in section 8.1.1.1, toxicities were noted at 100 and

500 mg/kg body weight of soot, but not when 1 and 10 mg/kg were administered.

10.1.4 Studies on rabbits

When the above-mentioned soot (or benzene extracts thereof) was applied dermally to New Zealand white rabbits (Silkworth et al., 1982) (see section 7.4.4.1), it produced no overt toxicity, weight loss, or histological changes in thymus, kidney, or skin, but centrilobular hypertrophy was found in both sexes. The soot extract gave rise to a reversible skin inflammation and hepatic centrilobular hypertrophy in females only. Histological examination showed no changes in kidney, thymus, and skin.

10.1.5 Studies on monkeys

The single oral LD_{50} value for TCDF in the young female rhesus monkey (Macaca mulatta) was found to be 1000 µg/kg in a 60-days study within the dose range 0, 500, 1000, and 1500 µg/kg and with two or four animals at each dose level (Moore et al., 1979). The two monkeys that received the sublethal dose developed skin lesions and had decreased body weight gain. With lethal doses the following overt signs occurred after 7 to 10 days: progressive weight loss, loss of body fat, facial oedema, loss of facial hair, loss of finger and toe nails, and thickening of skin. Death occurred within 2 to 4 weeks. Major histological findings included hyperkeratosis of the skin, thymic atrophy with lymphoid hypoplasia, and adverse effects on epithelial linings. No structural liver lesions were observed though the liver weight was increased. Increases in serum albumin and cholesterol were also recorded.

Three male rhesus monkeys given a single dose of 30.6 µg TCDF/kg body weight did not gain weight during the three following weeks, and they developed facial skin lesions, mainly of sebaceous glands (Birnbaum et al., 1981).

10.2 Short-Term Toxicity

10.2.1 Studies on rats

Male Sprague Dawley rats were fed 1 or 10 µg/kg of a PCDF mixture, containing two tetraCDFs, four pentaCDFs, and four hexaCDFs for 4 weeks (Oishi et al., 1978). Both diets gave rise to decreases in growth rate, food consumption, haemoglobin and haematocrit values, erythrocyte counts, serum levels of triglyceride, testosterone, glutamic pyruvic transaminase, and leucine aminopeptidase activities, as well as increases in serum cholesterol, cholinesterase, and glutamic oxaloacetic transaminase activities. Rats fed the 10 µg/kg diet developed chloracne-like lesions on the ears within 3 weeks. Furthermore, this diet decreased the relative weights of thymus, prostate, and seminal vesicles and increased the relative weights of liver, testes, spleen, adrenals, lung, heart, and brain. In another similar study, no effects were seen on total serum proteins or leukocyte counts (Oishi, 1977).

In studies by Hori et al. (1986), male Sprague Dawley rats (aged 5 weeks) were for 21 days given daily oral doses of a mixture of PCBs, PCQs, and PCDFs having a similar composition and isomeric ratio to those found in the contaminated rice oil causing "Yusho" (section 11.1). The toxicities noted included thymic atrophy, suppression of weight gain, hepatic enlargement, and an increased serum cholesterol level and a decrease in serum glutamic pyruvic transaminase activity. The mixture caused an induction of the AAH drug-metabolizing enzyme similar to that caused by PCDFs alone. These results support the hypothesis that the predominant etiology of "Yusho" involves PCDFs contained in the PCB-contaminated toxic rice oil.

10.2.2 Studies on mice

Mice (C57Bl/6), given TCDF orally 5 times per week for 30 days did not develop clinical signs of toxicity at doses of 30, 100, or 300 µg/kg body weight. However, thymus atrophy, liver hypertrophy, decreased leukocyte count, and slightly elevated total serum protein did occur in the high dose group at the end of the study (Moore et al., 1979). Daily doses of 10, 30, or 50 µg TCDF/kg body weight on gestation days 10-13 produced a dose-related increase in maternal liver weight in C57Bl/6 mice (Weber et al., 1984). Decreased thymus weight was recorded in ICR/JCL mice exposed to four weekly doses of a mixture (at 100 µg/kg) of 12% tetraCDF and 88% pentaCDF (Oishi & Hiraga, 1980). When PCDFs of unknown composition were given in the diet at 0.6 mg/kg to mice for 10 weeks, severe dermal lesions, hyperkeratosis, and dilated hair follicles filled with keratinous material occurred in 7 of 12 mice. Furthermore, hepatocytes had enlarged nuclei and vacuolations in the cytoplasm (Nagayama et al., 1979). Feeding female ddN mice 0.6 mg PCDFs/kg diet (48% tetraCDFs, 49% pentaCDFs, and 3% hexaCDFs) for 18 days after mating, or for 14 days after delivery, produced no overt toxic effects in dams or in offspring (Nagayama et al., 1980).

10.2.3 Studies on guinea-pigs

In studies by Luster et al. (1979b), oral administration of 0.05, 0.17, 0.5, or 1.0 μg 2,3,7,8-TCDF/kg body weight once weekly for 6 weeks to young female Hartley guinea-pigs produced 30% mortality in the high-dose group. The thymus weight was decreased in the 0.5 and 1.0 μg/kg dose groups, though histologically only a slight decrease in the density of thymic cortex was observable. Reduction in spleen weight or alterations in splenic morphology did not occur, neither was there a consistent decrease in body weight.

Four adult male Hartley guinea-pigs were given six or seven weekly doses of 1 μg TCDF/kg body weight (Decad et al., 1981a). The animals started to lose weight rapidly after the fifth or sixth dose, the cumulative dose then being comparable to the oral LD_{50} value for young guinea-pigs. At this time all animals were moribund and by day 44 the first animal died. Neither hepatomegaly nor thymic atrophy was observed in this study. Thus multiple sublethal doses of TCDF appear to have a cumulative effect, and may lead to a critical body burden that will result in irreversible and progressive weight loss eventually followed by death.

Weekly oral doses of 1 μg TCDF/kg body weight or biweekly doses of 2 μg TCDF/kg body weight (interrupted by a 4-week period of no dosing after the fourth dose) to young male Hartley guinea-pigs in groups of four resulted in deaths on days 47, 51, 84; 31, 38, 88; and 32, 70, 85, respectively (Ioannou et al., 1983). At each dosing schedule one animal was sacrificed at 101 days after exposure. Repeated small doses, with various intervals in between, resulted in a similar lethality but a less dramatic weight loss than with a high acute dose.

10.2.4 Studies on rabbits

The 25% ether-hexane extracts from two commercial polychlorinated biphenyl (PCB) preparations containing tetraCDFs and pentaCDFs produced hyperplasia and hyperkeratosis of the follicular epithelium of the rabbit ear skin when applied dermally weekly for 3 weeks in a dose corresponding to 200 mg PCB. Liver lesions or decreased weight gain were not observed. No dermal effects could be found when an ether-hexane extract from a PCB preparation lacking PCDF impurities was applied in the same manner (Vos & Beems, 1971).

A mixture of tetraCDFs and pentaCDFs was much less potent than was TCDD in producing hyperkeratosis when applied to the inside of depilated rabbit ears for 3 consecutive days (Nishizumi et al., 1975).

10.2.5 Studies on hamsters

No toxic effects were reported in male Golden Syrian hamsters (50-70 g) given a diet containing 2.5% HCl-pretreated fly ash from a municipal incinerator (Zaanstad, The Netherlands) for up to 95 days (van den Berg et al., 1986b).

10.2.6 Studies on monkeys

A two-month study with three young male rhesus monkeys (*Macaca mulatta*), serving as their own controls and fed a diet with 50 µg TCDF/kg, resulted in one case of illness after 1 month and one death after 2 months when the cumulative dose was calculated to be 300 µg/kg (McNulty et al., 1981, 1982a). Toxic changes observed after 1 month included periorbital oedema, reddening and thickening of the eyelids, enlargement of facial hair follicles, and decreased number and size of sebaceous glands in the skin. After 2 months these changes had become more severe and were accompanied by decreased physical activity and elevated (or eventual loss of) toe and finger nails. There were no changes in haematology or serum chemical values. The diseased and the surviving monkeys recovered rapidly when they were returned to uncontaminated food. Within 3 months, behaviour, clinical appearance, and histological structure of the skin were normal. The monkey that died had lost 23% of its initial weight and most of its body hair. Sebaceous glands were replaced by small squamous cysts. Severe lesions were confined to the skin, thymus, and the stomach epithelium, whereas liver lesions were modest. Decreased bone marrow cellularity was a postmortem finding which was not reflected in the peripheral blood count taken before death.

10.2.7 Studies on chickens

Mortality in one-day-old White Leghorn chickens given 1 or 5 µg TCDF/kg body weight orally for 3 weeks was 16% and 100%, respectively, with an average time to death of 19 and 11.5 days (McKinney et al., 1976). Body weight gain and food consumption were decreased during the third week post-treatment. Dose-related subcutaneous oedema, ascites, and hydropericardium, as well as thymus atrophy, occurred. Depletion of lymphatic cells was evident both in the spleen and thymus. Mild liver lesions were found only in the high-dose group. Total serum protein and serum albumin were reduced.

The significant difference in toxicity in chickens between three commercial PCB preparations (Vos & Koeman, 1970) was later demonstrated to be caused by the presence of tetra- and pentaCDFs in two of the three preparations (Vos et al.,

1970). The 25% ether-hexane extracts from these two PCB preparations were highly toxic in the chick embryo assay (Vos et al., 1970), whereas no effect could be produced by the extract from the PCB preparation lacking PCDF impurities.

10.3 Chronic Toxicity

10.3.1 Studies on monkeys

In studies by McNulty et al. (1981, 1982a), three young male rhesus monkeys (*Macaca mulatta*) were exposed for 6 months to 5 µg TCDF/kg diet, and one animal served as a control. One animal was killed after 6 weeks when moribund. Overt toxic signs in the two remaining animals started to appear after 3 months and the symptoms remained for the following 3 months. One of these animals died suddenly after 6 months. The remaining monkey was returned to normal food and rapidly recovered. Clinically and pathologically, chronic intake of small amounts of TCDF caused symptoms similar to those following a single large dose of TCDF (section 9.1.2.4) or acute or chronic ingestion of TCDD (see sections 7.1.1 and 7.3). The major histopathological changes in all cases were seen in the thymus, sebaceous glands, nail beds, bone marrow, and mucosa of the stomach and bile ducts. The toxic potency of TCDF when ingested chronically was approximately equal to that of TCDD. This contrasts with the acute toxic effect of TCDF, which is approximately 20 times less than that of its TCDD counterpart. The reason for death in the TCDF-poisoned monkeys was obscure; it was preceded by weight loss, anorexia, and depression. Only modest thymic and epithelial changes were present, and there was no evidence for liver damage. The quick recovery of animals returned to normal diet contrasted with the course of TCDD poisoning in which illness progressed to death, or recovery was much delayed, even after exposure had ended.

10.4 Effects Detected by Special Studies

10.4.1 Immunobiological effects

To date no studies have been performed on the effects of PCDFs on the developing immune system.

Comparative studies on humoral immune responses in mice have revealed that TCDF produces a pattern of responses similar to that found for TCDD but only at 30-fold higher doses. Furthermore the immunosuppressive effect of TCDD is much more persistent (Vecchi et al., 1983b).

10.4.1.1 Histopathology

During toxicity studies with pure isomers of PCDFs or with mixtures of PCDFs, thymus atrophy has been noted as a consistent effect in the mouse (Nishizumi et al., 1978; Moore et al., 1979), rat (Oishi, 1977; Oishi et al., 1978), guinea-pig (Moore et al., 1979), and monkey (Moore et al., 1979; McNulty et al., 1981). Studies aimed at investigating immunobiological effects revealed decreased thymic weights (Luster et al., 1979b; Vecchi et al., 1983). The histological findings are similar to those occurring after TCDD exposure, i.e., loss of lymphoid cells in the thymic cortex. A reduced number of spleen cells was obtained from mice treated with a single ip dose of 180 µg TCDF/kg body weight (Vecchi et al., 1983), but no splenic pathology was reported in mice given four weekly oral doses of a PCDF mixture (at 100 µg/kg) containing 12% tetraCDFs and 88% pentaCDFs (Oishi & Hiraga, 1980). Peritoneal cell and macrophage counts in mice were not modified by an ip dose of TCDF (180 µg/kg body weight) (Vecchi et al., 1983).

10.4.1.2 Humoral-mediated immunity

Adult female Hartley guinea-pigs exposed orally to 0.05, 0.17, and 0.5 µg TCDF/kg body weight once weekly for 6 weeks showed somewhat depressed serum IgG concentrations. A dose-related depression in splenic lymphocyte proliferation was seen in TCDF-treated animals after stimulation with the B-lymphocyte mitogen *Escherichia coli* 0127 lipopolysaccharide at 50 µg/ml medium. There were no effects on any of the major serum proteins, neither was there an effect on the antibody response towards bovine gamma globulin (BGG) (Luster et al., 1979b).

The antibody response to sheep red blood cells given 7 days after a single ip injection of 180 µg TCDF/kg body weight was inhibited by 85% and 35% in C57Bl/6 and DBA/2 mice, respectively (Vecchi et al., 1983), whereas a single ip dose of 10 µg TCDF/kg body weight to C57Bl/6 mice had no effect (Rizzardini et al., 1983). The suppression noted by Vecchi et al. (1983) was dose dependent as well as time dependent; by day 42 post-treatment a near-normal antibody response was obtained.

10.4.1.3 Cell-mediated immunity

Oral intubation of 10 or 100 µg PCDF (12% tetraCDFs and 88% pentaCDFs) per kg body weight once weekly for four weeks increased the sensitivity to endotoxin of ICR/JCL mice. Following an ip injection of 50, 250, or 500 µg endotoxin per mouse a dose-dependent increased mortality was noted two days after the final treatment with PCDF (Oishi & Hiraga, 1980). Only at high dose levels were there any effects on cell-mediated immunity functions in female Hartley guinea-pigs given 0.05, 0.17, 0.5, or 1.0 µg TCDF/kg body weight orally once weekly for six weeks (Luster et al., 1979b).

Both the depression in delayed hypersensitivity response to purified protein derivative and the ability of BGG-sensitized lymphocytes to release the macrophage inhibition factor were related to the dose of TCDF. Splenic lymphocytes from TCDF-treated animals, stimulated with the T-lymphocyte mitogen phyto-haemagglutinin (PHA), showed a decreased proliferation. On the other hand proliferation of splenic lymphocytes stimulated with concanavalin A (Con A), another T-lymphocyte mitogen, showed no TCDF-related effect. The increased proliferative response to Con A and PHA in thymocytes co-cultivated with thymus epithelial (TE) cells or cultivated in TE-conditioned medium was inhibited if the TE cells were pretreated with TCDF for 48 h, thus suggesting a direct effect on TE cells (Osborne et al., 1984).

10.4.2 Enzyme induction

Studies discussed below show that PCDFs are potent enzyme inducers, the enzyme-inducing potencies varying greatly depending on the position as well as on the number of chlorine atoms substituted. The structure-activity relationships of the PCDFs with regard to enzyme induction are similar to those for PCDDs, with TCDF and 2,3,4,7,8-pentaCDF being the most potent (Tables 56 and 61).

10.4.2.1 Studies on rats

Intraperitoneal doses of 2.5 µg TCDF/kg body weight given once daily for three days to female CD rats induced 38- and 3-fold increases, respectively, in AHH and UDPGT activities 24 h after the final dose. The cytochrome P-450 content was doubled but no effect was found on the aminopyrine *N*-demethylase activity (Goldstein et al., 1978).

Increased AHH and EROD activities were found in the hepatic microsomal fraction from immature male Wistar rats 5 days after ip injection of single doses of TCDF (1.7 µmol/kg body weight) or 2,3,4,7,8-pentaCDF (0.3, 1.5, 3.0 µmol/kg body weight) (Keys et al., 1985). This study also detected an alteration by TCDF in the hepatic metabolism of testosterone in these rats. Yoshihara et al. (1981) gave a single ip dose of 1, 5, or 10 mg PCDF/kg body weight of 13 individual PCDFs to young male Wistar rats five days prior to the determination of hepatic enzyme activities. Congeners having at least three chlorine atoms in the lateral positions typically showed increased AHH and DT-diaphorase activities, while those congeners having no more than two chlorine atoms in these positions were not inductive. The cytochrome P-448 content was increased by 5 of the 13 congeners whereas the benzphetamine- *N*-demethylase activity was depressed by 7 of the 13. The most potent isomers, TCDF and 2,3,4,7,8-pentaCDF, were effective at a single dose of 1 µg/kg body weight. The ranking of the potency for enzyme-inducing abilities did not coincide with the hepatic distribution of the test substances. Hepatic AHH activity in male Wistar rats was significantly enhanced only by TCDF and 2,3,4,7,8-pentaCDF among the 15 individual PCDF isomers tested, the dose administered intraperitoneally being 5 µg PCDF/kg body weight (Nagayama et al., 1983).

Eight of the 15 PCDF isomers tested increased the pulmonary AHH activity from 5-fold to 30-fold. In this study no PCDF-related AHH induction was present in the kidney, prostate, thymus, or spleen. Bandiera et al. (1984b) investigated the effect of three tetraCDFs and three pentaCDFs at doses of 500 and 1000 µg/kg body weight, respectively, on hepatic AHH, aminopyrine *N*-demethylase, 4-chlorobiphenyl hydroxylase, and EROD activities in male Wistar rats. The most active compounds, TCDF and 2,3,4,7,8-pentaCDF, were potent inducers of the cytochrome P-448-dependent monooxygenases. Some induction of microsomal AHH, EROD, and 4-chlorobiphenyl hydroxylase was observed also for the TCDF and 1,2,4,7,9-pentaCDF.

The ED_{50} values for hepatic AHH (Table 61) and 4-chlorobiphenyl hydroxylase induction were established for 15 individual PCDFs in immature male Wistar rats 14 days after a single ip injection (Mason et al., 1985).

Significant induction of hepatic AHH activity in male Sprague Dawley rats was given only by 3 out of 25 individual PCDFs given as single oral doses of 40 µg/kg body weight (Doyle & Fries, 1986). The active congeners were 2,7-diCDF, TCDF, and 2,3,4,7,8-pentaCDF.

A mixture of PCDFs, reconstituting the approximate composition found in the liver of Yusho victims (7.4% tetraCDF, 6.1% 1,2,4,7,8-pentaCDF, 19.0% 1,2,3,7,8-pentaCDF, 29.4% 2,3,4,7,8-pentaCDF and 39.1% 1,2,3,4,7,8-hexaCDF by weight) was given as a single ip injection to male Wistar rats 14 days before measuring the induction of cytochrome P-448-related enzyme activities (Bandiera et al., 1984a). A dose-related enhancement of AHH and EROD activities was found within the range 10 to 400 µg PCDF mixture/kg body weight.

10.4.2.2 Studies on mice

No induction of cytochrome P-448 content, or of ECOD activities, was found 12 days after a single ip injection of 10 µg TCDF/kg body weight to male C57Bl/6J mice (Rizzardini et al., 1983).

Nagayama et al. (1985) investigated the AHH-inducing potency of TCDF, 2,3,6,7- tetraCDF, 1,2,3,6,7-pentaCDF, 1,2,3,7,8-pentaCDF, 2,3,4,6,7-pentaCDF, 2,3,4,7,8-pentaCDF, 1,2,3,4,6,7-hexaCDF, and 1,2,3,4,7,8-hexaCDF in two strains of responsive (C57B1/6 and AKR/Qdj) and two strains of non-responsive (DBA/2 and DDD) mice. All congeners were given as single ip doses of 30 µg/kg body weight in olive oil. No single congener induced the AHH activity above the control level in the non-responsive mice. Significantly increased AHH activity was found in both responsive strains exposed to TCDF, 1,2,3,7,8-pentaCDF, and 2,3,4,7,8-pentaCDF. Mice (C57BL/6) treated with 2,3,4,6,7-pentaCDF and 1,2,3,4,7,8-hexaCDF also responded with increased AHH activity.

10.4.2.3 Studies on chickens

Hepatic AHH activity in chick embryos was inducible by TCDF, 2,3,4,7,8-pentaCDF, and 1,2,3,7,8-pentaCDF, with ED_{50} values of 0.015, 0.014, and 0.071 nmol/egg, respectively (Poland et al., 1976). No induction was produced by unchlorinated dibenzofuran, 2,8-diCDF, 2,4-diCDF, 2,4,8-triCDF or 1,3,6,7-tetraCDF at the doses tested. There were no effects on ALA synthetase, *p*-nitrophenol-UDPGT and testosterone-UDPGT activities. However, a modest increase in cytochrome P-450 content was present in one-day-old White Leghorn chickens 3 weeks after treatment with a single oral dose of 1 µg TCDF (Goldstein et al., 1976).

10.4.2.4 Studies on cell cultures

Exposure of primary hepatocytes isolated from adult male Wistar rats to TCDF for 72 h resulted in a 2-fold increase in AHH induction at 10^{-9} mol/litre and half-maximal induction at 3×10^{-10} mol/litre. However, no AHH induction was observed with 2,7-diCDF in the range 10^{-11} to 10^{-8} mol/litre in the same system (Jansing & Shain, 1985). A 59-fold increase in AHH activity and a 40-fold increase in EROD activity were obtained in rat hepatoma H-4-II E cells when exposed to 5×10^{-10} mol TCDF/litre for 3 days (Keys et al., 1986). In this same study it was demonstrated that TCDF had an additive effect, whereas 1,3,6,8-tetraCDF and 2,4,6,8-tetraCDF had counteracting effects on TCDD-induced enzyme induction.

The EC_{50} values for AHH and EROD induction (Table 61) have been established for 35 individual PCDFs in the rat hepatoma H-4-II E cell line (Bandiera et al., 1984b; Mason et al., 1985). AHH and EROD activities were determined after exposing the cells to optimal doses of PCDFs for 5 days. Unchlorinated dibenzofuran, or 2- and 3-chlorodibenzofuran did not induce these enzyme activities. EC_{50} values for all the remaining congeners varied between 10^{-4} and 1.3×10^{-10} mol/litre, the most active inducer being 2,3,4,7,8-PCDF.

Human lymphoblastoid cell lines, derived from the peripheral blood of healthy male and female volunteers of various ages, were exposed to eight individual PCDF isomers for 48 h (Nagayama et al., 1985b). The AHH inducibility was highly variable between individuals but less variable between isomers. In this system TCDF was about half as potent as 2,3,4,7,8-pentaCDF, 1,2,3,4,6,7-hexaCDF, or 1,2,3,4,7,8-hexaCDF, which were equally as potent as TCDD in inducing AHH.

A mixture of PCDFs, reconstituted on the basis of PCDF residues in the liver samples from Yusho victims (see section 10.4.2.1), had EC_{50} values for induction of AHH and EROD activities of 1.02×10^{-10} and 3.23×10^{-10} mol/litre, respectively, in the rat hepatoma H-4-II E assay (Sawyer & Safe, 1985). The calculated EC_{50} values based on the relative isomer content of the mixture were 3.07×10^{-10} and 4.43×10^{-10} mol/litre, respectively.

10.4.3 Receptor binding

The competitive binding of PCDFs to the TCDD receptor protein has been studied *in vitro* both in the hepatic cytosol (Poland et al., 1976; Bandiera et al., 1984b) and in the nucleus (Poellinger et al., 1982). Poland et al. (1974) investigated the ability of seven PCDF congeners to compete with TCDD in binding to the hepatic cytosol receptor from C57Bl/6J mice. They found the relative binding affinities for TCDF, 2,3,4,7,8-pentaCDF, and 1,2,3,7,8-pentaCDF to be 37%, 34%, and 38%, respectively, of the binding affinity between TCDD and the receptor. The EC_{50} values for the competitive binding of 33 individual PCDFs to the receptor from rat hepatoma H-4-II E cell cultures varied from less than 10^{-3} mol/litre for 4-chlorodibenzofuran to 1.5×10^{-8} mol/litre for the most active competitor, 2,3,4,7,8-pentaCDF, which had an EC_{50} value comparable to that for TCDD, i.e., 1.0×10^{-8} mol/litre (Table 61) (Bandiera et al., 1984b; Mason et al., 1985). Of the TCDD bound to the nuclear receptor *in vitro*, 58% was displaced by a 100-fold molar excess of TCDF. These nuclei were isolated from the liver of Sprague Dawley rats pretreated intravenously with 1 µg TCDF 2 h prior to the incubation (Poellinger et al., 1982).

10.5 Embryotoxicity and Reproductive Effects

TCDF has been found to be a potent teratogen in mice at doses that produce no overt toxic effects in dams. Malformations observed include cleft palate and kidney malformation similar to hydronephrosis. Dose-related increases in fetal mortality occur with single high doses. The teratogenic pattern of TCDF thus is strikingly similar to that of TCDD (see section 7.5).

Single doses of 100 to 1000 μg TCDF/kg body weight to pregnant C57Bl/6 mice on gestation days 10 to 13 produced dose-related increases in the number of cleft palates and kidney malformations; both the number of litters and the number of fetuses were affected (Hassoun et al., 1984a; Weber et al., 1984). No other treatment-related malformations were reported. A cleft palate incidence of 40% was obtained in NMRI mice offspring after sc treatment of the dams on gestation days 9 to 11 with 200 nmol TCDF/kg body weight (Krowke, 1986).

Palatal closure in mice occurs late on day 14 of gestation, and so it is somewhat peculiar that the peak sensitivity for cleft palate occurs on day 12 (Hassoun et al., 1984a). The peak sensitivity for kidney malformation in mice occurs on day 11 of gestation (Hassoun et al., 1984a). The quantitative data on this malformation somewhat conflict in the two studies. Weber et al. (1984) reported that 95.5% of the fetuses had kidney malformations after a dose of 500 μg/kg body weight on day 10 of gestation. However, only 17% of the fetuses per dam had this malformation after a single dose of 400 μg/kg body weight on the same day in the study of Hassoun et al. (1984a). The difference might be due to unequal judging of the malformation. Preliminary results (Weber et al., 1984), suggested that TCDF-induced kidney malformations, up to a certain degree, represent a reversible defect since no hydronephrotic kidneys were found in neonates, whereas in identically treated dams examined on day 18 of gestation over 80% of the fetuses/litter were affected. Fetal mortality increased in a dose-related manner with high single doses administered on days 10 to 12. Peak sensitivity occurred on day 10 (Hassoun et al., 1984a). Multiple low dosing on gestation days 10 to 13 was more effective in producing fetal malformations, but less effective in producing fetal deaths, than single high dosing on day 10 (Weber et al., 1984). No effect on fetal mortality (days 12, 13, and 14) was observed in C57BL/6N mice given a single oral dose of 800 μg TCDF/kg body weight on day 11 of gestation (Weber & Birnbaum, 1985).

Recombinant inbred strains of C57Bl/6 and DBA/2 mice segregating at the Ah locus respond differently to the teratogenic effect of TCDF (Hassoun et al., 1984b). Fetuses of Ah-responsive strains responded with a high frequency of cleft palates and kidney malformations after a single ip dose of 600 μg TCDF/kg body weight on day 12 of gestation. However, no cleft palates and only modestly increased numbers of kidney malformations in a few strains were found with the same treatment in Ah-nonresponsive strains.

A diet containing 0.6 mg PCDFs/kg (48% tetraCDFs, 49% pentaCDFs, and 3% hexaCDFs), fed to mice for 18 days after mating, had no effect on the number or body weight gain of the offspring, neither were there any malformations related to the diet (Nagayama et al., 1980).

Three PCDFs, namely 1,2,3,7,8-pentaCDF, 2,3,4,7,8-pentaCDF, and 1,2,3,4,7,8-hexa CDF, are teratogenic to C57BL/6N mice when administered orally by gavage on gestation days 10-13. A significant increase in hydronephrosis and cleft palate was found, with 2,3,4,7,8-PCDF being the most potent PCDF studied, having an ED_{50} of 36 µg/kg body weight for cleft palate and 7 µg/kg for hydronephrosis. For all three PCDFs, hydronephrosis occurred at a lower dose than did cleft palate (Birnbaum et al., 1987).

It has been pointed out by McNulty (1985) that chlorinated compounds such as 2,3,7,8-TCDD produce cystic periodontal lesions and squamous metaplasia of the ameloblasts surrounding unerupted teeth in rhesus monkeys. These findings are similar to those on the teeth development seen in Yusho patients (section 11.1).

10.6 Mutagenicity

When tested in *Salmonella typhimurium* strains KTA98 and TA100 with and without metabolic activation, no mutagenic activity was found for 2,9-diCDF, 3,6-diCDF, TCDF, or octaCDF (Schoeny, 1982). TCDF was also studied in *Saccharomyces cerevisiae* strain MP-1 and was found to be negative for forward mutation, mitotic crossing over, and mitotic gene conversion at concentrations up to 1000 mg/litre. Stationary phase cells were tested in the absence of exogenous activation (Fahrig et al., 1978).

10.7 Carcinogenicity

The hepatic tumour-promoting activity of a commercial polychlorinated biphenyl mixture, Aroclor 1254, with (Ar 1254) or without (Ar 1254-PCDF) PCDF impurities, was studied in Sprague Dawley rats pretreated with 66 µg diethylnitrosamine/ml drinking water for 5 weeks (Preston et al., 1981). Thereafter the rats were fed a diet supplemented with 100 mg Ar 1254/kg ($\geq$ 3 mg PCDF/kg) or Ar 1254-PCDF (<0.1 mg PCDF/kg) for 18 weeks. Examination of liver lesions by light microscopy demonstrated that Ar 1254 promotes formation of hepatocellular carcinomas in rats. The promoting incidence of 64% remained essentially unchanged when PCDF was removed from Ar 1254 by adsorption chromatography. Due to the high incidence of hepatocellular carcinomas produced by Ar 1254-PCDF itself, an additional effect of PCDF might have been difficult to measure in this study.

11. EFFECTS OF PCDFs ON HUMAN BEINGS

Braun (1955) was the first to report chloracne due to chlorinated dibenzofurans, subsequently experimentally proven by Bauer et al. (1961). Vos et al. (1970) identified by mass spectrometry the presence of chlorinated dibenzofurans in commercial PCB mixtures, accounting for their acnegenic properties.

11.1 Yusho and Yu-cheng

A mass outbreak of food poisoning occurred in western Japan in 1968 following ingestion of a commercial brand of rice oil contaminated with polychlorinated biphenyls (PCBs) and related hydrocarbons. The poisoning was named "Yusho" (oil disease). Epidemiological proof of the cause of the epidemic depended on the demonstration of a dose-response relationship between the consumption of the toxic rice oil and the incidence of the poisoning or between the oil consumption and the clinical severity of the reaction. Approximately 2000 cases were recognized. In 1969, Japanese scientists first reported that the toxic rice oil which caused Yusho was contaminated with polychlorinated biphenyls (Tsukamoto et al., 1969). A few years later, the oil was found also to be contaminated with a smaller quantity of PCDFs (Nagayama et al., 1976) and a relatively large amount of polychlorinated quaterphenyls (PCQs) (Masuda & Yoshimura, 1982).

In March 1979, an epidemic of a peculiar skin disease broke out in Taichung and Changhwa in Central Taiwan. The cause of the disease was later identified to be the ingestion of rice-bran oil contaminated with polychlorinated biphenyls (Chen et al., 1980, 1981; Hsu et al., 1984; Masuda et al., 1986). By the end of 1980, the total number of reported cases was about 2000. The local name for the disease was Yu-cheng. The mean consumption of total PCDFs of the Yusho and Yu-cheng patients has been estimated to be 3.3-3.8 mg/person or 400-500 µg of toxic 2,3,7,8-substituted PCDFs per person. (Hayabuchi et al., 1979). Hayabuchi et al. (1979) estimated the daily intake of total PCDFs in the Yusho intoxication to have been 0.9 µg/kg body weight. Analyses of liver samples taken from the Yusho patients about 18 months after the exposure showed a dramatic decrease in the number of PCDF isomers. Apparently most of the PCDF isomers were metabolized or excreted during the period between exposure and sampling (Rappe et al., 1979). A comparison between the PCDF isomers found in the Yusho oil and the liver samples revealed an interesting relationship. Most of the isomers retained had all lateral positions (2-, 3-, 7-, and 8-) substituted with chlorine (Rappe et al., 1979).

The rate of excretion of these toxic PCDF isomers is very slow. Rappe et al. (1983c) could detect 2,3,4,7,8-pentaCDF in blood plasma from Yusho patients when the samples were collected 11 years after exposure. Higher levels were found in blood from Yu-cheng patients one year after exposure and these analyses also showed a 15-20% reduction in one year (Rappe, 1984). PCDFs are selectively retained in the liver, with levels corresponding to the fatty level of the tissue. They are not found in unexposed controls or in PCB-exposed workers. PCB levels in Yusho patients were only about two times higher than those of normal people several years after the outbreak. PCB-exposed workers had more than 10 times greater PCB blood levels than Yusho patients, whereas the PCQ levels of these two groups were similar.

Generally a correlation between degree or severity of clinical signs and the amount of PCDFs retained in the blood exists, whereas there is no correspondence between the severity of disease and PCB concentrations in blood.

Mild dermal lesions seen in workers exposed to PCB disappeared quickly after discontinuation of PCB handling, in contrast to the persistence of Yusho and Yu-cheng symptoms. Everything thus suggests that the PCDF contaminant is the causative agent.

Immunological evaluation of patients exposed in 1979 in Taiwan (Yu-cheng) has been reported by Chang et al. (1981, 1982a, 1982b) and Wu et al. (1984). Serum immunoglobulin concentrations and lymphocyte subpopulations were determined in the peripheral blood of 30 patients exposed to PCBs and 23 healthy individuals. The groups were age and sex matched. In the patients, serum concentrations of IgA and IgM, but not of IgG, were significantly decreased. Also the percentages of total T lymphocytes and T-helper lymphocytes were significantly reduced, whereas the percentages of T-suppressor cells and B lymphocytes were not affected (Chang et al., 1981).

In a later report (Chang et al., 1982a), monocyte and polymorphonuclear lymphocyte (PMN) complement and Fc receptors were evaluated in peripheral blood from 30 Yu-cheng patients and 23 normal human subjects. Monocytes and PMNs from patients had significantly lower percentages of cells bearing immunoglobulin Fc and complement receptors. The immune system was further investigated by determining the delayed-type hypersensitivity skin response to streptokinase and streptodornase, as parameters of cellular immune function. The response was studied in 30 PCB-poisoned patients and 50 healthy volunteers. Results of the study showed that 80% of the controls had positive hypersensitivity skin tests, compared to only 43% of the patients. The significant suppression of cellular immunity correlated with the severity of the dermal lesions; the size of the hypersensitivity skin reaction was negatively correlated with the dermal lesions and also with PCB concentrations in whole blood (Chang et al., 1982b). More recently, the delayed-type hypersensitivity response to tuberculin was reported in 83 PCB-poisoned Yu-cheng patients and in 30 age- and sex-matched healthy controls. Compared to a positive response rate of 74% in the control group, the patients had a significantly lower skin response of 48% (40 out of 83 patients). In contrast to the delayed-type hypersensitivity response, the _in vitro_ proliferation responses of peripheral blood lymphocytes treated with phytohaemagglutinin and pokeweed mitogens, as well as tuberculin, were significantly enhanced (Wu et al., 1984).

There are also indications of immunosuppression in the Yusho poisoning. Serum IgA and IgM levels decreased considerably within 2 years after the onset of the disease. Respiratory involvement included bronchiolitis, and respiratory distress was often exacerbated by viral or bacterial infection (Shigematsu et al., 1978).

The symptomatology of Yusho has been summarized by Reggiani (1983b) and is to be found in Tables 72 and 73. It is similar to that of Yu-cheng, but there are differences such as the frequency of transient visual disturbances, hearing difficulties, and a persistent bronchitis.

Table 72. Clinical symptomatology of Yusho 1969-1972[a]

1. Skin (82-87%).
   Acneiform eruptions, districtive hair follicles, red plaques on limbs, dark brown pigmentation of nail, skin, and mucous membranes, itching, sweating of palms.

2. Ocular manifestations (83-88%).
   Increased eye discharge, swelling of the upper eyelids, hyperaemia of conjunctiva, transient visual disturbance.

3. Jaundice (10%).
   No abnormalities of liver function in the majority of cases.

4. Numbness of the limbs, feeling of weakness, muscular spasms (32-39%).
   Reduced sensory and motor nerve conduction velocity in a few cases (9%).

5. Hearing difficulties (18%).

6. Headaches, vomiting, diarrhoea (17-39%).

7. Chronic bronchitis (40%).
   Low serum IgA and IgM, PCB in the sputum.

8. Irregular menstrual cycles (60%).

9. Dark brown skin pigmentation (which gradually fades) of newborn, retarded growth, abnormal teeth number and shape.

[a] Numbers in brackets refer to per cent of patients exhibiting the symptoms.

Table 73. Changes in the clinical symptomatology of Yusho in the years 1968-1978

1. Skin lesions.
   All skin symptoms diminished gradually, subcutaneous cyst formation still present in some of the most severe cases.

2. Ocular manifestations.
   Eye discharge, oedema of the eyelids, pigmentation of eyelids and conjunctiva, and cyst formation of tarsal gland still present in some of the cases.

3. Stomatological alterations.
   Pigmentation of oral mucosa decreased gradually; anomalies in number of teeth and shape of the root still present.

4. Chronic bronchitis correlated in severity with concentration of PCBs in sputum and blood.

5. Serum triglycerides.
   The hyperglycidaemia observed in 1968-1970 returned to a normal level by 1973 in females and by 1975 in males.

6. Mortality.
   Of 737 cases in the Fukuoka region, 51 (6.92%) died between 1968 and 1978; there were 11 cancer deaths (3 stomach cancer, 2 lung cancer, 1 breast cancer, 1 liver cancer, 2 malignant lymphoma).

12. EVALUATION OF HEALTH RISKS FROM THE EXPOSURE TO CHLORINATED DIBENZO-P-DIOXINS (PCDDs) AND DIBENZOFURANS (PCDFs)

12.1 Introduction

In order to evaluate the human health risk of PCDDs and PCDFs, it is necessary to know both the levels of human exposure and the corresponding human health effects.

Human exposure assessment is complex. Several approaches may be taken to estimate it, such as the following.

(a) Use of standard physiological models of inhalation, ingestion, and dermal absorption. Data requirements include detailed information on ambient levels in environmental media and food, and on bioavailability.

(b) Intake estimates based on simple pharmacokinetic models and known levels in human tissue for accurate assessment of exposure. Detailed knowledge is also required of the uptake, distribution, metabolism, and elimination of PCDDs and PCDFs in humans.

12.2 Exposure Assessment

12.2.1 Sources of contamination

The main sources of PCDDs and PCDFs that have so far been identified are contaminated commercial chemicals (see section 3.3), emissions from combustion sources (see section 3.5), and disposal of industrial wastes containing PCDDs and PCDFs (sections 3.4, 3.5.9, and 3.5.10).

In some cases estimates of the relative contribution of these sources can be generated on a local basis. However, the data and methods available today do not allow firm conclusions with regard to the relative quantitative importance of these sources on a nation-wide or world-wide basis.

12.2.2 Ambient levels

The limited data available indicate very low (fg/m^3) background levels in ambient air of the 2,3,7,8-tetra-, penta-, and hexachlorinated PCDDs and PCDFs. (If hepta- and octachlorinated congeners are included, pg/m^3 levels are noted).

The few data available indicate that the 2,3,7,8-tetra-, penta-, and hexachlorinated PCDDs and PCDFs are unlikely to occur in finished drinking-water, even at a level of

1 pg/litre (see section 5.2). In all soil and sediment samples analyzed (both from industrialized and non-industrialized areas), PCDDs and PCDFs were identified at levels ranging from a few ng/kg to several hundred ng/kg (the latter in sediments and in urban soil).

There are no available data on background levels of PCDDs and PCDFs in vegetation in the general environment.

Levels of up to 50 ng/kg of the 2,3,7,8-tetra-, penta-, and hexachlorinated PCDDs and PCDFs (principally the tetra- and pentachlorinated congeners) have been found in fish from the general environment. For the most part these have been detected in fatty or bottom-feeding fish (see section 4.4.2).

Data from terrestrial organisms are inadequate for estimation of background levels (see section 4.4.3). Three samples of pooled cow's milk showed a maximum of 100 pg/kg of the 2,3,7,8-tetra-, penta-, and hexachlorinated PCDDs and PCDFs in whole milk (see section 5.4). Data on contamination of other commercial foods are also very limited. Analyses of several samples of chicken and pork have shown contamination with highly chlorinated congeners at about 5-30 ng/kg. The congener profile differs from that noted in aquatic organisms (see section 5.4).

The data available are not sufficient for assessing the total exposure of general populations. They are sufficient to perform a limited evaluation of exposure for local populations. Based on the environmental levels discussed above and the usual assumptions regarding intakes of foodstuffs, air, and water, food is more likely to be a significant source of PCDD/PCDF exposure than air, while drinking-water is likely to be of much less concern.

12.2.3 Routes of exposure

Human adipose tissue contains 2,3,7,8-tetra-, penta-, and hexachlorinated PCDDs and PCDFs. This contamination is presumably due to exposure at the ambient concentrations noted in the preceding sections.

In addition, infants may be exposed through breast milk, and small children may also be exposed through ingestion of contaminated soil. However, this latter route of exposure, in most instances, is likely to be of concern only in heavily contaminated areas.

Some populations have been at special risk through exposure in industrial accidents (and their clean-up) that have occurred during the normal production and use of chlorophenols and phenoxy herbicides and PCBs. In these situations inhalation and dermal contact are the exposure routes of greatest concern. However, quantitative information on the nature and concentration of contaminants is not available.

Based on the environmental levels discussed above and the usual assumptions regarding physiological and intake parameters, ingestion is likely to be the exposure route of greatest concern. Inhalation of ambient air is not likely to be a problem, although inhalation of heavily contaminated air may make a significant contribution to exposure. In general, it is not possible, at present, to estimate the relative contribution of dermal exposure.

12.2.4 Bioavailability

No bioavailability data from studies in humans are available. From animal studies, it is clear that bioavailability of PCDDs and PCDFs following ingestion depends on the matrix ingested. Table 46 summarizes the data available on oral intake.

Studies on hairless rats indicate that dermal exposure through intact skin from contact with contaminated soil is about 1 to 2%. No data are available for inhalation exposure.

12.3 Animal Data

12.3.1 Toxicokinetics of 2,3,7,8-TCDD

Studies on rodents given single or repeated oral doses of 2,3,7,8-TCDD have shown that 50% or more of the administered amount is absorbed from the gastrointestinal tract in rats, guinea-pigs, and hamsters, but less than 30% in mice (Table 40). The reported half-lives for elimination were in the ranges 12-31 days for rats, mice, and hamsters and 22-94 days for guinea-pigs (Table 41). However, most of these studies have been performed at toxic doses. The half-life of 2,3,7,8-TCDD in primates has not been well established, but available data for the rhesus monkey suggest an apparent half-life in the adipose tissue of about 1 year.

2,3,7,8-TCDD does accumulate in animal tissues. In rodents accumulation occurs predominantly in the liver and adipose tissue (Tables 42 to 44). In rhesus monkeys (Table 45), high levels of 2,3,7,8-TCDD are recovered from the adipose tissues, liver, skin, and muscles.

At a daily dose of 1 ng 2,3,7,8-TCDD/kg body weight for 2 years, rats accumulated 540 ng 2,3,7,8-TCDD/kg body weight in the liver where some morphological changes were also observed. Similar levels were found in beach mice that had been exposed to 2,3,7,8-TCDD soil levels ranging from 10-710 ng/kg. Total body exposure of animals to 2,3,7,8-TCDD in soil at such concentrations may thus result in tissue levels that have been demonstrated to cause effects in experimental animals.

TCDD is largely eliminated in the faeces, although some urinary excretion occurs. The hamster has a higher urinary elimination than other species studied.

Transformation of 2,3,7,8-TCDD to more polar metabolites occurs in all animal species investigated (see section 6.2 and Table 62). Elimination of metabolites from tissues into faeces and urine occurs rapidly in all of these species except in the case of the guinea-pig. Known metabolites are much less toxic than the parent compound.

12.3.2 Toxicokinetics of PCDDs and PCDFs, other than TCDD

Animal data on the toxicokinetics of pure PCDDs other than 2,3,7,8-TCDD are limited. PCDFs have been more extensively studied in this respect. The half-life for 2,3,7,8-TCDF has been reported to be in the range of 2-8 days for rats, mice, and rhesus monkeys and more than 20 days for guinea-pigs (Table 65). Studies on rats have shown that 2,3,4,7,8-pentaCDF is more highly retained than is 2,3,7,8-TCDF (65% and 3.8%, respectively, after 5 days).

Tissue retention data of PCDDs and PCDFs in various species exposed to synthetic mixtures or to environmental samples containing PCDDs and PCDFs show a high variability in retention time between congeners with or without chlorine substitution in all the positions 2,3,7, and 8.

12.3.3 Toxic effects of 2,3,7,8-TCDD

The toxic and biological effects resulting from exposure to 2,3,7,8-TCDD are dependent on a number of factors, including the species, strain, age, and sex of the animals used. The toxic responses observed in several animal species include body weight loss, hepatotoxicity, porphyria, dermal toxicity, gastric lesions, thymus atrophy and immunotoxicity, teratogenicity, reproductive effects, and carcinogenicity. TCDD induces a wide spectrum of biological effects including enzyme induction and vitamin A depletion. The complete spectrum of toxic and biological effects is not usually observed in any single animal species. The two most characteristic toxic effects observed in all laboratory animals are body weight loss and thymus atrophy and immunotoxicity. Chloracne and related dermal lesions are the most frequently noted signs of 2,3,7,8-TCDD toxicosis in humans; dermal lesions are also observed in rhesus monkeys, hairless mice, and rabbits. In contrast, rats, most strains of mice, guinea-pigs, and hamsters do not develop chloracne and related dermal toxic lesions after exposure to 2,3,7,8-TCDD. Many of the observed toxic lesions are either hyperplastic/metaplastic or hypoplastic, and primarily affect epithelial tissues.

Reproductive toxicity has been reported in rhesus monkeys: the lowest-observed-effect level (LOEL) was calculated to be 1 to 2 ng/kg body weight per day. A no-observed-effect level (NOEL), or possibly a LOEL, of 1 ng/kg body weight per day for reproductive effects in rats has been discussed (Murray et al., 1979; Nisbet & Paxton, 1982).

If the cancer studies in rats conducted by Kociba et al. (1978) and by the NIH (1982a, b) are compared, it is evident that the liver tumours, including hepatocellular carcinomas, are produced at similar dose levels. Although an increased incidence of tumours in other organs was observed by the NTP, and by Kociba et al. (1978), the other target organs varied in the two studies. This may be caused, in part, by differences in dosing (gavage versus exposure in ground feed) and by differences in strains. In the Kociba study, doses of 10 ng/kg body weight caused an increased incidence of neoplastic (hyperplastic) nodules in females, and doses of 1 ng/kg body weight resulted in foci or areas of hepatocellular alteration (swollen hepatocytes). At these dose rates in experimental groups, the incidence of certain hormone-dependent tumours was lower than in the control animals, suggesting endocrine changes induced by 2,3,7,8-TCDD. Based on these animal studies and on available human data IARC (1982 suppl. 4) concluded that TCDD showed sufficient evidence for carcinogenicity in animals, but inadequate evidence for carcinogenicity in humans.

TCDD does not appear to have mutagenic properties, and is, therefore, not likely to be genotoxic. Thus, it is assumed to be carcinogenic through an indirect (epigenetic) mechanism.

12.3.4 Toxic effects of PCDDs and PCDFs, other than TCDD

Several other PCDDs and PCDFs cause signs and symptoms similar to those of 2,3,7,8-TCDD, but there is a wide variation with regard to potency (Tables 56, 62). In summary, there are 12 isomers that display high toxicity, i.e., the tetra-, penta-, hexa-, and heptaCDDs and CDFs with four chlorine atoms in the symmetrical lateral positions 2,3,7, and 8. A mixture of two hexaCDDs (1,2,3,7,8,9- and 1,2,3,6,7,8-hexaCDD) has been demonstrated to possess carcinogenic properties in long-term animal studies, but at higher doses than those used in the study of TCDD. Unsubstituted dioxin and 2,7-diCDD failed to demonstrate carcinogenic properties.

The relative toxic and biological potencies of PCDDs and PCDFs have been estimated using short-term studies in rats and mammalian cell cultures. Endpoints used include inhibition of body weight gain, thymic atrophy, enzyme induction, teratogenicity, acnegenic response, and keratinization. In the absence of long-term toxicity data, results obtained from such short-term tests are at present the only source for ranking the toxicity for human risk assessment.

When investigated, mixtures of these compounds have shown additive or less than additive responses.

12.3.5 Review of species differences

There are marked species differences in the susceptibility to the biological and toxic effects elicited by 2,3,7,8-TCDD. For example, the oral LD_{50} values range from 0.6 µg/kg body weight in guinea-pigs, to 5051 µg/kg body weight in Golden Syrian hamsters (Table 47); moreover, pronounced differences in LD_{50} values have also been reported in different strains of the same species (e.g., rats and mice). The toxicity and toxicokinetics of TCDD in monkeys most closely resemble the effects observed in human beings. However, the tremendous variation in species and strain sensitivity to 2,3,7,8-TCDD and related compounds cannot be explained by the observed toxicokinetic differences. There is evidence in inbred mice, that the cellular levels of the Ah receptor correlate, in part, with susceptibility to the biological and toxic effects of these compounds. The receptor has also been identified in other species, including human beings. However, interspecies comparison of cellular Ah receptor levels do not explain their differences in sensitivity to 2,3,7,8-TCDD; this is consistent with complex as yet unknown mechanisms of toxicity that involve multiple factors in addition to the Ah receptor.

12.4 Human Health Effects

12.4.1 PCDDs

Exposure of the general population is to small amounts of PCDDs and PCDFs in complex mixtures and these have not been associated with disease. In a few incidents workers and others have been exposed to larger amounts of a limited number of these compounds, e.g., Seveso and in Yusho disease.

For occupational and accidental exposure the most prominent clinical effect has been chloracne. Other effects (Table 64) have been noted, but, apart from chloracne and perhaps minor functional disorders, none has been persistent.

In some, but not all mortality studies, an increased incidence of cancer at different sites has been claimed, but the small numbers of cases limit confidence in the findings.

The overall impression from the follow-up studies is that even severe acute systemic effects of TCDD are usually reversible, except for chloracne, or markedly improved over time following cessation of exposure. In Seveso, the only clear-cut adverse health effect recorded has been chloracne. 193 cases of chloracne occurred in 1976 and 1977, and 20 of those still presented active symptoms in 1984. Many studies have been performed to find possible links between exposure and health effects in civilians or military personnel exposed to Agent Orange in Viet Nam. However, the information available to date does not allow definite conclusions to be drawn with regard to effects on human reproduction or any other significant health effects (see section 9.2).

In a number of studies, exposed populations and various control groups have been compared by measuring serum lipids, liver function tests, and other variables. Although certain statistically significant differences have been reported there, and also in isolated case reports, lack of uniformity, various technical shortcomings, and the inability to exclude confounding factors means that the results have been inconclusive.

In the Missouri (USA) incident, children who showed acute illness when the contamination occurred in 1971 are now reportedly in good health. Epidemiological studies in Missouri on populations exposed to lower concentration over longer periods of time have so far not revealed any significant health effects. Although no clinical illness was observed, there were indications of an effect on the cell-mediated immune system.

The ranges of health effects produced by TCDD in human beings have yet to be defined. It can be concluded that the data from human exposure and effects, when taken together, do not allow any determinations of dose/effect or dose/response relationships in human beings.

In spite of many clinical and follow-up studies, no clearcut persistent systemic effects have been delineated, except for chloracne. In the light of present information, it seems unlikely that permanent, severe, and debilitating toxicological sequelae are inevitable after exposure to TCDD.

12.4.2 PCDFs

The only well documented intoxications with PCDFs in human beings are the two instances of contamination of rice oil with PCDFs, PCBs, and PCQs, i.e., Yusho in Japan (1968) and Yu-cheng in Taiwan (1979) (see section 11.1). In total, several thousand people were acutely intoxicated. The summarized data makes it most likely that the causative agent was PCDFs. The general symptomatology was similar to that found in intoxications with TCDD. The differences may reflect intensity in exposure and the ages and sex of the exposed human beings. Attempts to estimate the average daily intake of PCDFs over several months in Yusho patients indicated a figure of 0.9 µg/kg body weight of total PCDFs, 0.1-0.2 µg/kg of 2,3,7,8-substituted tetra-, penta-, and hexaPCDFs, together with 157 µg PCBs and 148 µg PCQs/kg body weight (Hayabuchi et al., 1979). The lowest dose causing disease was estimated to be 0.6 mg total PCDFs per person over 30 days, corresponding to a daily dose of 0.05-0.1 µg/kg body weight of 2,3,7,8-substituted PCDFs. However, the data available are not sufficient to permit any conclusions as to what dose might be safe for human intake.

12.4.3 Human body burden and kinetics

In human fat, background levels of TCDD up to 20 ng/kg have been found in the general population with no known specific exposure, but higher levels have been reported in some cases without evidence of disease. None of these populations have been randomly sampled. The more highly chlorinated other PCDDs and PCDFs, especially octaDD, also occur in these samples (see Tables 29, 30). Averages values seem to increase with age.

In special situations, higher levels (in the low µg/kg range) have been found that have not been associated with disease.

In the Yusho and Yu-cheng incidents, symptoms were noticed at higher levels of PCDFs, e.g., 2,3,4,7,8-pentaCDF was found at 6.9 µg/kg fat tissue one year after the exposure to contaminated rice oil.

Based on the very limited data available, the levels of, for instance, 2,3,4,7,8-pentaCDF in the general population, seem to be two orders of magnitude lower than the levels associated with the Yusho disease.

No such comparisons can be made for PCDDs.

Limited data indicate that those isomers chlorinated at the 2,3,7, and 8 positions are selectively retained, except for TCDF.

A half-life for TCDD in human beings of 5 years has been indicated by one experimental study. In another study half-lives in the range of 2-6 years were estimated for 1,2,3,6,7,8-hexaCDD, 1,2,3,4,6,7,8-heptaCDD, octaCDD, 1,2,3,4,6,7,8-heptaCDF, and octaCDF. These data need to be expanded since they are based on studies in only two subjects and since the toxicokinetics of these types of compounds may not simply be controlled by first-order kinetics. However, even if there are limitations in the present data, it is apparent that the half-lives of these compounds are in the range of one or more years.

These reported half-lives for human beings are very different from those reported in rodents. However, animal experiments have usually been performed with toxic doses.

Furthermore, animals with a short life span have a higher metabolic rate, thus shorter half-lives could be expected.

The PCDDs and PCDFs are predominantly stored in fat, but they are also excreted in milk (Table 39) and pass the placenta. They also appear in the blood and vital organs at lower concentrations. The distribution between different tissues in human beings is not at present clear, although it has been suggested that the ratio between fatty tissue and liver is higher in human beings than that in rodents. However, this conclusion is based on very limited data from autopsy specimens. Whether this is relevant for the general population remains to be seen.

The intake route for human beings is at present not very well delineated, but it has been assumed that intake from food is the main route. However, the human infant represents a special case; because of transplacental transfer of these compounds, the neonate might be expected to be exposed *in utero*. Levels measured so far in human milk suggest that this food might be an important source of these compounds.

No data are available regarding what dose of PCDDs is toxic to human beings. However, in the Yusho and Yu-cheng episodes, total intakes of total PCDFs in the range 3.3-3.8 mg/person and total intakes of 2,3,7,8-substituted PCDFs in the range 400-500 µg/person were associated with the disease. No good data are available as to what intakes occurred without causing disease.

12.5 General Conclusions

PCDDs and PCDFs occur throughout the environment and we all probably carry a body burden of them. They have sometimes produced complex toxic effects following occupational and accidental exposure.

Based on the Yusho disease and experiments in sensitive species of monkeys, and making assumptions about the relative potencies of PCDDs and PCDFs, human beings and certain monkey species may have comparable sensitivity to these compounds. However, the uncertainties related to the real dose received by human beings and the difficulties of assessing toxic effects other than chloracne in our species prevent a firm conclusion as to the relative resistance of human beings to the toxic effects of these compounds. Exposure should be reduced to levels as low as are reasonably practicable.

13. RECOMMENDATIONS

1. Analytical interlaboratory validation and round-robin studies using standardized quality assurance and quality control procedures are needed to improve analytical methodology.
   Sampling strategy and analytical procedures and data interpretation should be optimized and standardized before undertaking surveys.

2. Further information is required about the origins and environmental distribution and fate of PCDDs and PCDFs.
   Further monitoring data, including time trends and determinations of isomer patterns, are required for environmental levels of PCDDs and PCDFs, especially for food, ambient air, and sediments.

3. Data should be obtained about the effects of PCDDs and PCDFs on environmental biota.

4. More information is required about the bioavailability of PCDDs and PCDFs from different matrices in the environment and from the diet. Exposure from these sources should be correlated with agricultural and industrial practices.

5. Simpler and less expensive methods suitable for screening should be developed and validated.

6. Studies to determine the mechanisms of toxicity of PCDDs and PCDFs are needed to support an evaluation of the differences in effects between species and to allow extrapolation to human beings.

7. Further investigation of immunotoxicity is important, including cytotoxic T lymphocyte function. Studies of the effects of perinatal exposure and of the duration of actions on the immune system are important.

8. Long-term toxicity studies, including multigeneration reproductive studies, in different species with three of the most widespread PCDDs and PCDFs, namely 2,3,4,7,8-pentaCDF, 1,2,3,7,8-pentaCDD, and octaCDD, should be carried out.

9. Because humans are exposed to complex mixtures of PCDDs and PCDFs, test systems, including techniques applicable to evaluating human tissues, should be further developed

and validated for the toxic potency of these compounds and other mixtures. These systems can be used to study mechanisms of action, structure activity relationships, and interactive effects.

10. Investigations to examine the body burden and to correlate it with clinical effects and laboratory findings are indicated. Follow-up studies of previously exposed groups are important.

14. EVALUATIONS BY INTERNATIONAL BODIES AND THE CONCEPT OF TCDD EQUIVALENTS

14.1 International Evaluations

IARC evaluated the carcinogenic risk of TCDD to man (IARC, 1977, 1982) and concluded that there was sufficient evidence that it was carcinogenic to animals, but that the data for carcinogenicity to human beings was inadequate. None of the other PCDDs or PCDFs have been evaluated by IARC.

Regulatory standards for TCDD and mixtures containing TCDD, established by national bodies in different countries and the European Economic Community, are summarized in the Legal File of the International Register of Potentially Toxic Chemicals (IRPTC, 1987).

14.2 Methodologies Used in Assessment of Risk from PCDDs and PCDFs

14.2.1 Individual Congeners

As shown in this monograph, sufficient high quality data for assessing human health risks exist only for TCDD. For the other congeners and isomers where data do exist, they are generally derived from studies using acute exposures in experimental animals and/or from *in vitro* tests.

The several risk evaluations on TCDD from various countries have utilized the long-term ocogenic rat studies (Kociba et al., 1978) or the reproduction studies on rats (Murray et al., 1979) or monkeys (Schantz et al., 1979). Mathematical models have been applied to the cancer data and "virtually safe doses" between 0.006 and 0.028 pg/kg body weight per day have been calculated (Kimbrough, 1984). The biological relevance of such models has been questioned, since TCDD has not been shown to be genotoxic, and has been found to be a strong promoter of liver tumours in a two-stage pre-carcinogenesis study (Pitot et al., 1980) To avoid the use of mathematical models, several evaluations have used safety factors in the range of 100 to 1000 applied to the assumed no-effect, or lowest-observed-effect levels in the cancer study of Kociba et al. (1978) or the reproduction studies of Murray et al. (1979) or Schantz et al. (1978). Using this methodology "tolerable daily intakes" have been calculated for human beings in the range of 1-10 pg/kg body weight (Denmark, 1984; Ontario, 1985; US EPA, 1985; Ahlborg & Victorin, 1987).

14.2.2 Mixtures of PCDD and PCDF congeners and isomers - concept of TCDD toxic equivalents.

The results of recent isomer-specific analyses of such diverse environmental samples as emissions from the combustion of hazardous industrial and municipal wastes, soil, industrial process wastes, human adipose tissue, and milk indicate that the majority of the 75 CDD and 135 CDF isomers can be detected. Humans are therefore exposed to complex mixtures of these environmental contaminants (sometimes 2,3,7,8-tetraCDD is only a minor component), and the level of risk from such exposures must be assessed.

In the absence of long-term whole animal tests on complex mixtures of PCDDs and PCDFs, as well as similar studies on individual isomers and/or congeners, several models have been proposed to relate the toxicity of environmental mixtures to the well studied isomer 2,3,7,8-TCDD. The results from these models are presented as "TCDD Toxic Equivalents". A summary of some models which have been published is given in Table 74. The toxic potencies used, relative to TCDD, are shown. The scientific basis for deriving these relative toxicities is somewhat different for each model. The Swiss (Switzerland, 1982) and Danish (Denmark, 1984) models are based essentially on the relative potency for AHH induction, whereas the German (Germany, 1985) and Canadian models (Ontario, 1985) are based on a weighting of all available quantitative data. The USA model (US EPA, 1987) utilizes primarily the relative carcinogenic potencies of TCDD and hexaCDD, with consideration given to other relevant quantitative data. A discussion of the structure-activity relationships and relative biological activities of many PCDD and PCDF isomers is given in sections 7 and 10.

Data requirements, and assumptions made in the application of these models to various environmental mixtures have been reviewed by US EPA (1987) and Ontario (1985). Suter-Hofmann & Schlatter (1985) fed toluene extracts of acid-washed particulates from a municipal waste incinerator to Sprague Dawley rats at levels in the diet corresponding to 4, 12, and 24% of particulates. The calculated daily TCDD intakes at these doses were 4.8, 14.4, and 28.8 ng/kg body weight. Depending upon which model was used from Table 74, the estimated intake of PCDDs and PCDFs would be 48-300 (4% particulates), 144-900 (12% particulates), and 288-1800 ng TCDD-equivalents/kg body weight per day (24% particulates). No mortality was noted in the groups fed 24% particulates, but at this dose body weight gain was depressed in females and depressed thymus and increased liver weights were noted in both sexes. No adverse affects were seen at the 4% and 12% dose levels. From the known toxicity of TCDD, more severe effects would have

Table 74. Examples of TCDD-equivalence models

Compound	Relative PCDD and PCDF toxicities in model					
	Olie et al. (1983)	Switzerland (1982)	Germany (1985)	Denmark (1984)	Ontario (1985)	United States (US EPA 1987)
MonoCDD	0				0.001	0
DiCDD	0				0.001	0
TriCDD	0				0.01	0
TetraCDD-2,3,7,8	1.0	1.0	1.0	1.0	1.0	1.0
-non 2,3,7,8	1.0	0.01	0.01		0.01	0.01
PentaCDD-1,2,3,7,8	0.1			0.01		
-all 2,3,7,8	0.1	0.1	0.1		0.1	0.5
-non 2,3,7,8	0.1	0.1	0.01		0.1	0.005
HexaCDD-1,2,3,4,7,8				0.1		
-1,2,3,6,7,8				0.01		
-1,2,3,7,8,9				0.01		
-all 2,3,7,8	0.1	0.1	0.1		0.1	0.04
-non 2,3,7,8	0.1	0.1	0.01		0.1	0.0004
HeptaCDD-1,2,3,4,6,7,8				0.01		
-all 2,3,7,8	0.1	0.1	0.01		0.01	0.001
-non 2,3,7,8	0.1	0.1	0.001		0.01	0.00001
OctaCDD	0		0.001		0.0001	0
MonoCDF					0.0001	
DiCDF					0.0001	
TriCDF					0.01	

Table 74 (contd).

TetraCDF-2,3,7,8	0.1	0.1	0.1	0.1	0.5	0.1
-non 2,3,7,8	0.1	0.1	0.01		0.5	0.001
PentaCDF-1,2,3,7,8				0.2		
-2,3,4,7,8				0.2		
-all 2,3,7,8	0.1	0.1	0.1		0.5	0.1
-non 2,3,7,8	0.1	0.1	0.01		0.5	0.001
HexaCDF-1,2,3,4,7,8				0.2		
-1,2,3,6,7,8				0.05		
-1,2,3,7,8,9						
-2,3,4,6,7,8				0.1		
-all 2,3,7,8	0.1	0.1	0.1		0.1	0.01
-non 2,3,7,8	0.1	0.1	0.01		0.1	0.0001
HeptaCDF-1,2,3,4,6,7,8				0.01		
-1,2,3,4,7,8,9						
-all 2,3,7,8	0.1	0.1	0.01		0.01	0.00001
-non 2,3,7,8	0.1		0.001		0.01	0.00001
OctaCDF	0		0.001		0.0001	0

been expected from the calculated dose of between 288 and 1800 ng TCDD-equivalents/kg body weight per day. These data support the conclusion that the application of TCDD-equivalence models may over-estimate the inherent risk from exposures to dioxin-containing environmental mixtures, depending largely upon the assumptions used in deriving the model. However, a definitive conclusion on this point awaits further research (US EPA, 1987) (see section 13).

It must be recognized that an approach such as the use of "TCDD-equivalents" must be regarded as an interim procedure for the measurement of the toxicity of environmental samples in the absence of long-term toxicity data on specific PCDD and PCDF isomers and mixtures of these compounds. At present it is an imprecise evaluation methodology with many data gaps in the supporting data base.

The TCDD-equivalent models have two major sources of uncertainty, i.e., firstly, the unanswered scientific questions related to the toxicity of TCDD itself, and secondly, the lack of data on the other PCDD and PCDF congeners and isomers that would permit a more accurate determination of the potency of these chemicals relative to TCDD. The research recommendations in this document address some of these concerns. As such data become available, TCDD-equivalent models must be continuously updated and risk assessments based on the present models (Table 74) considered only as interim evaluations.

REFERENCES

ABATE, L., BASSO, P., BELLONI, A., BISANTI, L., BORGNA, C., BRUZZI, P., DORIGOTTI, G., FALLIVA, L., FANUZZI, A., FORMIGARO, M., MAGGIORE, G., MARNI, E., MEAZZA, L., MERLO, F., PUNTONI, R., ROSA, A., STAGNARO, E., & VERCELLI, M. (1982) Mortality and birth defects from 1976 to 1979 in the population living in the TCDD polluted area of Seveso. In: Hutzinger, O., ed. Chlorinated dioxins and related compounds. Impact on the environment, Oxford, New York, Pergamon Press, pp. 571-598.

ABERNETHY, D.J., GREENLEE, W.F., HUBAND, J.C., & BOREIKO, C.J. (1985) 2,3,7,8-tetrachlorodibenzo-p-dioxin (TCDD) promotes the transformation of C3H/10T1/2 cells. Carcinogenesis, 6: 651-653.

ADAMS, E.M., IRISH, D.D., SPENCER, H.C., & ROWE, V.K. (1941) The response of rabbit skin to compounds reported to have caused acneform dermatits. Ind. Med., 2: 1-4.

AHLBORG, U.G. & VICTORIN, K. (1987) Impact on health and environment from trace organic emissions. Waste Manage. Res., 5: 203-224.

AHLBORG, U.G., WAERN, F., & HAKANSSON, H. (1987) Interactive effects of PCDDs and PCDFs occurring in human mother's milk. Chemosphere, 16(8/9): 1701-1706.

AHLING, B., BJORSETH, A., & LUNE, G. (1978) Formation of chlorinated hydro- carbons during combustion of poly(vinyl chloride). Chemosphere, 8(10): 799-806.

AHLING, B., LINDSKOG, A., JANSSON, B., & SUNDSTROM, G. (1977) Formation of polychlorinated dibenzo-p-dioxins and dibenzofurans during combustion of a 2,4,5-T formulation. Chemosphere, 6(8): 461-468.

AITIO, A. & PARKKI, M.G. (1978) Organ specific induction of drug metabolizing enzymes by 2,3,7,8-tetrachlorodibenzo-p-dioxin in the rat. Toxicol. appl. Pharmacol., 44: 107-114.

AITIO, A., PARKKI, M.G., & MARNIEMI, J. (1979) Different effect of 2,3,7,8-tetrachlorodibenzo-p-dioxin on glucuronide conjugation of various aglycones. Studies in Wistar and Gunn rats. Toxicol. appl. Pharmacol., 47: 55-60.

AKERMARK, B. (1978) Photochemical reactions of phenoxy acids and dioxins. Chlorinated phenoxy acids and their dioxins. Ecol. Bull., 21: 75-81.

ALBRO, P.W. & CORBETT, B.J. (1977) Extraction and clean-up of animal tissues for subsequent determination of mixtures of chlorinated dibenzo-p-dioxins and dibenzofurans. Chemosphere, 7: 381-385.

ALBRO, P.W., CORBETT, J.T., HARRIS, M., & LAWSON, L.D. (1978) Effects of 2,3,7,8-tetrachlorodibenzo-p-dioxin on lipid profiles in tissue of the Fisher rat. Chem.-biol. Interact., 23: 315-330.

ALBRO, P.W., CRUMMETT, W.B., DUPUY., A.E., Jr, GROSS, M.L., HANSON, M., HARLESS, R.L., HILEMAN, F.D., HILKER, D., JASON, C., JOHNSON, J.L., LAMPARSKI, L.L., LAU, B.P.Y., MCDANIEL, D.D., MEEHAN, J.L., NESTRICK, T.J., NYGREN, M., O'KEEFE, P., PETERS, T.L., RAPPE, C., RYAN, J.J., SMITH, L.M., STALLING, D.L., WEERASINGHE, N.C.A., & WENDLING, J.M. (1985) Methods for the quantitative determination of multiple, specific polychlorinated dibenzo-p-dioxin and dibenzofuran isomers in human adipose tissue in the parts-per-trillion range. An interlaboratory study. Anal. Chem., 57: 2717-2725.

ALBRO, P.W., CORBETT, J.T., & SCHROEDER, J.L. (1986) Effects of 2,3,7,8-tetrachlorodibenzo-p-dioxin on lipid peroxidation in microsomal systems in vitro. Chem.-biol. Interact., 57: 301-313.

ALLEN, J.R. (1964) The role of "toxic fat" in the production of hydro- pericardium and ascites in chickens. Am. J. vet. Res., 25: 1210-1219.

ALLEN, J.R. & CARSTENS, L.A. (1967) Light and electron microscopic observations in Macaca mulatta monkeys fed toxic fat. Am. J. vet. Res., 28: 1513-1526.

ALLEN, J.R. & LALICH, J.J. (1962) Response of chickens to prolonged feeding of crude "toxic fat". Proc. Soc. Exp. Biol. Med., 109: 48-51.

ALLEN, J.R., VAN MILLER, J.P., & NORBACK, D.H. (1975) Tissue distribution, excretion and biological effects of (^{14}C) tetrachlorodibenzo-p-dioxin in rats. Food Cosmet. Toxicol., 13: 501-505.

ALLEN, J.R., BARSOTTI, D.A., VAN MILLER, J.P., ABRAHAMSON, L.J., & LALICH, J.J. (1977) Morphological changes in monkeys consuming a diet containing low levels of 2,3,7,8-tetrachlorodibenzo-p-dioxin. Food Cosmet. Toxicol., 15(5): 401-410.

ALLEN, J.R., HARGRAVES, W.A., HSIA, M.T.S., & LIN, F.S.D. (1979a) Comparative toxicology of chlorinated compounds on mammalian species. Pharmacol. Ther., 7: 513-547.

ALLEN, J.R., BARSOTTI, D.A., LAMBRECHT, L.K., & VAN MILLER, J.P. (1979b) Reproductive effects of halogenated aromatic hydrocarbons on nonhuman primates. Ann. N.Y. Acad. Sci., 320: 19-27.

ANDERSSON, K., BOSSHARDT, H.P., BUSER, H.R., MARKLUND, S., & RAPPE, C. (1978) Chlorinated phenoxy acids and their dioxins: Chemistry-summary. Ecol. Bull., 27: 19-27.

ARSTILA, A.U., REGGIANI, G., SORVARI, T.E., RAISANEN, S., & WIPF, H.K. (1981) Elimination of 2,3,7,8-tetrachlorodibenzo-p-dioxin in goat milk. Toxicol. Lett., 9: 215-219.

ASHE, W.F. & SUSKIND, R.R. (1949) Clinical Report on four patients from Monsanto Chemical Company in Nitro, West Virginia, USA, 14 pp. (Submitted December 1949).

ASHE, W.F. & SUSKIND, R.R. (1950) Clinical report on six patients from Monsanto Chemical Company in Nitro, West Virginia, USA, 16 pp. (Submitted April 1950).

BAADER, E.W. & BAUER, H.J. (1951) Industrial intoxication due to pentachlorophenol. Ind. Med. Surg., 20(6): 286-290.

BAARS, A.J., MUKHTAR, H., JANSEN, M., & BREIMER, D.D. (1982) Induction of rat hepatic glutathione-s-tranferase activities by 2,3,7,8-tetrachlorodibenzo- p-dioxin, Oxford, New York, Pergamon Press, pp. 393-401 (Pergamon Series on Environmental Science, Vol. 5).

BALK, J.L. & PIPER, W.N. (1984) Altered blood levels of corticosteroids in the rat after exposure to 2,3,7,8-tetra-chlorodibenzo-p-dioxin. Biochem. Pharmacol., 33(15): 2531-2534.

BALL, L.M. & CHABRA, R.S. (1981) Intestinal absorption of nutrients in rats treated with 2,3,7,8-tetrachlorodibenzo-p-dioxin (TCDD). J. Toxicol. environ. Health, 8: 629-638.

BANDIERA, S., FARRELL, K., MASON, G., KELLEY, M., ROMKES, M., BANNISTER, R., & SAFE, S. (1984a) Comparative toxicities of the polychlorinated dibenzofuran (PCDF) and biphenyl (PCB) mixtures which persist in yusho victims. Chemosphere, 13(4): 507-512.

BANDIERA, S., SAWYER, T., ROMKES, M., ZMUDZKA, B., SAFE, L., MASON, G., KEYS, B., & SAFE, S. (1984b) Polychlorinated dibenzofurans (PCDFs): Effects of structure on binding to the 2,3,7,8-TCDD cytosolic receptor protein, AHH induction and toxicity. Toxicology, 32: 131-144.

BANNISTER, R. & SAFE, S. (1987) Aroclor 1254 as a 2,3,7,8-tetrachlorodibenzo-p-dioxin antagonist in C57BL/6J and DBA/2J mice - effects of enzyme induction. Toxicologist, 7: 160.

BANNISTER, R., MASON, G., KELLEY, M., & SAFE, S. (1986) The effects of cytosolic receptor modulation on the AHH-inducing activity of 2,3,7,8-TCDD. Chemosphere, 15: 1909-1911.

BARSOTTI, D.A., ABRAHAMSON, L.J., & ALLEN, J.R. (1979) Hormonal alterations in female rhesus monkeys fed a diet containing 2,3,7,8-tetrachlorodibenzo-p-dioxin. Bull. environ. Contam. Toxicol., 21: 463-469.

BARTELSON, F.D., HARRISON, D.D., & MORGAN, J.D. (1975) Field studies of wildlife exposed to TCDD contaminated soil, Florida, Airforce Armament Laboratory, Eglin Air Force Base (AFATL-TR-75-49).

BASTOMSKY, C.H. (1977) Enhanced thyroxine metabolism and high uptake goiters in rats after a single dose of 2,3,7,8-tetrachlorodibenzo-p-dioxin. Endocrinology, 101(1): 292-296.

BAUER, H., SCHULZ, K.H., & SPIEGELBERG, U. (1961) [Occupational poisoning in the manufacture of chlorophenol compounds.] Arch. Gewerbepathol. Gewerbehyg., 18: 538-555 (in German).

BAUGHMAN, R.W. (1974) Tetrachlorodibenzo-p-dioxins in the environment. High resolution mass spectrometry of the picogram level, Cambridge, Massachussets, Harvard University (Thesis).

BAUGHMAN, R.W. & MESELSON, M. (1973) An analytical method for detecting TCDD (dioxin): Levels of TCDD in samples from Vietnam. Environ. Health Perspect., 5: 27-35.

BEALE, M.G., SHEARER, W.T., KARL, M.M., & ROBSON, A.M. (1977) Long-term effects of dioxin exposure. Lancet, 1: 748.

BEATTY, P.W. & NEAL, R.A. (1977) Factors affecting the induction of DT-diaphorase by 2,3,7,8-tetrachlorodibenzo-p-dioxin. Biochem. Pharmacol., 27: 505-510.

BEATTY, P.W., LEMBACH, K.J., HOLSCHER, M.A., & NEAL, R.A. (1975) Effects of 2,3,7,8-tetrachlorodibenzo-p-dioxin (TCDD) on mammalian cells in tissue cultures. Toxicol. appl. Pharmacol., 31: 309-312.

BEATTY, P.W., VAUGHN, W.K., & NEAL, R.A. (1978) Effect of alteration of rat hepatic mixed-function oxidase (MFO) activity on the toxicity of 2,3,7,8- tetrachlorodibenzo-p-dioxin (TCDD). Toxicol. appl. Pharmacol., 45: 513-519.

BECK, H., ECKART, K., KELLERT, M., MATHAR, W., RUHL, CH.-S., & WITTOWSKI, R. (1987) Levels of PCDF and PCDD in samples of human origin and food in the Federal Republic of Germany. Chemosphere, 16: 1977-1982.

BELL, R.A. & GARA, A. (1985) Synthesis and characterization of the isomers of polychlorinated dibenzofurans, tetra- through octa-. In: Keith, L.H., Rappe, C., & Choudhary, C.G., ed. Chlorinated dioxins and dibenzofurans in the total environment, Boston, Butterworth Publishers, pp. 3-16.

BERGMAN, A., HAGMAN, A., JACOBSSON, S., JANSSON, B., & AHLMAN, M. (1984) Thermal degradation of polychlorinated alkanes. Chemosphere, 13: 237-250.

BERLIN, A., BURRATTA, A., & VAN DER VENNE, M.-T. (1967) Proceedings of the Expert Meeting on the Problems raised by TCDD-Pollution, Milan, Italy, Luxembourg, Commission of the European Communities, p. 179.

BERRY, D.L., ZACHARIAH, P.K., NAMKUNG, M.J., & JUCHAU, M.R. (1976) Transplacental induction of carcinogen-hydroxylating systems with 2,3,7,8- tetrachlorodibenzo-p-dioxin. Toxicol. appl. Pharmacol., 36: 569-548.

BERRY, D.L., SLAGA, T.J., WILSON, N.M., ZACHARIAH, P.K., NAMKUNG, M.J., BRACKEN, W.M., & JUCHAU, M.R. (1977) Tranplacental induction of mixed- function oxygenases in extra-hepatic tissues by 2,3,7,8-tetrachlorodibenzo-p-dioxin. Biochem. Pharmacol., 26: 1383-1388.

BERRY, D.L., SLAGA, T.J., DIGIOVANNI, J., & JUCHAU, M.R. (1979) Studies with chlorinated dibenzo-p-dioxins, polybrominated biphenyls, and poly chlorinated biphenyls in a two-stage system of mouse skin tumorigenesis: potent anticarcinogenic effects. Ann. N.Y. Acad. Sci., 320: 405-414.

BERTONI, G., BROCCO, D., DI PALO, V., LIBERTI, A., POSSANZINI, M., & BRUNER, F. (1978) Gas chromatographic determination of 2,3,7,8-tetra chloro- dibenzodioxin in the experimental decontamination of Seveso soil by ultraviolet radiation. Anal. Chem., 50: 732-735.

BIRNBAUM, L.S. (1986) Distribution and excretion of 2,3,7,8-tetra- chlorodibenzo-p-dioxin in congenic strains of mice which differ at the Ah locus. Drug Metab. Disp., 14(1): 34-40.

BIRNBAUM, L.S., DECAD, G.M., & MATTHEWS, H.B. (1980) Disposition and excretion of 2,3,7,8-tetrachlorodibenzofuran in the rat. Toxicol. appl. Pharmacol., 55: 342-352.

BIRNBAUM, L.S., DECAD, G.M., MATTHEWS, H.B., & MCCONNELL, E.E. (1981) Fate of 2,3,7,8-tetrachlorodibenzofuran in the monkey. Toxicol. appl. Pharmacol., 57: 189-196.

BIRNBAUM, L.S., WEBER, H., HARRIS, M.W., LAMB, J.C., IV, & MCKINNEY, J.D. (1985) Toxic interaction of specific polychlorinated biphenyls and 2,3,7,8-tetrachlorodibenzo-p-dioxin: Increased incidence of cleft palate in mice. Toxicol. appl. Pharmacol., 77: 292-302.

BIRNBAUM, L.S., HARRIS, M.W., MILLER, C.P., PRATT, R.M., & LAMB, J.C. (1986) Synergistic interaction of 2,3,7,8-tetra-chlorodibenzo-p-dioxin and hydro-cortisone in the induction of cleft palate in mice. Teratology, 33: 29-35.

BIRNBAUM, L.S., HARRIS, M.W., BARNHART, E.R., & MORRISSEY, R.E. (1987) Teratogenicity of three polychlorinated dibenzo-furans in C57BL/6N mice. Toxicol. appl. Pharmacol., 90: 206-216.

BLEIBERG, J., WALLEN, M., BRODKIN, R., & APPLEBAUM, I.L. (1964) Industrially acquired porphyria. Arch. Dermatol., 89: 793-797.

BLOMHOFF, R., HELGERUD, P., RASMUSSEN, M., BERG, T., & NORUM, K.R. (1982) In vivo uptake of chylomicron (3H)retinyl ester by rat liver: Evidence for retinol transfer from parenchymal to nonparenchymal cells. Proc. Natl Acad. Sci. (USA), 79: 7326-7330.

BOER, F.P., NEUMAN, M.A., VAN REMOORTERE, F.P., NORTH, P.P., & RINN, H.W., (1973) X-Ray diffraction studies of chlorinated dibenzo-p-dioxins. Chlorodioxins - origin and fate. Adv. Chem. Ser., 120, 14-25.

BOMBICK, D.W., MATSUMURA, F., & MADHUKAR, B.V. (1984) TCDD (2,3,7,8-Tetrachlorodibenzo-p-dioxin) causes reduction in the low density lipoprotein (LDL) receptor activities in the hepatic plasma membrane of the guinea pig and rat. Biochem. biophys. Res. Commun., 118: 548-554.

BOMBICK, D.W., MADHUKAR, B.V., BREWSTER, D.W., & MATSUMURA, F. (1985) TCDD (2,3,7,8-tetrachlorodibenzo-p-dioxin) causes increases in protein kinases particularly protein kinase C in the hepatic plasma membrane of the rat and the guinea pig. Biochem. biophys. Res. Commun., 127(1): 296-302.

BONACCORSI, A., DI DOMENICO, A., FANELLI, R., MERLI, F., MOTTA, R., VANZATI, R., & ZAPPONI, G.A. (1984) The influence of soil particle adsorption on 2,3,7,8-tetrachlorodibenzo-p-dioxin biological uptake in the rabbit. Arch. Toxicol., 7: 431-434.

BOTRE, C., MEMOLI, A., & ALHAIQUE, F. (1978) TCDD solubilization and photodecomposition in aqueous solutions. Environ. Sci. Technol., 12: 335-336.

BOWES, G.W., MULVIHILL, M.J., DECAMP, M.R., & KENDE, A.S. (1975) Gas chromatographic characteristics of authentic chlorinated dibenzofurans; identification of two isomers in American and Japanese polychlorinated biphenyls. J. agric. food Chem., 23(6): 1222-1223.

BRADLAW, J.A. & CASTERLINE, J.L., Jr (1979) Induction of enzyme activity in cell culture: a rapid screen for detection of planar polychlorinated organic compounds. J. Assoc. Off. Anal. Chem., 62(4): 904-916.

BRADLAW, J.A., GARTHOFF, L.H., HURLEY, N.E., & FIRESTONE, D. (1980) Comparative induction of aryl hydrocarbon hydroxylase activity in vitro by analogues of dibenzo-p-dioxin. Food Cosmet. Toxicol., 18: 627-635.

BRAUN, W. (1955) [Chloracne. Monographs with the Journal Berufsdermatosen,] Aulendorf i. Wurtt., Editio Cantor, Vol. 1. (in German).

BREWSTER, D.W., MADHUKAR, B.V., & MATSUMURA, F. (1982) Influence of 2,3,7,8-TCDD on the protein composition of the plasma membrane of hepatic cells from the rat. Biochem. biophys. Res. Commun., 107: 68-74.

BRONZETTI, G., BAUER, C., CORSI, C., DEL CARRATORE, R., NIERI, R., & PAOLINI, M. (1983) Mutagenicity study of TCDD and ashes from urban incinerator "in vitro" and "in vivo" using yeast D7 strain. Chemosphere, 12(4/5): 549-553.

BROWN, E.F. & MORGAN, A.F. (1948) The effect of vitamin A deficiency upon the nitrogen metabolism of the rat. J. Nutr., 35: 425-438.

BUMB, R.R., CRUMMETT, W.B., CUTIE, S.S., GLADHILL, R.H., VAGEL, R.O., LAMPAVSKI, L.L., LUOMA, E.V., MILLER, D.L., NESTRIDE, T.J., SHADOFF, L.A., STEHL, R.H., & WOODS, J.S., (1980) Trace chemistries of fire: A source of chlorinated dioxins. Science, 210: 385-390.

BURKHARD, L.P. & KUEHL, D.W. (1986) N-Octanol/water partition coefficients by reverse phase liquid chromatography/mass spectrometry for eight tetrachlorinated planar molecules. Chemosphere, 15: 163-167.

BUS, J.S. & GIBSON, J.E. (1979) Lipid peroxidation and its role in toxicology. Rev. Biochem. Toxicol., 1: 125-149.

BUSER, H.R. (1975) Polychlorinated dibenzo-p-dioxins. Separation and identification of isomers by gas chromotagrophy mass spectrometry. J. Chromatogr., 114: 95-108.

BUSER, H.R. (1979) Formation of polychlorinated dibenzofurans (PCDFs) and dibenzo-p-dioxins (PCDDs) from the pyrolysis of chlorobenzenes. Chemosphere, 6: 415-424.

BUSER, H.R. & BOSSHARDT, H.P. (1976) Determination of polychlorinated dibenzo-p-dioxins and dibenzofurans in commercial pentachlorophenols by combined gas chromatography - mass spectrometry. J. Assoc. Off. Anal. Chem., 59: 562-569.

BUSER, H.R. & BOSSHARDT, H.P. (1978) [Polychlorinated dibenzo-p-dioxin, dibenzofuran and benzene in the ashes from municipal and industrial incinerators.] Mitt. Geb. Lebensm. Hyg., 69: 191-199 (in German).

BUSER, H.R. & RAPPE, C. (1978) Identification of substitution patterns in polychlorinated dibenzo-p-dioxins (PCDDs) by mass spectrometry. Chemosphere, 7: 199-211.

BUSER, H.R. & RAPPE, C. (1979) Formation of polychlorinated dibenzofurans (PCDFs) from the pyrolysis of individual PCB isomers. Chemosphere, 3: 157-174.

BUSER, H.R. & RAPPE, C. (1980) High-resolution gas chromatography of the 22 tetrachlorodibenzo-p-dioxin isomers. Anal. Chem., 52: 2257-2262.

BUSER, H.R. & RAPPE, C. (1984) Isomer-specific separation of 2,3,7,8- substituted polychlorinated dibenzo-p-dioxins by high-resolution gas chromatography/mass spectrometry. Anal. Chem., 56: 442-448.

BUSER, H.R., BOSSHARDT, H.P., & RAPPE, C. (1978a) Formation of polychlorinated dibenzofurans (PCDFs) from the pyrolysis of PCBs. Chemosphere, 1: 109-119.

BUSER, H.R., BOSSHARDT, H.P., & RAPPE, C. (1978b) Identification of polychlorinated dibenzo-p-dioxin isomers found in fly ash. Chemosphere, 7(2): 165-172.

BUSER, H.R., BOSSHARDT, H.P., RAPPE, C., & LINDAHL, R. (1978c) Identification of polychlorinated dibenzofuran isomers in fly ash and PCB pyrolysis. Chemosphere, 5: 419-429.

BUSER, H.R., RAPPE, C., & GARA, A. (1978d) Polychlorinated dibenzofurans (PCDFs) found in Yosho oil and in used Japanese PCB. Chemosphere, 5: 439-449.

BUSER, H.R., RAPPE, C., & BERGQVIST, P.-A. (1985) Analysis of polychlorinated dibenzofurans, dioxins, and related compounds in environmental samples. Environ. Health Perspect., 60: 293-302.

BUU-HOI, N.P., HIEN, D.P., SAINT-RUF, G., & SERVOIN-SIDOINE, J. (1971a) Propriétés canc̄éromimétiques de la tétrachloro-2,3,7,8 dibenzo-p-dioxin. C. R. Acad. Sci. Paris, 272: 1447-1450.

BUU-HOI, N.P., SAINT-RUF, G., BIGOT, P., & MANGANE, M. (1971b) Préparation, propriétés et identification de la "dioxine" (tétrachloro-2,3,7,8- dibenzo-p-dioxine) dans les pyrolysats de défoliants à base d'acide trichloro-2,4,5 phénoxyacétique et de ses esters et des végétaux contaminés. C. R. Acad. Sci. Paris, 273: 708-711.

BUU-HOI, N.P., CHANH, P.H., SESQUE, G., AZUM-GELADE, M.C., & SAINT-RUF, G. (1972a) Organs as targets of "dioxin" (2,3,7,8-tetrachlorodibenzo-p-dioxin) intoxication. Naturwissenschaften, 59: 174-175.

BUU-HOI, N.P., CHANH, P.H., SESQUE, G., AZUM-GELADE, M.C., & SAINT-RUF, G. (1972b) Enzymatic functions as targets of the toxicity of "dioxin" (2,3,7,8-tetrachlorodibnzo-p-dioxin. Naturwissenschaften, 59: 173-174.

CANTONI, L., SALMONA, M., & RIZZARDINI, M. (1981) Porphyrogenic effect of chronic treatment with 2,3,7,8-tetrachlorodibenzo-p-dioxin in female rats. Dose-effect relationship following urinary excretion of porphyrins. Toxicol. appl. Pharmacol., 57: 156-163.

CANTONI, L., DAL FIUME, D., FERRAROLI, A., SALMONA, M., & RUGGIERI, R. (1984a) Different susceptibility of mouse tissues to porphyrogenic effect of 2,3,7,8-tetrachlorodibenzo-p-dioxin. Toxicol. Lett., 20: 201-210.

CANTONI, L., DAL FIUME, D., RIZZARDINI, M., & RUGGIERI, R. (1984b) In vitro inhibitory effect on porphyrinogen carboxylase of liver extracts from TCDD treated mice. Toxicol. Lett., 20: 211-217.

CARLSTEDT-DUKE, J.M.B. (1979) Tissue distribution of the receptor for 2,3,7,8-tetrachlorodibenzo-p-dioxin in the rat. Cancer Res., 39: 3172-3176.

CARLSTEDT-DUKE, J.M.B, ELFSTROEM, G., HOEGBERG, B., & GUSTAFSSON, J.-A. (1979) Oncogeny of the rat hepatic receptor for 2,3,7,8-tetrachlorodibenzo-p-dioxin and its endocrine independence. Cancer Res., 39: 4653-4656.

CARLSTEDT-DUKE, J.M.B., HARNEMO, U.-B., HOEGBERG, B., & GUSTAFSSON, J.-A. (1981) Interaction of the hepatic receptor protein for 2,3,7,8-tetrachlorodibenzo-p-dioxin with DNA. Biochim. Biophys. Acta, 672: 131-141.

CARLSTEDT-DUKE, J.M.B., KURL, R., POELLINGER, L., GILLNER, M., HANSSON, L.-A., TOFTGARD, R., HOEGBERG, B., & GUSTAFSSON, J.-A. (1982) The detection and function of the cytosolic receptor for 2,3,7,8-tetrachlorodibenzo-p-dioxin (TCDD) and related cocarcinogens. In: Hutzinger, O., ed. Chlorinated dioxins and related compounds. Impact on the environment, Oxford, New York, Pergamon Press, pp. 355-365

CARTER, C.D., KIMBROUGH, R.D., LIDDLE, J.A., CLINE, R.E., ZACH, M.M., Jr, BARTHEL, W.F., KOEHLER, R.E., & PHILLIPS, P.E. (1975) Tetrachlorodibenzo-dioxin: An accidental poisoning episode in horse arenas. Science, 188: 738-740.

CAVALLARO, A., BANDI, G., INVERNIZZI, G., LUCIANI, L., MONGINI, E., & GORNI, G. (1982) Negative ion chemical ionization ms as a structure tool in the determination of small amounts of PCDD and PCDF. In: Hutzinger, O., ed. Chlorinated dioxins and related compounds, Oxford, New York, Pergamon Press, Vol. 5, pp. 55-65.

CECIL, H.C., HARRIS, S.J., BITMAN, J., & FRIES, G.F. (1973) Polychlorinated biphenyl-induced decrease in liver vitamin A in Japanese Quail and rats. Bull. environ. Contam. Toxicol., 9: 179-185.

CHANG, K.J., HSIEH, K.H., LEE, T.P., TANG, S.Y., & TUNG, T.C. (1981) Immunologic evaluation of patients with polychlorinated biphenyl poisoning: determination of lymphocyte subpopulations. Toxicol. appl. Pharmacol., 61: 58-63.

CHANG, K.J., HSIEH, K.H., LEE, T.P., & TUNG, T.C. (1982a) Immunologic evaluation of patients with polychlorinated biphenyl poisoning: determination of phagocyte Fc and complement receptors. Environ. Res., 28: 329-334.

CHANG, K.J., HSIEH, K.H., TANG, S.Y., TUNG, T.C., & LEE, T.P. (1982b) Immunologic evaluation of patients with polychlorinated biphenyl poisoning: evaluation of delayed-type skin hypersensitive response and its relation to clinical studies. J. Toxicol. environ. Health, 9: 217-223.

CHAPMAN, D.E. & SCHILLER, C.M. (1985) Dose-related effects of 2,3,7,8-tetrachlorodibenzo-p-dioxin (TCDD) in C57BL/6J and DBA/2J mice. Toxicol. appl. Pharmacol., 78: 147-157.

CHASTAIN, J.E. & PAZDERNIK, T.L. (1985) 2,3,7,8-Tetrachlorodibenzo-p-dioxin (TCDD)-induced immunotoxicity. Int. J. Immunopharmacol., 7(6): 849-856.

CHEN, P.H. & HITES, R.A. (1983) Polychlorinated biphenyls and dibenzofurans retained in the tissues of a deceased patient with Yu-Cheng in Taiwan. Chemosphere, 12: 1507-1516.

CHEN, P.H., GAW, J.M., WONG, C.K., & CHEN, C.J. (1980) Levels and gas chromatographic patterns of polychlorinated biphenyls in the blood of patients after PCB poisoning in Taiwan. Bull. environ. Contam. Toxicol., 25: 325-329.

CHEN, P.H., CHANG, K.T., & LU, Y.D. (1981) Polychlorinated biphenyls and polychlorinated dibenzofurans in the toxic rice-bran oil that caused PCB poisoning in Taichung. Bull. environ. Contam. Toxicol., 26, 489-495.

CHEN, P.H., WONG, C.K., RAPPE, C., & NYGREN, M. (1985) Polychlorinated biphenyls, dibenzofurans and quaterphenyls in toxic rice-bran oil and in the blood and tissues of patients with PCB poisoning (Yu-Cheng) in Taiwan. Environ. Health Perspect., 59: 59-65.

CHEUNG, M.O., GILBERT, E.F., & PETERSON, R.E. (1981) Cardiovascular teratogenicity of 2,3,7,8-tetrachlorodibenzo-p-dioxin in the chick embryo. Toxicol. appl. Pharmacol., 61: 197-204.

CHRISTIAN, B.J., INHORN, S.L., & PETERSON, R.E. (1986a) Relationship of the wasting syndrome to lethality in rats treated with 2,3,7,8-tetrachloro- dibenzo-p-dioxin. Toxicol. appl. Pharmacol., 82: 239-255.

CHRISTIAN, B.J., MENAHAN, L.A., & PETERSON, R.E. (1986b) Intermediary metabolism of the mature rat following 2,3,7,8-tetrachlorodibenzo-p-dioxin treatment. Toxicol. appl. Pharmacol., 83: 360-378.

CLARK, D.A., GAULDIE, J., SZEWCZUK, M.R., & SWEENEY, G. (1981) Enhanced suppressor cell activity as a mechanism of immunosuppression by 2,3,7,8-tetrachlorodibenzo-p-dioxin (41275). Proc. Soc. Exp. Biol. Med., 168: 290-299.

CLARK, D.A., SWEENEY, G., SAFE, S., HANCOCK, E., KILBURN, D.G., & GAULDIE, J. (1983) Cellular and genetic basis for suppression of cytotoxic T-cell generation by haloaromatic hydrocarbons. Immunopharmacology, 6: 143-153.

CLEMENT, R.E., TOSINE, H.M., & ALI, B. (1985) Levels of polychlorinated dibenzo-p-dioxins and dibenzofurans in wood burning stoves and fireplaces. Chemosphere, 14: 815-819.

COCCIA, P., CROCI, T., & MANARA, L. (1981) Less TCDD persists in liver 2 weeks after a single dose to mice fed chow with added charcoal or cholic acid. Br. J. Pharmacol., 72: 181-182.

COCHRANE, W.P., SINGH, J., MILES, W., WAKEFORD, B., & SCOTT, J. (1981) Analysis of technical and formulated products of 2,4-dichlorophenoxy acid for the presence of chlorinated dibenzo-p-dioxins. In: Hutzinger, O., Frei, R.W., Merian, E., & Pocchiari, F., ed. Impact of chlorinated dioxins and related compounds on the environment, Oxford, New York, Pergamon Press, pp. 209-213.

COHEN, G.M., BRACKEN, W.M., IYER, R.P., BERRY, D.L., SELKIRK, J.K., & SLAGA, T.J. (1979) Anticarcinogenic effects of 2,3,7,8-tetrachlorodibenzo-p-dioxin on benzo(a)pyrene and 7,12-dimethylbenz(a)anthracene tumor initiation and its relationship to DNA binding. Cancer Res., 39: 4027-4033.

CONAWAY, C.C. & MATSUMURA, F. (1975) Alteration of cellular utilization of thymidine by TCDD (2,3,7,8-tetrachlorodibenzo-p -dioxin). Bull. environ. Contam. Toxicol., 12: 52-56.

CONSTABLE, J.D. & HATCH, M.C. (1985) Reproductive effects of herbicide exposure in Vietnam: Recent studies by the Vietnamese and others. Teratog. Carcinog. Mutagen., 5: 231-250.

COOK, R.R. (1981) Dioxin, chloracne, and soft tissue sarcoma. Lancet, 1: 618-619.

COOK, R.R., TOWNSEND, J.C., OTT, M.G., & SILVERSTEIN, L.G. (1980) Mortality experience of employees exposed to 2,3,7,8-tetrachlorodibenzo-p-dioxin (TCDD). J. occup. Med., 22: 530-532.

COURTNEY, K.D. (1976) Mouse teratology studies with chlorodibenzo-p-dioxins. Bull. environ. Contam. Toxicol., 16: 674-681.

COURTNEY, K.D. & MOORE, J.A. (1971) Teratology studies with 2,4,5-trichlorophenoxy-acetic acid and 2,3,7,8-tetrachloro-dibenzo-p-dioxin. Toxicol. appl. Pharmacol., 20: 396-403.

COURTNEY, K.D., GAYLOR, D.W., HOGAN, M.D., FALK, H.L., BATES, R.R., & MITCHEL, I. (1970) Teratogenic evaluation of 2,4,5-T. Science, 168: 864-866.

COURTNEY, K.D., PUTNAM, J.P., & ANDREWS, J.E. (1978) Metabolic studies with TCDD (Dioxin) treated rats. Arch. environ. Contam. Toxicol., 7: 385-396.

COWARD, K.H. (1947) The determination of vitamin A. In: The biological standardisation of the vitamins, London, Baillière, Tindall and Cox, pp. 23-58.

CROSBY, D.G. & WONG, A.S. (1976) Photochemical generation of chlorinated dioxins. Chemosphere, 5: 327-332.

CROSBY, D.G. & WONG, A.S. (1977) Environmental degradation of 2,3,7,8-tetrachlorodibenzo-p-dioxin (TCDD). Science, 195: 1337-1338.

CROSBY, D.G., WONG, A.S., PLIMMER, J.R., & WOOLSON, E.A. (1971) Photodecomposition of chlorinated dibenzo-p-dioxins. Science, 173: 748-749.

CROSBY, D.G., MOILANEN, K.W., & WONG, A.S. (1973) Environmental generation and degradation of dibenzodioxins and dibenzofurans. Environ. Health Perspect., 5: 259-266.

CROW, K.D. (1970) Chloracne. A critical review including a comparison of two series of cases of acne from chlornaphtalene and pitch fumes. Trans. St. John's Hosp. Dermatol. Soc., 56: 79-99.

CRUMMETT, W.B. & STEHL, R.H. (1973) Determination of chlorinated dibenzo-p-dioxins and dibenzofurans in various materials. Environ. Health Perspect., 5: 15-25.

CRUMMETT, W.B., NESTRICK, T.J., & LAMPARSKI, L.L., (1985) Analytical methodology for the determination of PCDDs in environmental samples: an overview and critique. In: Kamrin, M.A. & Rodgers, P.W., ed. Dioxins in the environment, Washington, DC, Hemisphere Publishing, pp. 57-83.

CUNNINGHAM, H.M. & WILLIAMS, D.T. (1972) Effect of tetrachlorodibenzo-p-dioxin on growth rate and the synthesis of lipids and proteins in rats. Bull. environ. Contam. Toxicol., 7: 45-51.

CZUCZWA, J.M. & HITES, R.A. (1985) Historical record of polychlorinated dioxins and furans in Lake Huron sediments. In: Keith, L.H., Rappe, C., & Choudhary, G., ed. Chlorinated dioxins and dibenzofurans in the total environment, Stoneham, Maine, Butterworth Publishers, pp. 59-63.

DALDERUP, L.M. (1974a) Safety measures for taking down buildings contaminated with toxic material I. T. Soc. Geneeskd., 52: 582-588.

DALDERUP, L.M. ((1974b) Safety measures for taking down buildings contaminated with toxic material II. T. Soc. Geneeskd., 52: 616-623.

D'ARGY, R., HASSOUN, E., & DENCKER, L. (1984) Teratogenicity of TCDD and the congener 3,3',4,4'-tetrachloroazoxybenzene in sensitive and nonsensitive mouse strains after reciprocal blastocyst transfer. Toxicol. Lett., 21: 197-202.

DAVISON, K.L. & COX, J.H. (1976) Methoxychlor effects on hepatic storage of vitamin A in rats. Bull. environ. Contam. Toxicol., 16: 145-148.

DECAD, G.M., BIRNBAUM, L.S., & MATTHEWS, H.B. (1981a) 2,3,7,8-tetrachlorodibenzofuran tissue distribution and excretion in guinea pigs. Toxicol. appl. Pharmacol., 57: 231-240.

DECAD, G.M., BIRNBAUM, L.S., & MATTHEWS, H.B. (1981b) Distribution and excretion of 2,3,7,8-tetrachlorodibenzofuran in C57BL/6J and DBA/2J mice. Toxicol. appl. Pharmacol., 59: 564-573.

DECAPRIO, A.P., MCMARTIN, D.N., SILKWORTH, J.B., REJ, R., PAUSE, R., & KAMINSKY, L.S. (1983) Subchronic oral toxicity in guinea pigs of soot from a polychlorinated biphenyl-containing transformer fire. Toxicol. appl. Pharmacol., 68: 308-322.

DECAPRIO, A.P., MCMARTIN, D.N., O'KEEFE, P.W., REJ, R., SILKWORTH, J.B., & KAMINSKY, L.S. (1986) Subchronic oral toxicity of 2,3,7,8-tetrachlorodibenzo-p-dioxin in the guinea pig: comparisons with a PCB-containing transformer fluid pyrolysate. Fundam. appl. Toxicol., 6: 454-463.

DEITRICH, R.A., BLUDEAU, P., ROPER, M., & SCHMUCK, J. (1978) Induction of aldehyde dehydrogenases. Biochem. Pharmacol., 27: 2343-2347.

DENCKER, L. & PRATT, R.M. (1981) Association between the presence of the Ah receptor in embryonic murine tissues and sensitivity to TCDD-induced cleft palate. Teratog. Carcinog. Mutagen., 1: 399-406.

DENCKER, L., HASSOUN, E., D'ARGY, R., & ALM, G. (1985) Fetal thymus organ culture as an in vitro model for the toxicity of 2,3,7,8-tetrachlorodibenzo-p-dioxin and its congeners. Mol. Pharmacol., 27: 133-140.

DENISON, M.S., VELLA, L.M., & OKEY, A.B. (1986a) Structure and function of the Ah receptor for 2,3,7,8-tetrachlorodibenzo-p-dioxin. Species difference in molecular properties of the receptors from mouse and rat hepatic cytosols. J. biol. Chem., 261: 3987-3995.

DENISON, M.S., WILKINSON, C.F., & OKEY, A.B. (1986b) Ah receptor for 2,3,7,8-tetrachlorodibenzo-p-dioxin: comparative studies in mammalian and nonmammalian species. Chemosphere, 15: 1665-1672.

DENISON, M.S., HARPER, P.A., & OKEY, A.B. (1986c) Ah receptor for 2,3,7,8-tetrachlorodibenzo-p-dioxin. Codistribution of unoccupied receptor with cytosolic marker enzymes during fractionation of mouse liver, rat liver and cultured Hepa-1c1 cells. Eur. J. Biochem., 155: 223-229.

DENMARK (1984) [Formation and emission of dioxins especially in connection with waste incineration: supplement,] Copenhagen, Miljöstyrelsen (in Danish).

DICKINS, M., SEEFELD, M.D., & PETERSON, R.E. (1981) Enhanced liver DNA synthesis in partially hepatectomized rats pre-treated with 2,3,7,8-tetrachlorodibenzo-p-dioxin. Toxicol. appl. Pharmacol., 58: 389-398.

DIDOMENICO, A., SILANO, V., VIVIANO, G., & ZAPPONI, G. (1980) Accidental release of 2,3,7,8-tetrachlorodibenzo-p-dioxin (TCDD) at Seveso, Italy. II. TCDD distribution in the soil surface layer. Ecotoxicol. environ. Saf., 4: 298-320.

DIGIOVANNI, J., VIAJE, A., BERRY, D.L., SLAGA, T.J., & JUCHAU, M.R. (1977) Tumor-initiating ability of 2,3,7,8-tetrachlorodibenzo-p-dioxin (TCDD) and arochlor 1254 in the two-stage system of mouse skin carcinogenesis. Bull. environ. Contam. Toxicol., 18: 552-557.

DIGIOVANNI, J., BERRY, D.L., JUCHAU, M.R., & SLAGA, T.J. (1979) 2,3,7,8-Tetra-chlorodibenzo-p-dioxin: potent anticarcinogenic activity in CD-1 mice. Biochem. biophys. Res. Commun., 86: 577-584.

DIGIOVANNI, J., BERRY, D.L., GLEASON, G.L., KISHORE, G.S., & SLAGA, T.J. (1980) Time dependent inhibition by 2,3,7,8-tetrachlorodibenzo-p-dioxin of skin tumorogenesis with polycyclic hydrocarbons. Cancer Res., 40: 1580-1587.

DOBLES, A.J. & GRANT, C. (1979) Photolysis of highly chlorinated dibenzo-p-dioxins by sunlight. Nature (Lond.), 278: 162-165.

DOHMEIER, H.J. & JANSON, E. (1983) [Killing flies and people: Dioxin - the poison of Seveso and Viet Nam and how we come into daily contact with it.] Reinbek, Aktuell Rororo, p. 25.

DONOVAN, J.W., MACLENNAN, R., & ADENA, N. (1984) Vietnam service and the risk of congenital anomalies: a case-control study. Med. J. Aust., 140: 394-397.

DOYLE, B.W., DRUM, D.A., & LAUDER, J.D. (1985) The smoldering question of hospital wastes. Pollut. Eng., 17: 35-39.

DOYLE, E.A. & FRIES, G.F. (1986) Induction of aryl hydrocarbon hydroxylase by chlorinated dibenzofurans in rats. Chemosphere, 15: 1745-1748.

DRINKER, C.K., FIELD WARREN, M., & GRANVILLE, A. (1937) The problem of possible systemic effects from certain chlorinated hydrocarbons. J. ind. Hyg. Toxicol., 19: 283-311.

DUGOIS, P. & COLOMB, L. (1956) Acné chlorique au 2-4-5 trichlorophénol. J. Méd. Lyon, 88: 446-447.

DUGOIS, P. & COLOMB, L. (1957) Remarques sur l'acné chlorique. A propos d'une éclosion de cas provoqués par la préparation du 2,4,5-trichlorophénol. J. Méd. Lyon, 38: 899-903.

DUGOIS, P., MARECHAL, J., & COLOMB, L. (1958) Acné chlorique au 2,4,5-tri-chlorophénol. Arch. Mal. prof. Hyg. Toxicol. ind., 19: 626-627.

DUGOIS, P., AMBLARD, P., AIMARD, M., & DESHORS, G. (1967) Acné chlorique collective et accidentelle d'un type nouveau. Bull. Soc. Dermatol., 75: 260-261.

DUVERNE, J., THIVOLET, J., & BERARD, J. (1964) Acné chlorique profuse avec épanchement pleural récidivant chez un sujet à réactions tuberculiniques négatives. Bull. Soc. Fr. Dermatol. Syphiligr., 71: 649-652.

EATON, D.L. & KLAASSEN, C.D. (1979) Effects of 2,3,7,8-tetra-chlorodibenzo-p-dioxin, kepone, and polybrominated biphenyls on transport systems in isolated rat hepatocytes. Toxicol. appl. Pharmacol., 51: 137-144.

EDULJEE, G.H., ATKINS, D.H.F., & EGGLETON, A.E. (1986) Observations and assessment relating to incineration of chlorinated chemical wastes. Chemosphere, 15: 1577-1584.

ELDER, D.G., LEE, G.B., & TOVEY, J.A. (1978) Decreased activity of hepatic uroporphyrinogen decarboxylase in sporadic porphyria cutanea tarda. New Engl. J. Med., 299: 274-278.

ELDER, G.H. & SHEPPARD, D.M. (1982) Immunoreactive uroporphyrinogen decarboxylase is unchanged in porphyria caused by TCDD and hexachlorobenzene. Biochem. biophys. Res. Commun., 109: 113-120.

ELDER, G.H., EVANS, J.O., & MATLIN, S.A. (1976) The effect of porhyrogenic compound, hexachlorobenzene, on the activity of hepatic uroporphyrinogen decarboxylase in the rat. Clin. Sci. mol. Med., 51: 71-80.

ERICKSON, J.D., MULINARE, J., MCCLAIN, P.W., FITCH, T.G., JAMES, L.M., MCCLEARN, A.B., & ADAMS, M.J. (1984) Vietnam veterans' risks for fathering babies with birth defects. J. Am. Med. Assoc., 252: 903-937.

ESPOSITO, G., FAELLI, A., & CAPRARO, V. (1967) Metabolism and transport phenomena in isolated intestine of normal and semi-starved rats. Arch. int. Physiol. Biochim., 75: 601-608.

ESPOSITO, M.P., TIERNAN, T.O., & DRYDEN, F.E. (1980) Dioxins, Cincinnati, Ohio, US Environmental Protection Agency, Office of Research and Development (EPA-600/2-80-197).

FACCHETTI, S., BALASSO, A., FICHTNER, C., FRARE, G., LEONI, A., MAURI, C., & VASCONI, M. (1986) Studies on the absorption of TCDD by plant species. In: Rappe, C., Choudhary, G., & Keith, L.H., ed. Chlorinated dioxins and dibenzofurans in perspective, Chelsea, Michigan, Lewis Publishers, pp. 225-239.

FAHRIG, R., NILSSON, C.-A., & RAPPE, C. (1978) Genetic activity of chlorophenols and chlorophenol impurities. Environ. Sci. Res., 12: 325-338.

FAITH, R.E. & LUSTER, M.I. (1979) Investigations on the effects of 2,3,7,8-tetrachlorodibenzo-p-dioxin (TCDD) on parameters of various immune functions. Ann. N.Y. Acad. Sci., 320: 564-571.

FAITH, R.E. & MOORE, J.A. (1977) Impairment of thymus-dependent immune functions by exposure of the developing immune system to 2,3,7,8-tetrachlorodibenzo-p-dioxin (TCDD). J. Toxicol. environ. Health, 3: 451-464.

FARA, G.M., DEL CORNO, G., BONETTI, F., CARAMASHI, F., DARDANONI, L., FAVARETTI, C., GIAMBELLUCA, S.E., MARNI, E., MOCARELLI, P., MONTESARCHIO, E., PUCCINELLI, V., & VOLPATO, C. (1976) Chloracne after release of TCDD at Seveso, Italy. In: Hutzinger, O., Frei, R., Merian, E., & Pocchiari, F. ed. Chlorinated dioxins and related compounds. Impact on the environment, Oxford, New York, Pergamon Press, pp. 545-559.

FARRELL, K. & SAFE, S. (1986) 2,3,7,8-tetrachlorodibenzo-p-dioxin: Relationship between toxicity and the induction of aryl hydrocarbon hydroxylase and ornithine decarboxylase. Chemosphere, 15: 1971-1976.

FEDERAL REGISTER (1980) Storage and disposal of waste material: Prohibition of disposal of tetrachlorodibenzo-p-dioxin. Fed. Reg., 45(98): 32676.

FILIPPINI, G., BORDO, B., CRENNA, P., MASSETTO, N., MUSICCO, M., & BOERI, R. (1981) Relationship between clinical and electrophysiological findings and indicators of heavy exposure to 2,3,7,8-tetrachlorodibenzo-dioxin. Scand. J. Work Environ. Health, 7: 257-262.

FINGERHUT, M.A., HALPERIN, W.E., HONCHAR, P.A., SMITH, A.B., GROTH, D.H., & RUSSELL, W.O. (1984) Review of exposure and pathology data for seven cases reported as soft tissue sarcoma among persons occupationally exposed to dioxin-contaminated herbicides. In: Lowrance, W.W., ed. Public health risks of the dioxins. Proceedings of a Symposium held at the Rockefeller University, New York, 19-20 October, 1983, Los Altos, California, William Kaufmann, pp. 187-203.

FIRESTONE, D. (1973) Etiology of chick edema disease. Environ. Health Perspect., 5: 59-66.

FIRESTONE, D., (1978) The 2,3,7,8-tetrachlorodibenzo-para-dioxin problem: A review. Proceedings of a Conference on Chlorinated Phenoxyacids and their Dioxins, Stockholm, 1977. Ecol. Bull., 27: 39-52.

FIRESTONE, D., CLOWER, M., Jr, BORSETTI, A.P., TESKE, R.H., & LONG, P.E. (1979) Polychlorodibenzo-p-dioxin and pentachlorophenol residues in milk and blood of cows fed technical pentachlorophenol. J. agric. food Chem., 27: 1171-1177.

FIRESTONE, D., NIEMANN, R.A., SCHNIDER, L.F., GRIDLEY, J.R., & BROWN, D.E., (1986) Dioxin residues in fish and other food. In: Rappe, C., Choudhary, G., & Keith, L., ed. Chlorinated dioxins and dibenzofurans in perspective, Chelsea, Michigan, Lewis Publishers.

FLICK, D.F., FIRESTONE, D., & HIGGINBOTHAM, G.R. (1972) Studies of the chick edema disease. 9. Response of chicks fed or singly administered synthetic edema-producing compounds. Poult. Sci., 51: 2026-2034.

FLICK, D.F., FIRESTONE, D., RESS, J., & ALLEN, J.R. (1973) Studies of the chick edema disease. 10. Toxicity of chick edema factors in the chick, chick embryo, and monkey. Poult. Sci., 52: 1637-1641.

FORTH, W. (1977) [The Seveso Disaster.] Dtsch. Arztebl., 44: 2617-2626 (in German).

FOWLER, B.A., LUCIER, G.W., BROWN, H.W., & MCDANIEL, O.S. (1973) Ultrastructural changes in rat liver cells following a single oral dose of TCDD. Environ. Health Perspect., 5: 141-148.

FRAENKEL, C. (1902) [Reports of associations and congresses. Medical Association of Hall: Meeting of 23 October.] Münchener Med. Wochenschr., October: 39-41.

FREEDMAN, H.J., PARKER, N.B., MARINELLO, A.J., GURTOO, H.L., & MINOWADA, J. (1979) Induction, inhibition and biological properties of aryl hydrocarbon hydroxylase in a stable human B-lymphocyte cell line, RPMI-1788. Cancer Res., 39: 4612-4619.

FREEMAN, R.A., SCHROY, J.M., HILEMAN, F.D., & NOBLE, R.W. (1986) Environmental mobility of 2,3,7,8-TCDD and companion chemicals in a roadway soil matrix. In: Rappe, C., Choudhary, G., & Keith, L., ed. Chlorinated dioxins and dibenzofurans in perspective, Chelsea, Michigan, Lewis Publishers, pp. 171-183.

FRIES, G.F. & MARROW, G.S. (1975) Retention and excretion of 2,3,7,8-tetrachlorodibenzo-p-dioxin by rats. J. agric. food Chem., 23: 265-269.

FRIESEN, K.J., SARNA, L.P., & WEBSTER, G.R.B. (1985) Aqueous solubility of polychlorinated dibenzo-p-dioxins determined by high pressure liquid chromatography. Chemosphere, 14: 1267-1274.

FUCHS, E. & GREEN, H. (1981) Regulation of terminal differentiation of cultured human keratinocytes by vitamin A. Cell, 25: 617-625.

FUNG, D., BOYD, R.K., SAFE, S., & CHITTIM, B.G. (1985) Gas chromatographic/mass spectrometric analysis of specific isomers of polychlorodibenzofurans. Biomed. mass Spectrom., 12: 247-253.

FURST, P., MEEMKEN, H.-A. KRUGER, Chr., & GROEBEL, W. (1987) Polychlorinated dibenzodioxins and dibenzofurans in human milk samples from Western Germany. Chemosphere, 16: 1983-1988.

FURUHASHI, N., KURL, R.N., WONG, J., & VILLEE, C.A. (1986) A cytosolic binding protein for 2,3,7,8-tetrachlorodibenzo-p-dioxin (TCDD) in the uterus and deciduoma of rats. Pharmacology, 33: 110-120.

GALLO, M.A., HESSE, E.J., MACDONALD, G.J., & UMBREIT, T.H. (1986) Interactive effects of estradiol and 2,3,7-8-tetrachlorodibenzo-p-dioxin on hepatic cytochrome P-450 and mouse uterus. Toxicol. Lett., 32: 123-132.

GASIEWICZ, T.A. & NEAL, R.A. (1979) 2,3,7,8-Tetrachlorodibenzo-p-dioxin tissue distribution, excretion, and effects on clinical chemical parameters in guinea pigs. Toxicol. appl. Pharmacol., 51: 329-339.

GASIEWICZ, T.A. & RUCCI, G. (1984) Cytosolic receptor for 2,3,7,8-tetrachlorodibenzo-p-dioxin. Evidence for a homologous nature among various mammalian species. Mol. Pharmacol., 26: 90-98.

GASIEWICZ, T.A., HOLSCHER, M.A., & NEAL, R.A. (1980) The effect of total parenteral nutrition on the toxicity of 2,3,7,8-tetrachlorodibenzo-p-dioxin in the rat. Toxicol. appl. Pharmacol., 54: 469-488.

GASIEWCICZ, T.A., OLSON, J.R., GEIGER, L.H., & NEAL, R.A. (1983a) Absorption, distribution and metabolism of 2,3,7,8-tetrachlorodibenzodioxin (TCDD) in experimental animals. Environ. Sci. Res., 26: 495-525.

GASIEWICZ, T.A., GEIGER, L.E., RUCCI, G., & NEAL, R.A. (1983b) Distribution, excretion, and metabolism of 2,3,7,8-tetrachlorodibenzo-p-dioxin in C57Bl/6J, DBA/2J, and B6O2F,/J mice. Drug Metab. Disp., 11: 397-403.

GASIEWICZ, T.A., NESS, W.C., & RUCCI, G. (1984) Ontogeny of the cytosolic receptor for 2,3,7,8-tetrachlorodibenzo-p-dioxin in rat liver, lung, and thymus. Biochem. biophys. Res. Commun., 118: 183-190.

GASIEWICZ, T.A., RUCCI, G., HENRY, E.C., & BAGGS, R.B. (1986) Changes in hamster hepatic cytochrome P-450, ethoxycoumarin o-deethylase, and reduced NAD(P): Menadione oxidoreductase following treatment with 2,3,7,8-tetrachlorodibenzo-p-dioxin. Biochem. Pharmacol., 35: 2737-2742.

GEBEFUGI, I., BAUMANN, R., & KORTE, F. (1977) [Photochemical breakdown of 2,3,7,8-tetrachlorodibenzo-p-dioxin (TCDD) under stimulated environmental conditions.] Naturwissenschaften, 64: 486-487 (in German).

GEIGER, L.E. & NEAL, R.A. (1981) Mutagenicity testing of 2,3,7,8-tetrachlorodibenzo-p-dioxin in histidine auxotrophs of Salmonella typhimurium. Toxicol. appl. Pharmacol., 59: 125-129.

GERMANY (1985) [Review of dioxins], Berlin, Erich Schmidt Verlag, pp. 257-266 (Federal Office for the Environment, Report 5/85, November 1984) (in German).

GIAVINI, E., PRATI, M., & VISMARA, C. (1982a) Effects of 2,3,7,8-tetrachlorodibenzo-p-dioxin administered to pregnant rats during the pre-implantation period. Environ. Res., 29: 185-189.

GIAVINI, E., PRATI, M., & VISMARA, C. (1982b) Rabbit teratology study with 2,3,7,8-tetrachlorodibenzo-p-dioxin. Environ. Res., 27: 74-78.

GIAVINI, E., PRATI, M., & VISMARA, C. (1983) Embryotoxic effects of 2,3,7,8-tetrachlorodibenzo-p-dioxin administered to female rats before mating. Environ. Res., 31: 105-110.

GIERTHY, J.F. & CRANE, D. (1984) Reversible inhibition of in vitro epithelial cell proliferation by 2,3,7,8-tetrachlorodibenzo-p-dioxin. Toxicol. appl. Pharmacol., 74: 91-98.

GIERTHY, J.F. & CRANE, D. (1985a) In vitro bioassay for dioxin-like activity based on alterations in epithelial cell proliferation and morphology. Fundam. appl. Toxicol., 5: 754-759.

GIERTHY, J.F. & CRANE, D. (1985b) Development of in vitro bioassays for chlorinated dioxins and dibenzofurans. In: Keith, L.H., Rappe, C., & Choudhary, G., ed. Chlorinated dioxins and dibenzofurans in the total environment II, Stoneham, Maine, Butterworth Publishers, pp. 267-284.

GIERTHY, J.F., CRANE, D., & FRENKEL, G.D. (1984) Application of an in vitro keratinization assay to extracts of soot from a fire in a polychlorinated biphenyl-containing transformer. Fundam. appl. Toxicol., 4: 1036-1041.

GILBERT, P., SAINT-RUF, G., PONCELET, F., & MERCIER, M. (1980) Genetic effects of chlorinated anilines and azobenzenes on salmonella typhimurium. Arch. environ. Contam. Toxicol., 9: 533-541.

GOLDMANN, P.J. (1972) [Very severe acute chloracne caused by trichlorophenol decomposition products.] Arbeitsmed. Sozialmed. Arbeitshyg., 7: 12-18 (in German).

GOLDMANN, P.J. (1973) [Very severe acute chloracne: mass poisoning by 2,3,6,7-tetrachlorodibenzodioxin.] Hautarzt, 24: 149-152 (in German).

GOLDSTEIN, J.A. & LINKO, P. (1984) Differential induction of two 2,3,7,8-tetrachlorodibenzo-p-dioxin-inducible forms of cytochrome P-450 in extrahepatic versus hepatic tissues. Mol. Pharmacol., 25: 185-191.

GOLDSTEIN, J.A., HICKMAN, P., BERGMAN, H., & VOS, J.G. (1973) Hepatic porphyria induced by 2,3,7,8-tetrachlorodibenzo-p-dioxin in the mouse. Res. Commun. chem. Pathol. Pharmacol., 6: 919-928.

GOLDSTEIN, J.A., MCKINNEY, J.D., LUCIER, G.W., HICKMAN, P., BERGMAN, H., & MOORE, J.A. (1976) Toxicological assessment of hexachlorobiphenyl isomers and 2,3,7,8-tetrachlorodibenzofuran in chicks. II. Effects on drug metabolism and porphyrin accumulation. Toxicol. appl. Pharmacol., 36: 81-92.

GOLDSTEIN, J.A., HASS, J.R., LINKO, P., & HARVAN, D.J. (1978) 2,3,7,8-Tetrachlorodibenzofuran in a commercially available 99% pure polychlorinated biphenyl isomer identified as the inducer of hepatic cytochrome P-448 and aryl hydrocarbon hydroxylase in the rat. Drug Metab. Disp., 6: 258-264.

GOLDSTEIN, J.A., LINKO, P., & BERGMAN, H. (1982) Induction of porphyria in the rat by chronic versus acute exposure to 2,3,7,8-tetrachlorodibenzo-p-dioxin. Biochem. Pharmacol., 31: 1607-1613.

GONZALES, F.J., TUKEY, R.H., & NEBERT, D.W. (1984) Structural gene products of the Ah locus. Transcriptional regulation of cytochrome P1-450 and P3-450mRNA levels by 3-methylcholanthrene. Mol. Pharmacol., 26: 117-121.

GORSKI, T., KONOPKA, L., & BRODZKI, M. (1984) Persistence of some polychlorinated dibenzo-p-dioxins and polychlorinated dibenzofurans of pentachlorophenol in human adipose tissue. Rocz. Pzh, XXXV(4): 297-301.

GOTHE, R. & WACHTMEISTER, C.A. (1972) Synthesis of 1,2,4,5,7,8-hexa-chloroxanthene. Acta chem. Scand., 26: 2523-2576.

GOTZ, R. (1986) Chlorinated dioxins and dibenzofurans in leachate and sediments of the sanitary landfill in Hamburg-Georswerder. Chemosphere, 15: 1981-1984.

GRAY, A.P., STEVEN, P.C., & CANTRELL, J.S. (1975) Intervention of the Smiles rearrangement in synthesis of dibenzo-p-dioxins: 1,2,3,6,7,8- and 1,2,3,7,8,9-hexachlorodibenzo-dioxin. Tetrahydron Lett., 33: 2873-2876.

GRAY, A.P., STEVEN, P.C., SOLOMON, I.J., & ANILINE, O. (1976) Synthesis of specific polychlorinated dibenzo-p-dioxins. J. org. Chem., 41: 2435-2437.

GREEN, S. & MORELAND, F.S. (1975) Cytogenetic evaluation of several dioxins in the rat. Toxicol. appl. Pharmacol., 33: 161.

GREEN, S., MORELAND, F., & SHEU, C. (1977) Cytogenetic effect of 2,3,7,8-tetrachlorodibenzo-p-dioxin on rat bone marrow cells. FDA By-lines, 6: 292-294.

GREENBURG, L., MAYERS, M.R., & SMITH, A.R. (1939) The systemic effects resulting from exposure to certain chlorinated hydrocarbons. J. ind. Hyg. Toxicol., 21: 29-38.

GREENLEE, W.F. & POLAND, A. (1978) An improved assay of 7-ethoxycoumarin O-deethylase activity: induction of hepatic enzyme activity in C57BL/6J and DBA/2J mice by phenobarbital, 3-methylcholanthrene and 2,3,7,8-tetrachlorodibenzo-p-dioxin. J. Pharmacol. exp. Ther., 205: 596-605.

GREENLEE, W.F. & POLAND, A. (1979) Nuclear uptake of 2,3,7,8-tetrachlorodibenzo-p-dioxin in C57BL/6J and DBA/2J mice. Role of the hepatic cytosol receptor protein. J. biol. Chem., 254: 9814-9821.

GREENLEE, W.F., DOLD, K.M., IRONS, R.D., & OSBORNE, R. (1985) Evidence for direct action of 2,3,7,8-tetrachlorodidibenzo-p-dioxin (TCDD) on thymic epithelium. Toxicol. appl. Pharmacol., 79: 112-120.

GREIG, J.B. (1972) Effect of 2,3,7,8-tetrachlorodibenzo-1, 4-dioxin on drug metabolism in the rat. Biochem. Pharmacol., 21: 3196-3198.

GREIG, J.B. & OSBORNE, G. (1981) Biochemical and morphological changes induced by 2,3,7,8-tetrachlorodibenzo-p-dioxin in the rat liver cell plasma membrane. J. appl. Toxicol., 1(6): 334-338.

GREIG, J.B., JONES, G., BUTLER, W.H., & BARNES, J.M. (1973) Toxic effects of 2,3,7,8-tetrachlorodibenzo-p-dioxin. Food Cosmet. Toxicol., 11: 585-595.

GREIG, J.B., TAYLOR, D.M., & JONES, J.D. (1974) Effects of 2,3,7,8-tetrachlorodibenzo-p-dioxin on stimulated DNA synthesis in the liver and kidney of the rat. Chem.-biol. Interact., 8: 31-39.

GREIG, J.B., FRANCIS, J.E., KAY, S.J.E., LOVELL, D.P., & SMITH, A.G. (1984) Incomplete correlation of 2,3,7,8-tetrachlorodibenzo-p-dioxin hepatotoxicity with Ah phenotype in mice. Toxicol. appl. Pharmacol., 74: 17-25.

GROSS, M.L., LAY, J.O., Jr, LYON, P.A., LIPPSTREU, D., KANGAS, N., HARLESS, R.L., TAYLOR, S.E., & DUPUY, A.E. Jr (1984) 2,3,7,8-Tetrachlorodibenzo-p-dioxin levels in adipose tissue of Vietnam veterans. Environ. Res., 33: 261-268.

GUENTHNER, T.M., FYSH, J.M., & NEBERT, D.W. (1979) 2,3,7,8-Tetrachlorodibenzo-p-dioxin: covalent binding of reactive metabolic intermediates principally to protein in vitro. Pharmacology, 19: 12-22.

GUPTA, B.N., VOS, J.G., MOORE, J.A., ZINKL, J.G., & BULLOCK, B.C. (1973) Pathologic effects of 2,3,7,8-tetrachlorodibenzo-p-dioxin in laboratory animals. Environ. Health Perspect., 5: 125-140.

GURTOO, H.L., PARKER, N.B., PAIGEN, B., HAVENS, M.B., MINOWADA, J., & FREEDMAN, H.J. (1979) Induction, inhibition and some enzymological properties of aryl hydrocarbon hydroxylase in fresh mitogen-activated human lymphocytes. Cancer Res., 39: 4620-4629.

GUSTAFSSON, J.-A. & INGELMAN-SUNDBERG, M. (1979) Changes in steroid hormone metabolism in rat liver microsomes following administration of 2,3,7,8-tetrachlorodibenzo-p-dioxin (TCDD). Biochem. Pharmacol., 28: 497-499.

HAAPARANTA, T., GLAUMANN, H., & GUSTAFSSON, J.-A. (1983) Induction of cytochrome P-450 dependent reactions in the rat ventral prostate by beta-naphthoflavone and 2,3,7,8-tetrachlorodibenzo-p-dioxin. Toxicology, 29: 61-75.

HAGENMAIER, H. & BRUNNER, H. (1987) Isomer specific analysis of PCDD and PCDF in pentachlorophenol and sodium pentachlorophenate samples in the sub-PPB range. Chemosphere, 16: 1759-1764.

HAGENMAIER, H., DRAFT, M., JAGER, W., MAYER, U., LUETZKE, K., & SIEGAL, D. (1986) Comparison of various sampling methods for PCDDs and PCDFs in stack gas. Chemosphere, 15(9-12): 1187-1192.

HAKANSSON, H. (1988) Effect of 2,3,7,8-tetrachlorodibenzo-p-dioxin of the fate of vitamin A in rodents, Stockholm, Department of Toxicology and Institute of Environmental Medicine, Karolinska Institute (Ph.D. Thesis).

HAKANSSON, H. & AHLBORG, U.G. (1985) The effect of 2,3,7,8-tetrachlorodibenzo-p-dioxin (TCDD) on the uptake, distribution and excretion of a single oral dose of 11,12, 3H-retinylacetate and on the vitamin A status in the rat. J. Nutr., 115: 759-771.

HAKANSSON, H., AHLBORG, U.G., & GOTTLING, L. (1986) The effect of 2,3,7,8-tetrachlorodibenzo-p-dioxin (TCDD) on the distribution and excretion of the endogenous pool of vitamin A in rats with low liver vitamin A stores. Chemosphere, 15: 1715-1723.

HAKANSSON, H., WAERN, F., & AHLBORG, U.G. (1987) Effects of 2,3,7,8-tetrachlorodibenzo-p-dioxin (TCDD) in the lactating rat on maternal and neonatal vitamin A status. J. Nutr., 117: 580-586.

HANNAH, R.R., LUND, J., POELLINGER, L., GILLNER, M., & GUSTAFSSON, J.-A. (1986) Characterization of the DNA-binding properties of the receptor for 2,3,7,8-tetrachlorodibenzo-p-dioxin. Eur. J. Biochem., 156: 237-242.

HARDELL, L. (1981) Relation of soft-tissue sarcoma, malignant lymphoma and colon cancer to phenoxy acids, chlorophenols and other agents. Scand. J. Work Environ. Health, 7: 119-130.

HARDELL, L. & ERIKSSON, M. (1981) Soft-tissue sarcomas, phenoxy herbicides, and chlorinated phenols. Lancet, 2: 250.

HARDELL, L. & SANDSTROM, A. (1979) Case-control study: soft-tissue sarcomas and exposure to phenoxyacetic acids or chlorophenols. Br. J. Cancer, 39: 711-717.

HARDELL, L., ERIKSSON, M., LENNER, P., & LUNDGREN, E. (1981) Malignant lymphoma and exposure to chemicals, especially organic solvents, chlorophenols and phenoxy acids: a case-control study. Br. J. Cancer, 43: 169-176.

HARLESS, R.L. & LEWIS, R.G. (1982) Quantitative determination of 2,3,7,8-tetrachlorodibenzo-p-dioxin residues by gas chromatography/mass spectrometry. In: Hutzinger, O., ed. Chlorinated dioxins and related compounds, Oxford, London, Pergamon Press, pp. 25-36.

HARLESS, R.L., OSWALD, E.O., LEWIS, R.G., DUPUY, A.E., MCDANIEL, D.D., & TAI, H. (1982) Determination of 2,3,7,8-tetrachlorodibenzo-p-dioxin in fresh water fish. Chemosphere, 11, 193-198.

HARLESS, R.L., LEWIS, R.G., DUPUY, A.E., & MCDANIEL, D.D. (1983) Analyses for 2,3,7,8-tetrachlorodibenzo-p-dioxin residues in environmental samples. In: Tucker, R.E., ed. Human and environmental risks of chlorinated dioxins and related compounds, New York, London, Plenum Press, pp. 161-172.

HARRIS, M.W., MOORE, J.A., VOS, J.G., & GUPTA, B.N. (1973) General biological effects of TCDD in laboratory animals. Environ. Health Perspect., 5: 101-109.

HASSAN, M.Q., STOHS, S.J., & MURRAY, W.J. (1983) Comparative ability of TCDD to induce lipid peroxidation in rats, guinea pigs and syrian golden hamsters. Bull. environ. Contam. Toxicol., 31: 649-657.

HASSAN, M.Q., STOHS, S.J., & MURRAY, W.J. (1985a) Inhibition of TCDD-induced lipid peroxidation, glutathione peroxidase activity and toxicity by BHA and glutathione. Bull. environ. Contam. Toxicol., 34: 787-796.

HASSAN, M.Q., STOHS, S.J., & MURRAY, W.J. (1985b) Effects of vitamins E and A on 2,3,7,8-tetrachlorodibenzo-p-dioxin (TCDD)-induced lipid peroxidation and other biochemical changes in the rat. Arch. environ. Contam. Toxicol., 14: 437-442.

HASSAN, M.Q., STOHS, S.J., MURRAY, W.J., & BIRT, D.F. (1985c) Dietary selenium, glutathione peroxidase activity, and toxicity of 2,3,7,8-tetrachlorodibenzo-p-dioxin. J. Toxicol. environ. Health, 15: 405-415.

HASSOUN, E.M. & DENCKER, L. (1982) TCDD embryotoxicity in the mouse may be enhanced by beta-naphtoflavone, another ligand of the Ah-receptor. Toxicol. Lett., 12: 191-198.

HASSOUN, E.M., D'ARGY, R., & DENCKER, L. (1984a) Teratogenicity of 2,3,7,8-tetrachlorodibenzofuran in the mouse. J. Toxicol. environ. Health, 14: 337-351.

HASSOUN, E.M., D'ARGY, R., DENCKER, L., LUNDING, L.G., & BORWELL, P. (1984b) Teratogenicity of 2,3,7,8-tetrachlorodibenzofuran in BXD recombinant inbred strains. Toxicol. Lett., 23: 37-42.

HAY, A. (1984) Experimental toxicology and cytogenetics: an overview. In: Westing, A.N., ed. Herbicides in war, the long-term ecological and human consequences, London, Taylor & Francis, pp. 161-166.

HAY, A.W.M. (1977) Tetrachlorodibenzo-p-dioxin release at Seveso. Disasters, 1: 289-308.

HAYABUCHI, H., YOSHIMURA, T., & KURATSUNE, M. (1979) Consumption of toxic rice oil by Yusho patients and its relation to the clinical response and latent period. Food Cosmet. Toxicol., 17: 455-461.

HAYES, K.C. (1971) On the pathophysiology of vitamin a deficiency. Nutr. Rev., 29: 3-6.

HELLING, C.S., ISENSEE, A.R., WOOLSON, E.A., ENZOR, P.D.J., JONES, G.E., PLIMMER, J.R., & KEARNEY, P.C. (1973) Chlorodioxins in pesticides, soils and plants. J. environ. Qual., 2: 171-178.

HENCK, J.M., NEW, M.A., KOBICA, R.J., & RAO, K.S. (1981) 2,3,7,8-tetrachlorodibenzo-p-dioxin: acute oral toxicity in hamsters. Toxicol. appl. Pharmacol., 59: 405-407.

HERXHEIMER, K. (1899) [Chloracne.] Münchenere med. Wochenschr., 46: 278 (in German).

HERZBERG, J.J. (1947) [Chloracne after ingestion of chlorinated paraffin.] Dermatol. Wochenschr., 7: 425-433 (in German).

HINSDILL, R.D., COUCH, D.L., & SPEIRS, R.S. (1980) Immunosuppression in mice induced by dioxin (TCDD) in feed. J. environ. Pathol. Toxicol., 3: 401-425.

HIROSAWA, K. & YAMADA, E. (1973). The localization of the vitamin A in the mouse liver as revealed by electron microscope radioautography. J. electron. Microsc., 22: 337-346.

HOFFMAN, R.E., STEHR-GREEN, P.A., WEBB, K.B., EVANS, R.G., KNUTSEN, A.P., SCHRAMM, W.F., STAAKE, J.L., GIBSON, B.B., & STEINBERG, K.K. (1986) Health effects of long-term exposure to 2,3,7,8-tetrachlorodibenzo-p-dioxin. J. Am. Med. Assoc., 255: 2031-2038.

HOFMANN, H.Th. (1957) [Recent findings with highly toxic chlorinated hydrocarbons.] Arch. exp. Pathol. Pharmakol., 232: 228-230 (in German).

HOFMANN, M.F. & MENEGHINI, C.L. (1962) [Folliculosis from chlorine-substituted hydrocarbons (chloracne).] G. Ital. Dermatol., 103: 427-450 (in Italian).

HOLMSTEDT, B. (1980) Prolegomena to Seveso. Arch. Toxicol., 44: 211-230.

HONCHAR, P.A. & HALPERIN, W.E. (1981) 2,4,5-trichlorophenol and soft-tissue sarcoma. Lancet, 21: 268-269.

HOOK, G.E.R., HASEMAN, J.K., & LUCIER, G.W. (1975a) Induction and suppression of hepatic and extrahepatic microsomal foreign-compound-metabolizing enzyme systems by 2,3,7,8-tetrachlorodibenzo-p-dioxin. Chem.-biol. Interact., 10: 199-214.

HOOK, G.E.R., ORTON, T.C., MOORE, J.A., & LUCIER, G.W. (1975b) 2,3,7,8-Tetrachlorodibenzo-p-dioxin-induced changes in the hydroxylation of biphenyl by rat liver microsomes. Biochem. Pharmacol., 24: 335-340.

HORI, S., OBANA, H., TANAKA, R., & KASHIMOTO, T. (1986) Comparative toxicity in rats of polychlorinated biphenyls (PCBs), polychlorinated quaterphenyls (PCQs) and polychlorinated dibenzofurans (PCDFs) present in rice oil causing "Yusho". Eisei Kagaku, 32: 13-21.

HRYHORCZUK, D.O., WITHROW, W.A., HESSE, C.S., & BEASLEY, V.R. (1981) A wire reclamation incinerator as a source of environmental contamination with tetrachlorodibenzo-p-dioxins and tetrachlorodibenzofurans. Arch. environ. Health, 36: 228-234.

HSU, S., MA, C., HSU, S.K., WU, S., HSU, N.H., & YEH, C. (1984) Discovery and epidemiology of PCB poisoning in Taiwan. Am. J. ind. Med., 5: 71-79.

HUDSON, L.G., SHAIKH, R., TOSCANO, W.A., Jr, & GREENLEE, W.F. (1983) Induction of 7-ethoxycoumarin o-deethylase activity in cultured human epithelial cells by 2,3,7,8-tetrachlorodibenzo-p-dioxin (TCDD): Evidence for TCDD receptor. Biochem. biophys. Res. Commun., 115: 611-617.

HUDSON, L.G., TOSCANO, W.A., Jr, & GREENLEE, W.F. (1985) Regulation of epidermal growth factor binding in a human keratinocyte cell line by 2,3,7,8-tetrachlorodibenzo-p-dioxin. Toxicol. appl. Pharmacol., 77: 251-259.

HUDSON, L.G., TOSCANO, W.A., Jr, & GREENLEE, W.F. (1986) 2,3,7,8-Tetrachorodibenzo-p-dioxin (TCDD) modulates epidermal growth factor (EGF) binding to basal cells from a human keratinocyte cell line. Toxicol. appl. Pharmacol., 82: 481-492.

HUFF, J.E., MOORE, J.A., SARACCI, R., & TOMATIS, L. (1980) Long-term hazards of polychlorinated dibenzodioxins and polychlorinated dibenzofurans. Environ. Health Perspect., 36: 221-240.

HUQUE, T. (1981) Excretion of radioactive metabolites of retinal as an index of vitamin A status in rats. Nutr. Rep. Int., 24: 171-179.

HUSSAIN, S., EHRENBERG, L., LOFROTH, G., & GEJVALL, T. (1972) Mutagenic effects of TCDD on bacterial systems. Ambio, 1: 32-33.

HUTZINGER, O., SAFE, S., WENTZELL, B.R., & ZITKO, V. (1973) Photochemical degradation of di- and octachlorodibenzofuran. Environ Health Perspect., 5: 267-271.

HWANG, S.W. (1973) Effect of 2,3,7,8-tetrachlorodibenzo-p-dioxin on the biliary excretion of indocyanine Green in rat. Environ. Health Perspect., 5: 227-231.

IARC (1977) Some fumigants, the herbicides 2,4-D and 2,4,5-T, chlorinated dibenzodioxins and miscellaneous industrial chemicals, Lyon, France, International Agency for Research on Cancer, pp. 41-102 (IARC Monographs on the Evaluation of the Carcinogenic Risk of Chemicals to Humans, Vol. 15).

IARC (1982) Chemicals, industrial processes and industries associated with cancer in humans, Lyon, France, International Agency for Research on Cancer (IARC Monograph on the Evaluation of the Carcinogenic Risk of Chemicals to Humans, Suppl. No. 4).

IARC (1986) Some halogenated hydrocarbons and pesticide exposures, Lyon, International Agency for Research on Cancer (IARC Monographs on the Evaluation of the Carcinogenic Risk of Chemicals to Humans, Vol. 41).

IDEO, G., BELLATI, G., BELLOBUONO, A., MOCARELLI, P., MAROCCHI, A., & BRAMBILLA, P. (1982) Increased urinary D-glucaric acid excretion by children living in an area polluted with tetrachlorodibenzo-para-dioxin (TCDD). Clin. Chim. Acta, 120: 273-283.

IDEO, G., BELLATI, G., BELLOBUONO, A., & BISSANTI, L. (1985) Urinary d-glucaric acid excretion in the Seveso area, polluted by tetrachlorodibenzo-p-dioxin (TCDD): Five years of experience. Environ. Health Perspect., 60: 151-157.

INNAMI, S.I., NAKAMURA, A., MIYAZAKI, M., NAGAYAMA, S., & NISHIDE, E. (1976) Further studies on the reduction of vitamin A content in the liver of rats given polychlorinated biphenyls. J. nutr. Sci. Vitaminol., 22: 409-418.

IOANNOU, Y.M., BIRNBAUM, L.S., & MATTHEWS, H.B. (1983) Toxicity and distribution of 2,3,7,8-tetrachlorodibenzofuran in male guinea pigs. J. Toxicol. environ. Health, 12: 541-553.

IRPTC (1987) IRPTC Legal file 1986, Geneva, International Register of Potentially Toxic Chemicals, United Nations Environment Programme, Geneva, Switzerland, Vol. I (Data Profile Series No. 7).

ISENSEE, A.R. (1978) Bioaccumulation of 2,3,7,8-tetrachloro-dibenzo-para-dioxin. Ecol. Bull. (Stockholm), 27: 255-262.

ISENSEE, A.R. & JONES, G.E. (1971) Absorption and translocation of root and foliage applied 2,4-dichlorophenol, 2,7-dichlorodibenzo-p-dioxin and 2,3,7,8-tetrachlorodibenzo-p-dioxin. J. agric. food. Chem., 19: 1210-1214.

ISENSEE, A.R. & JONES, G.E. (1975) Distribution of 2,3,7,8-tetrachlorodibenzo-p-dioxin (TCDD) in aquatic model ecosystem. Environ. Sci. Technol., 9: 668-672.

ISRAEL, D.I. & WHITLOCK, J.P., Jr (1983) Induction of mRNA specific for cytochrome P1-450 in wild type and variant mouse hepatoma cells. J. biol. Chem., 258: 10390-10394.

ISRAEL, D.I. & WHITLOCK, J.P., Jr (1984) Regulation of cytochrome P1-450 gene transcription by 2,3,7,8-tetrachloro-dibenzo-p-dioxin in wild type and variant mouse hepatoma cells. J. biol. Chem., 259: 5400-5402.

JANSING, R.L. & SHAIN, W. (1985) Aryl hydrocarbon hydroxylase induction in adult rat hepatocytes in primary culture by several chlorinated aromatic hydrocarbons including 2,3,7,8-tetrachloridibenzo-p-dioxin. Fundam. appl. Toxicol., 5: 713-720.

JENSEN, D.J. & HUMMEL, R.A. (1982) Secretion of TCDD in milk and cream following the feeding of TCDD to lactating dairy cows. Bull. environ. Contam. Toxicol., 29: 440-446.

JENSEN, D.J., GETZENDANER, M.E., HUMMEL, R.A., & TURLEY, J. (1983) Residue studies for (2,4,5-trichlorophenoxy)acetic acid and 2,3,7,8-tetrachlorodibenzo-p-dioxin in grass and rice. J. agric. food Chem., 31: 118-122.

JENSEN, N.E. & WALKER, A.E. (1972) Chloracne: Three cases. Proc. R. Soc. Med., 65: 687-688.

JIRASEK, L., KALENSKY, J., & KUBEC, K. (1973) [Acne chlorine and porphyria-cutanea tarda by the production of herbicides.] Cs. dermatol., 48: 306-317 (in Czech).

JIRASEK, L., KALENSKY, J., KUBEC, K., PAZDEROVA, J., & LUKAS, E. (1976) [Chloracne, porphyria-cutanea tarda and other intoxication by herbicides.] Hautarzt, 27: 328-333 (in German).

JOHANSSON, G., GILLNER, M., HOGBERG, B., & GUSTAFSSON, J.-A. (1982) The TCDD receptor in rat intestinal mucosa and its possible dietary ligands. Nutr. Cancer, 3: 134-143.

JOHNSON, E.F. & MULLER-EBERHARD, U. (1977a) Purification of the major cytochrome P-450 of liver microsomes from rabbits treated with 2,3,7,8-tetrachlorodibenzo-p-dioxin (TCDD). Biochem. biophys. Res. Commun., 76: 652-659.

JOHNSON, E.F. & MULLER-EBERHARD, U. (1977b) Resolution of two forms of cytochrome P-450 from liver microsomes of rabbits treated with 2,3,7,8-tetrachlorodibenzo-p-dioxin. J. biol. Chem., 252: 2839-2845.

JOHNSON, E.F., SCHWAB, G.E., & MULLER-EBERHARD, U. (1979) Multiple forms of cytochrome P-450: Catalytic differences exhibited by two homogeneous forms of rabbit cytochrome P-450. Mol. Pharmacol., 15: 708-718.

JOHNSON, F.E., KUGLER, N.A., & BROWN, S.M. (1981) Soft tissue sarcomas and chlorinated phenols. Lancet, 1: 40.

JONES, D., SAFE, S., MORCOM, E., HOLCOMB, C., COPPOCK, C., & IVIE, W. (1987) Bioavailability of tritiates 2,3,7,8-tetrachlorodibenzo-p-dioxin administered to Holstein dairy cows. Chemosphere, 16: 1743-1748.

JONES, E.L. & KRIZEK, H. (1962) A technic for testing acnegenic potency in rabbits, applied to the potent acnegen, 2,3,7,8-tetrachlorodibenzo-p-dioxin. J. invest. Dermatol., 39: 511-517.

JONES, G. (1975) A histochemical study of the liver lesion induced by 2,3,7,8-tetrachlorodibenzo-p-dioxin (dioxin) in rats. J. Pathol., 116: 101-105.

JONES, G. & BUTLER, W.H. (1974) A morphological study of the liver lesion induced by 2,3,7,8-tetrachlorodibenzo-p-dioxin in rats. J. Pathol., 112: 93-97.

JONES, G. & GREIG, J.B. (1975) Pathological changes in the liver of mice given 2,3,7,8-tetrachlorodibenzo-p-dioxin. Experientia (Basel), 31: 1315-1317.

JONES, K.G. & SWEENEY, G.D. (1977) Association between induction of aryl hydrocarbon hydroxylase and depression of uroporphyrinogen decarboxylase activity. Res. Commun. chem. Pathol. Pharmacol., 17: 631-637.

JONES, K.G. & SWEENEY, G.D. (1980) Dependence of the porphyrogenic effect of 2,3,7,8-tetrachlorodibenzo(p)dioxin upon inheritance of aryl hydrocarbon hydroxylase responsiveness. Toxicol. appl. Pharmacol., 53: 42-49.

JONES, P.A. (1981) Chlorophenols and their impurities in the Canadian environment, Ottawa, Environment Canada (EPS 3-EC-81-2).

JONES, P.A. (1984) Chlorophenols and their impurities in the Canadian environment: 1983 supplement, Ottawa, Environment Canada (EPS 3-EP-84-3).

JONES, P.B.C., MILLER, A.G., ISRAEL, D.I., GALEAZZI, D.R., & WHITLOCK, J.P., Jr (1984) Biochemical and genetic analysis of variant mouse hepatoma cells which overtranscribe the cytochrome P1-450 gene in response to 2,3,7,8-tetrachlorodibenzo-p-dioxin. J. biol. Chem., 259: 12357-12363.

JONES, P.B.C., GALEAZZI, D.R., & WHITLOCK, J.P., Jr (1985) Control of cytochrome P1-450 gene expression by dioxin. Science, 227: 1499-1502.

JONES, P.B.C., DURRIN, L.K., GALEAZZI, D.R., & WHITLOCK, J.P., Jr (1986) Control of cytochrome P1-450 gene expression: Analysis of a dioxin-responsive enhancer system. Proc. Natl Acad. Sci. (USA), 83: 2802-2806.

JONES, R.E. & CHELSKY, M. (1986) Further discussion concerning porphyria cutanea tarda and TCDD exposure. Arch. environ. Health, 41: 100-103.

JOSEPHSON, J. (1983) Chlorinated dioxins and furans in the environment. Environ. Sci. Technol., 17: 124A-128A.

JUNK, G.A. & RICHARD, J. (1981) Dioxins not detected in effluents from coal/refuse combustion. Chemosphere, 10: 1237-1241.

KARASEK, F.W. & ONUSKA, F.I. (1982) Trace analysis of the dioxins. Anal. Chem., 54: 309A-324A.

KARENLAMPI, S.O., EISEN, H.J., HANKINSON, O., & NEBER, D.W. (1983) Effects of cytochrome P1-450 inducers on the cell-surface receptors for epidermal growth factor, phorbol 12,13-dibutyrate, or insulin of cultured mouse hepatoma cells. J. biol. Chem., 17: 10378-10383.

KEARNEY, P.C., WOOLSON, E.A., & ELLINGTON, C.P., Jr (1972) Persistence and metabolism of chlorodioxins in soils. Environ. Sci. Technol., 6: 1017-1019.

KEESEY, R.E., BOYLE, P.C., KEMNITZ, J.W., & MITCHEL, J.S. (1976) The role of the lateral hypothalamus in determining the body weight set point. In: Novin, D., Wyrwicks, W., & Bray, G., ed. Hunger: Basic mechanisms and clinical implications, New York, Raven Press, pp. 243-255.

KELLING, C.K., CHRISTIAN, B.J., INHORN, S.L., & PETERSON, R.E. (1985) Hypophagia-induced weight loss in mice, rats, and guinea pigs treated with 2,3,7,8-tetrachlorodibenzo-p-dioxin. Fundam. appl. Toxicol., 5: 700-712.

KENDE, A.S., WADE, J.J., RIDGE, D., & POLAND, A. (1974) Synthesis and fourier transform carbon - 13 nuclear magnetic resonance spectroscopy of new toxic polyhalodibenzo-p-dioxins. J. org. Chem., 39: 931-937.

KERKVLIET, N.I., BRAUNER, J.A., & MATLOCK, J.P. (1985) Humoral immunotoxicity of polychlorinated diphenyl ethers, phenoxyphenols, dioxins and furans present as contaminants of technical grade pentachlorophenol. Toxicology, 36: 307-324.

KEYS, B., HLAVINKA, M., MASON, G., & SAFE, S. (1985) Modulation of rat hepatic microsomal testosterone hydroxylases by 2,3,7,8-tetrachlorodibenzo-p-dioxin and related toxic isostereomers. Can. J. Pharmacol., 63: 1537-1542.

KEYS, B., PISKORSKA-PLISZCZYNSKA, J., & SAFE, S. (1986) Polychlorinated dibenzofurans as 2,3,7,8-TCDD antagonists: in vitro inhibition of monooxygenase enzyme induction. Toxicol. Lett., 31: 151-158.

KHERA, K.S. & RUDDICK, J.A. (1973) Polychlorodibenzo-p-dioxins: Perinatal effects and the dominant lethal test in Wistar rats. Adv. Chem. Ser., 120: 70-84.

KIMBLE, B.J. & GROSS, M.L. (1980) Tetrachlorodibenzo-p-dioxin quantitation in stack-collected coal fly ash. Science, 207: 59-61.

KIMBROUGH, R.D. (1974) The toxicity of polychlorinated polycyclic compounds and related chemicals. CRC Crit. Rev. Toxicol., 2: 445-498.

KIMBROUGH, R.D. (1979) The carcinogenic and other chronic effects of persistent halogenated organic compounds. Ann. N.Y. Acad. Sci., 320: 415-418.

KIMBROUGH, R.D. (1984) The epidemiology and toxicology of TCDD. Bull. environ. Contam. Toxicol., 33: 636-647.

KIMBROUGH, R.D., GAINES, T.B., & LINDER, R.E. (1974) 2,4-Dichlorophenyl-p-nitrophenyl ether (TOK). Effects on the lung maturation of rat fetus. Arch. environ. Health, 28: 316-319.

KIMBROUGH, R.D., CARTER, C.D., LIDDLE, J.A., CLINE, R.E., & PHILLIPS, P.E. (1977) Epidemiology and pathology of a tetrachlorodibenzodioxin poisoning episode. Arch. environ. Health, 32: 77-86.

KIMBROUGH, R.D., FALK, H., & STEHR, P. (1984) Health implications of 2,3,7,8-tetrachlorodibenzodioxin (TCDD) contamination of residential soil. J. Toxicol. environ. Health, 14: 47-93.

KIMMIG, J. & SCHULZ, K.H. (1957a) [Occupational acne (so called chloracne) caused by chlorinated aromatic cyclic ethers.] Dermatologica, 115: 540-546 (in German).

KIMMIG, J. & SCHULZ, K.H. (1957b) [Chlorinated aromatic cyclic ethers as cause of chloracne.] Naturwissenschaften, 11: 337-338 (in German).

KIMURA, S., GONZALEZ, F.J., & NEBERT, D.W. (1986) Tissue-specific expression of the mouse dioxin-inducible P1450 and P3450 genes: Differential transcriptional activation and mRNA stability in liver and extrahepatic tissues. Mol. cell. Biol., 6: 1471-1477.

KING, F.G., DEDRICK, R.L., & COLLINS, J.M. (1983) Physiological model for the pharmacokinetics of 2,3,7,8-tetrachlorodibenzofuran in several species. Toxicol. appl. Pharmacol., 67: 390-400.

KITCHIN, K.T. & WOODS, J.S. (1979) 2,3,7,8-Tetrachlorodibenzo-p-dioxin (TCDD) effects on hepatic microsomal cytochrome P-448-mediated enzyme activities. Toxicol. appl. Pharmacol., 47: 537-546.

KLEU, G. & GOLTZ, R. (1971) [Late and lasting damage resulting from the chronic occupational action of chlorophenol compounds.] Med. Klin., 66: 53-58 (in German).

KNUTSON, J.C. & POLAND, A. (1980a) 2,3,7,8-Tetrachlorodibenzo-p-dioxin: failure to demonstrate toxicity in twenty-three cultured cell types. Toxicol. appl. Pharmacol., 54: 377-383.

KNUTSON, J.C. & POLAND, A. (1980b) Keratinization of mouse teratoma cell line XB produced by 2,3,7,8-tetrachlorodibenzo-p-dioxin: an in vitro model of toxicity. Cell, 22: 27-36.

KNUTSON, J.C. & POLAND, A. (1982) Response of murine epidermis to 2,3,7,8-tetrachlorodibenzo-p-dioxin: Interaction of the Ah and hr Loci. Cell, 30: 225-234.

KNUTSON, J.C. & POLAND, A. (1984) 2,3,7,8-Tetrachlorodibenzo-p-dioxin: Examination of biochemical effects involved in the proliferation and differentiation of XB cells. J. cell. Physiol., 121: 143-151.

KOCHER, C.W., MAHLE, N.H., HUMMEL, R.A., & SHADOFF, L.A. (1978) A search for the presence of 2,3,7,8-tetrachlorodibenzo-p-dioxin in beef fat. Bull. environ. Contam. Toxicol., 19: 229-236.

KOCHMAN, S., BERNARD, J., CAZABAT, A., LAVAUD, F., LORTON, C., & RAPPE, C. (1986) Phenotypical dissection of immunoregulatory T cell subsets in human after furan exposure. Chemosphere, 15: 1799-1804.

KOCIBA, R.J., KEELER, P.A., PARK, C.N., & GEHRING, P.J. (1976) 2,3,7,8-Tetrachlorodibenzo-p-dioxin (TCDD): Results of a 13-week oral toxicity study in rats. Toxicol. appl. Pharmacol., 35: 553-574.

KOCIBA, R.J., KEYES, D.G., BEYER, J.E., CARREON, R.M., WADE, C.E., DITTENBER, D., KALNINS, R., FRAUSON, L., PARK, C.N., BARNARD, S., HUMMEL, R., & HUMISTON, C.G. (1978) Results of a two year chronic toxicity and oncogenicity study of 2,3,7,8-tetrachlorodibenzo-p-dioxin (TCDD) in rats. Toxicol. appl. Pharmacol., 46: 279-303.

KOCIBA, R.J., KEYES, D.G., LISOWE, R.W., KALNINS, R.P., DITTENBER, D.D., WADE, C.E., GORZINSKI, S.J., HAHLE, N.H., & SCHWETZ, B.A. (1979a) Results of a two-year chronic toxicity and encogenic study of rats ingesting diets containing 2,4,5-trichlorophenoxyacetic acid (2,4,5-T). Food Cosmet. Toxicol., 17: 205-221.

KOCIBA, R.J., KEYES, D.G., BEYER, J.E., CARREON, R.M., & GEHRING, P.J. (1979b) Long-term toxicologic studies of 2,3,7,8-tetrachlorodibenzo-p-dioxin (TCDD) in laboratory animals. Ann. N.Y. Acad. Sci., 320: 397-404.

KOHLI, K.K. & GOLDSTEIN, J.A. (1981) Effects of 2,3,7,8-tetrachlorodibenzo-p-dioxin on hepatic and renal prostaglandin synthetase. Life Sci., 29: 299-305.

KONDOROSI, A., FEDORCSAK, I., SOLYMOSY, F., EHRENBERG, L., & OSTERMAN-GOLKAR, S. (1973) Inactivation of Q-beta RNA by electrophiles. Mutat. Res., 17: 149-161.

KOSHAKJI, R.P., HARBISON, R.D., & BUSH, M.T. (1984) Studies on the metabolic fate of (^{14}C)2,3,7,8-tetrachlorodibenzo-p-dioxin (TCDD) in the mouse. Toxicol. appl. Pharmacol., 73: 69-77.

KOURI, R.E., RATRIE, H., III, ATLAS, C.A., NIWA, A., & NEBERT, D.W. (1974) Aryl hydrocarbon hydroxylase induction in human lymphocyte cultures by 2,3,7,8-tetrachlorodibenzo-p-dioxin. Life Sci., 15: 1585-1595.

KOURI, R.E., RUDE, T.H., & JOGLEKAR, R. (1978) 2,3,7,8-Tetrachlorodibenzo-p-dioxin as cocarcinogen causing 3-methylcholantrene-initiated subcutaneous tumors in mice genetically "non responsive" at Ah locus. Cancer Res., 38: 2777-2783.

KRAUSE, L., VON & BRASSOW, H. (1978) [Contamnestic study of chloracne cases from the year 1954/55.] Arbeitsmed. Socialmed. Präventivmed., 13: 19-21 (in German).

KROWKE, R. (1986) Studies on distribution and embryotoxicity of different PCDD and PCDF in mice and marmosets. Chemosphere, 15: 2011-2022.

KUNITA, N., KASHIMATO, T., MIYATA, H., FUKUSHIMA, S., HARI, S., & OBANA, H. (1984) Causal agents of Yusho. Am. J. ind. Med., 5: 45-58.

KUNTZMAN, D., LAWRENCE, D., & CONNEY, A.H. (1965) Michaelis constants for the hydroxylation of steroid hormones and drugs by rat liver microsomes. Mol. Pharmacol., 1: 163-167.

KURL, R.N. & VILLEE, C.A. (1985) A metabolite of riboflavin binds to the 2,3,7,8-tetrachlorodibenzo-p-dioxin (TCDD) receptor. Pharmacology, 30: 241-244.

KURL, R.N., LUND, J., POELLINGER, L., & GUSTAFSSON, J-A. (1982) Differential effect of 2,3,7,8-tetrachlorodibenzo-p-dioxin on nuclear RNA polymerase activity in the rat liver and thymus. Biochem. Pharmacol., 31: 2459-2462.

KURL, R.N., LORING, J.M., & VILLEE, C.A. (1985) Control of 2,3,7,8-tetrachlorodibenzo-p-dioxin binding protein(s) in the hamster kidney. Pharmacology, 30: 245-254.

KUROKI, H., MASUDA, Y., YOSHIHARA, S., & YOSHIMURA, H. (1980) Accumulation of polychlorinated dibenzofurans in the livers of monkeys and rats. Food Cosmet. Toxicol., 18: 387-392.

KUROKI, H., HARAGUCHI, K., & MASUDA, Y. (1984) Synthesis of polychlorinated dibenzofuran isomers and their gas chromatographic profiles. Chemosphere, 13: 561-573.

KUROKI, J., KOGA, N., & YOSHIMURA, H. (1986) High affinity of 2,3,4,7,8-pentachloridibenzofuran to cytochrome P-450 in the hepatic microsomes of rats. Chemosphere, 15: 731-738.

LAHANIATIS, E.S., PARLAR, H., & KORTE, F. (1977) [Contributions to ecological chemistry CXXXII. On the occurrence of chlorinated hydrocarbons in the flue dust of refuse incinerators.] Chemosphere, 7: 11-16 (in German).

LAMB, J.C., MARKS, T.A., GLADEN, B.C., ALLEN, J.W., & MOORE, J.A. (1981) Male fertility, sister chromatid exchange, and germ cell toxicity following exposure to mixtures of chlorinated phenoxy acids containing 2,3,7,8-tetrachlorodibenzo-p-dioxin. J. Toxicol. environ. Health, 8: 825-834.

LAMB, J.C., IV, HARRIS, M.W., MCKINNEY, J.D., & BIRNBAUM, L.S. (1986) Effects of thyroid hormones on the induction of cleft palate by 2,3,7,8-tetrachlorodibenzo-p-dioxin (TCDD) in C57Bl/6N mice. Toxicol. appl. Pharmacol., 84: 115-124.

LAMPARSKI, L.L. & NESTRICK, T.J. (1981) Synthesis and identification of the 10 hexachlorodibenzo-p-dioxin isomers by high performance liquid and packed column gas chromatography. Chemosphere, 10: 3-18.

LAMPARSKI, L.L., NESTRICK, T.J., & STEHL, R.H. (1979) Determination of part-per-trillion concentration of 2,3,7,8-tetrachlorodibenzo-p-dioxin in fish. Anal. Chem., 51: 1453-1458.

LAMPARSKI, L.L., NESTRICK, T.J., FRAWLEY, N.N., HUMMEL, R.A., KOCKER, C.W., MAHLE, N.H., MCCOY, J.W., MILLER, D.L., PETERS, T.L., PILLIPICH, J.L., SMITH, W.E., & TOBEY, S.W. (1986) Perspectives of a large scale environmental survey for chlorinated dioxins: Water analyses. Chemosphere, 15: 1445-1452.

LANGER, H.G., BRADEY, T.P., & BRIGGS, P.R. (1973) Formation of dibenzodioxins and other condensation products from chlorinated phenols and derivatives. Environ. Health Perspect., 5: 3-7.

LATHROP, G.D., WOLFE, W.H., ALBANESE, R.A., & MOYANAHAN, P.M. (1984) An epidemiologic investigation of health effects in air force personnel following exposure to herbicides. Baseline morbidity study results, San Antonio, Texas, USAF School of Aerospace Medicine (EK), Aerospace Medical Division, Brooks Air Force Base.

LEE, P. & SUZUKI, K. (1980) Induction of aryl hydrocarbon hydroxylase activity in the rat prostate glands by 2,3,7,8-tetrachlorodibenzo-p-dioxin. J. Pharmacol. exp. Ther., 215: 601-605.

LIEM, H.H., MULLER-EBERHARD, U., & JOHNSON, E.F. (1980) Differential induction by 2,3,7,8-tetrachlorodibenzo-p-dioxin of multiple forms of rabbit microsomal cytochrome P-450: Evidence for tissue specificity. Mol. Pharmacol., 18: 565-570.

LIGON, W.V., Jr & MAY, R.J. (1986) Determination of selected chlorodibenzofurans and chlorodibenzodioxins using two-dimensional gas chromatography/mass spectrometry. Anal. Chem., 58: 558-561.

LINDAHL, R., RAPPE, C., & BUSER, H.R. (1980) Formation of polychlorinated dibenzofurans (PCDFs) and polychlorinated dibenzo-p-dioxins (PCDDs) from the pyrolysis of polychlorinated diphenyl ethers. Chemosphere, 9: 351-361.

LINDAHL, R., ROPER, M., & DIETRICH, R.A. (1978) Rat liver aldehyde dehydrogenase-immunochemical identity of 2,3,7,8-tetrachlorodibenzo-p-dioxin inducible normal liver and 2-acetylaminofluorene inducible hepatoma isozymes. Biochem. Pharmacol., 27: 2463-2465.

LOPRIENO, N., SBRANA, I., RUSCIANO, D., LASCIALFARI, D., & LARI, T. (1982a) In vivo cytogenetic studies on mice and rats exposed to 2,3,7,8-tetrachlorodibenzo-p-dioxin. In: Hutzinger, O., Frei, R.W., Merian, E., & Pocchiari, P., ed. Chlorinated dioxins and related compounds. Impact on the environment, Oxford, New York, Pergamon Press, pp. 419-428.

LOPRIENO, N., SBRANA, I., RUSCIANO, D., LASCIALFARI, D., LARI, T., STRETTI, G., & FREZZA, D. (1982b) In vitro and in vivo genotoxicity studies on 2,3,7,8-tetrachlorodibenzo-p-dioxin (TCDD). In: Report of the 5th Meeting of the Seveso International Scientific Advisory Committee, Milan, Regione Lombardia (Report No. 32).

LOVATI, M.R., GALBUSSERA, M., FRANCESCHINI, G., WEBER, G., RESI, L., TANGANELLI, P., & SIRTORI, C.R. (1984) Increased plasma and aortic triglycerides in rabbits after acute administration of 2,3,7,8-tetrachlorodibenzo-p-dioxin. Toxicol. appl. Pharmacol., 75: 91-97.

LU, C.-J.H., BAGGS, R.B., REDMOND, D., HENRY, E.C., SCHECTER, A., & GASIEWICZ, T.A. (1986) Toxicity and evidence for metabolic alterations in 2,3,7,8-tetrachlorodibenzo-p-treated guinea pigs fed by total parenteral nutrition. Toxicol. appl. Pharmacol., 84: 439-453.

LUCIER, G.W., MCDANIEL, O.S., HOOK, G.E.R., FOWLER, B.A., SONAWANE, B.R., & FAEDER, E. (1973) TCDD-induced changes in rat liver microsomal enzymes. Environ. Health Perspect., 5: 199-209.

LUCIER, G.W., MCDANIEL, O.S., & HOOK, G.E.R. (1975a) Nature of the enhancement of hepatic uridine diphosphate gluburonyltransferase activity by 2,3,7,8-tetrachlorodibenzo-p-dioxin in rats. Biochem. Pharmacol., 24: 325-334.

LUCIER, G.W., SONAWANE, B.R., MCDANIEL, O.S., & HOOK, G.E.R. (1975b) Postnatal stimulation of hepatic microsomal enzymes following administration of TCDD to pregnant rats. Chem.-biol. Interact., 11: 15-26.

LUCIER, G.W., RUMBAUGH, R.C., MCCOY, Z., HASS, R., HARVAN, D., & ALBRO, P. (1986) Ingestion of soil contaminated with 2,3,7,8-tetrachlorodibenzop-dioxin (TCDD) alters hepatic enzyme activities in rats. Fundam. appl. Toxicol., 6: 364-371.

LUSTENHOUWER, J.W.A., OLIE, K., & HUTZINGER, O. (1980) Chlorinated dibenzo-p-dioxins and related compounds in incinerator effluents: A review of measurements and mechanisms of formation. Chemosphere, 9: 501-522.

LUSTER, M.I., CLARK, G., LAWSON, L.D., & FAITH, R.E. (1979a) Effects of brief in vitro exposure to 2,3,7,8-tetrachlorodibenzo-p-dioxin (TCDD) on mouse lymphocytes. J. environ. Pathol. Toxicol., 2: 965-977.

LUSTER, M.I., FAITH, R.E., & LAWSON, L.D. (1979b) Effects of 2,3,7,8-tetrachlorodibenzofuran (TCDF) on the immune system in guinea pigs. Drug chem. Toxicol., 2: 49-60.

LUSTER, M.I., BOORMAN, G.A., DEAN, J.H., HARRIS, M.W., LUEBKE, R.W., PADARATHSINGH, M.L., & MOORE, J.A. (1980) Examination of bone marrow, immunologic parameters and host susceptibility following pre- and postnatal exposure to 2,3,7,8-tetrachlorodibenzo-p-dioxin (TCDD). Int. J. Immunopharmacol., 2: 301-310.

LUSTER, M.I., TUCKER, A.N., HONG, L., BOORMAN, G.A., & PATTERSON, R. (1984) In vivo and in vitro effects of TCDD on stem cell and B cell differentiation. In: Biological mechanisms of dioxin action, Cold Spring Harbor, New York, Cold Spring Harbor Laboratory, pp. 411-417 (Banbury Report No. 18).

LUSTER, M.I., HONG, L.H., BOORMAN, G.A., CLARK, G., HAYES, H.T., GREENLEE, W.F., DOLD, K., & TUCKER, A.N. (1985) Acute myelotoxic responses in mice exposed to 2,3,7,8-tetrachlorodibenzo-p-dioxin (TCDD). Toxicol. appl. Pharmacol., 81: 156-165.

MCCONNELL, E.E. (1980) Acute and chronic toxicity, carcinogenesis, reproduction, teratogenesis and mutagenesis in animals. In: Kimbrough, R.D., ed. Halogenated biphenyls, perphenyls, naphthalenes, dibenzodioxins and related products, Amsterdam, Oxford, New York, Elsevier Science Publishers, pp. 109-150.

MCCONNELL, E.E. & MOORE, J.A. (1979) Toxicopathology characteristis of the halogenated aromatics. Ann. N.Y. Acad. Sci., 320: 138-150.

MCCONNELL, E.E., MOORE, J.A., & DALGARD, D.W. (1978a) Toxicity of 2,3,7,8-tetrachlorodibenzo-p-dioxin in Rhesus monkeys (Macaca mulatta) following a single oral dose. Toxicol. appl. Pharmacol., 43: 175-187.

MCCONNELL, E.E., MOORE, J.A., HASEMAN, J.K., & HARRIS, M.W. (1978b) The comparative toxicity of chlorinated dibenzo-p-dioxins in mice and guinea pigs. Toxicol. appl. Pharmacol., 44: 335-356.

MCCONNELL, E.E., LUCIER, G.W., RUMBAUGH, R.C., ALBRO, P.W., HARVAN, D.J., HASS, J.R., & HARRIS, M.W. (1984) Dioxin in soil: bioavailability after ingestion by rats and guinea pigs. Science, 223: 1077-1079.

MCCUNE, E.L., SAVAGE, J.E., & O'DELL, B.L. (1962) Hydropericardium and ascites in chicks fed a chlorinated hydrocarbon. Poult. Sci., 41: 295-299.

MCKINNEY, J., ALBRO, P., LUSTER, M., CORBETT, B., SCHROEDER, J., & LAWSON, L. (1982) Development and reliability of a radioimmunoassay for 2,3,7,8-tetrachlorodibenzo-p-dioxin. In: Hutzinger, O., ed. Chlorinated dioxins and related compounds: Impact on the environment, Oxford, New York, Pergammon Press, pp. 67-77.

MCKINNEY, J.D. (1978) Analysis of 2,3,7,8-tetrachlorodibenzo-para-dioxin in environmental samples. Ecol. Bull. (Stockholm), 27: 53-66.

MCKINNEY, J.D., CHAE, K., GUPTA, B.N., MOORE, J.A., & GOLDSTEIN, J.A. (1976) Toxicological assessment of hexachlorobiphenyl isomers and 2,3,7,8-tetrachlorodibenzofuran in chicks. I. Relationship of chemical parameters. Toxicol. appl. Pharmacol., 36: 65-80.

MCKINNEY, J.D., FAWKES, J., JORDAN, S., CHAE, K., OATLEY, S., COLEMAN, R.E., & BRINER, W. (1985) 2,3,7,8-Tetrachlorodibenzo-p-dioxin (TCDD) as a potent and persistent thyroxine agonist: a mechanistic model for toxicity based on molecular reactivity. Environ. Health Perspect., 61: 41-53.

MCLAUGHLIN, D.L. & PEARSON, R.G. (1984) Concentrations of PCDD and PCDF in soil from the vicinity of the SWARU incinerator, Stoney Creek, July, 1983, Toronto, Ontario, Air Resources Branch, Ontario Ministry of the Environment, 22 pp.

MCNULTY, W.P. (1984) Fetotoxicity of 2,3,7,8-tetrachlorodibenzo-p-dioxin (TCDD) for rhesus macaques (Macaca mulatta). Am. J. Primatol., 6: 41-47.

MCNULTY, W.P. (1985) Toxicity and fetotoxicity of TCDD, TCDF and PCB isomers in rhesus macaques (Macaca mulatta). Environ. Health Perspect., 60: 77-78.

MCNULTY, W.P., POMERANTZ, I., & FARRELL, T. (1981) Chronic toxicity of 2,3,7,8-tetrachlorodibenzofuran for rhesus macaques. Food Cosmet. Toxicol., 19: 57-65.

MCNULTY, W.P., POMERANTZ, L.H., & FARRELL, T.J. (1982a) Chronic toxicity of 2,3,7,8-tetrachlorodibenzofuran for rhesus macaques. In: Hutzinger, O., ed. Chlorinated dioxins and related compounds: Impact on the environment, Oxford, New York, Pergamon Press, pp. 411-418.

MCNULTY, W.P., NIELSEN-SMITH, K.A., & LAY, J.O., Jr (1982b) Persistence of TCDD in monkey adipose tissue. Food Cosmet. Toxicol., 20: 985-987.

MADGE, D.S. (1977) Effects of trichlorophenoxyacetic acid and chlorodioxins on small intestinal function. Gen. Pharmacol., 8: 319-324.

MADHUKAR, B.V. & MATSUMURA, F. (1981) Differences in the nature of induction of mixed-function oxidase systems of the rat liver among phenobarbital, DDT, 3-methylcholanthrene, and TCDD. Toxicol. appl. Pharmacol., 61: 109-118.

MADHUKAR, B.V., BREWSTER, D.W., & MATSUMURA, F. (1984) Effects of in vivo-administered 2,3,7,8-tetrachlorodibenzo-p-dioxin on receptor binding of epidermal growth factor in the hepatic plasma membrane of rat, guinea pig, mouse, and hamster. Proc. Natl Acad. Sci. (USA), 81: 7407-7411.

MANARA, L., COCCIA, P., & CROCI, T. (1982) Persistent tissue levels of TCDD in the mouse and their reduction as related to prevention of toxicity. Drug Metab. Rev., 13(3): 423-446.

MANARA, L., COCCIA, P., & CROCI, T. (1984) Prevention of TCDD toxicity in laboratory rodents by addition of charcoal or cholic acids to chow. Food chem. Toxicol., 22(10): 815-818.

MANIS, J. & APAP, R. (1979) Intestinal organic anion transport, glutathione transferase and aryl hydrocarbon hydroxylase activity: effect of dioxin. Life Sci., 24: 1373-1380.

MANIS, J. & KIM, G. (1977) Induction of intestinal iron transport by 2,3,7,8-tetrachlorodibenzo-p-dioxin on environmental pollutant and potent inducer of aryl hydrocarbon hydroxylase. Clin. Res., 25: 468A.

MANIS, J. & KIM, G. (1979) Introduction of iron transport by a potent inducer of aryl hydrocarbon hydroxylase, 2,3,7,8-tetrachlorodibenzo-p-dioxin. Arch. environ. Health, 34(3): 141-145.

MANTOVANI, A., VECCHI, A., LUINI, W., SIRONI, M., CANDIANI, G.P., SPREAFICO, F., & GARATTINI, S. (1980) Effects of 2,3,7,8-tetrachlorodibenzo-p-dioxin on macrophage and natural killer cell-mediated cytotoxicity in mice. Biomedicine, 32: 200-204.

MARKLUND, S., KJELLER, L.-O., HANSSON, M., TYSKLIND, M., RAPPE, C., RYAN, C., COLLAZO, H., & DOUGHERTY, R. (1986) Determination of PCDDs and PCDFs in incineration samples and pyrolytic products. In: Rappe, C., Choudhary, G., & Keith, L., ed. Chlorinated dioxins and dibenzofurans in perspective, Chelsea, Michigan, Lewis Publishers, pp. 79-92.

MARKLUND, S., RAPPE, C., TYSKLIND, M., & EGEBACK, K. (1987) Identification of polychlorinated dibenzofurans and dioxins in exhausts from cars run on unleaded gasoline. Chemosphere, 16: 29-36.

MARPLE, L., BRUNCK, R., & THROOP, L. (1986a) Water solubility of 2,3,7,8-tetrachlorodibenzo-p-dioxin. Environ. Sci. Technol., 20: 180-182.

MARPLE, L., BERRIDGE, B., & THROOP, L. (1986b) Measurement of the water-octanol partition coefficient of 2,3,7,8-tetrachlorodibenzo-p-dioxin. Environ. Sci. Technol., 20: 397-399.

MASON, G. & SAFE, S. (1986) Synthesis, biologic and toxic effects of the major 2,3,7,8-tetrachlorodibenzo-p-dioxin metabolites in the rat. Toxicology, 41: 153-159.

MASON, G., SAWYER, T., KEYS, B., BANDIERA, S., ROMKES, M., PISKORSKA-PLISZCZYNSKA, J., ZMUDZKA, B., & SAFE, S. (1985) Polychlorinated dibenzofurans (PCDFs): correlation between in vivo and in vitro structure-activity relationships. Toxicology, 37: 1-12.

MASON, G., FARRELL, K., KEYS, B., PISKORSKA-PLISZCZYNSKA, J., SAFE, L., & SAFE, S. (1986) Polychlorinated dibenzo-p-dioxins: Quantitative in vitro and in vivo structure-activity relationships. Toxicology, 41: 21-31.

MASON, M.E. & OKEY, A.B. (1982) Cytosolic and nuclear binding of 2,3,7,8-tetrachlorodibenzo-p-dioxin to the Ah receptor in extra-hepatic tissues of rats and mice. Eur. J. Biochem., 123: 209-215.

MASUDA, Y., KUROKI, H., HARAGUCHI, K., & NAGAYAMA, J. (1985) PCB and PCDF congeners in the blood and tissues of Yusho and Yu-Cheng patients. Environ. Health Perspect., 59: 53-58.

MASUDA, Y., KUROKI, H., HARAGUCHI, K., & NAGAYAMA, J. (1986) PCDFs and related compounds in humans from Yusho and Yu-Cheng incidents. Chemosphere, 15: 1621-1628.

MATSUMURA, F. & BENEZET, H.J. (1973) Studies on the bioaccumulation and microbial degradation of 2,3,7,8-tetrachlorodibenzo-p-dioxin. Environ. Health Perspect., 5: 253-258.

MATSUMURA, F., QUENSEN, J., & TSUSHIMOTO, G. (1983) Microbial degradation of TCDD in a model ecosystem. In: Tucker, R.E., Young, A.L., & Gray, A.P., ed. Human and environmental risks of chlorinated dioxins and related compounds, New York, London, Plenum Press, pp. 191-220.

MATSUMURA, F., BREWSTER, D.W., MADHUKAR, B.V., & BOMBICK, D.W. (1984) Alteration of rat hepatic plasma membrane functions by 2,3,7,8-tetrachlorodibenzo-p-dioxin (TCDD). Arch. environ. Contam. Toxicol., 13: 509-515.

MATTISON, D.R. & THORGEIRSSON, S.S. (1978) Gonadal aryl hydrocarbon hydroxylase in rats and mice. Cancer Res., 38: 1368-1373.

MAY, G. (1973) Chloracne from the accidental production of tetrachlorodibenzodioxin. Br. J. ind. Med., 30: 276-283.

MAY, G. (1982) Tetrachlorodibenzodioxin: a survey of subjects ten years after exposure. Br. J. ind. Med., 39: 128-135.

MAZER, T., HILEMAN, F.D., NOBLE, R.W., & BROOKS, J.J. (1983) Synthesis of the 38 tetrachlorodibenzofuran isomers and identification by capillary column gas chromatography/mass spectrometry. Anal. Chem., 55: 104-110.

MEYNE, J., ALLISON, D.C., BOSE, K., JORDAN, S.W., RIDOLPHO, P.F., & SMITH, J. (1985) Hepatotoxic doses of dioxin do not damage mouse bone marrow chromosomes. Mutat. Res., 157: 63-69.

MILES, W.F., SINGH, J., GURPRASAD, N.P., & MALIS, G.P. (1985) Isomer specific determination of hexachlorodioxins in technical pentachlorophenol (PCP) and its sodium salt. Chemosphere, 14(6/7): 807-810.

MILLER, A.G., ISRAEL, D., & WHITLOCK, J.P., Jr (1983) Biochemical and genetic analysis of variant mouse hepatoma cells defective in the induction of benzo(a)pyrene-metabolizing enzyme. J. biol. Chem., 258: 3523-3527.

MILNES, M.H. (1971) Formation of 2,3,7,8-tetrachlorodibenzodioxin by thermal decomposition of sodium 2,4,5-trichlorophentane. Nature (Lond.), 232: 395-396.

MILSTONE, L.M. & LAVIGNE, J.F. (1984) 2,3,7,8-Tetrachlorodibenzo-p-dioxin induces hyperplasia in confluent cultures of human keratinocytes. J. invest. Dermatol., 82: 532-534.

MITCHUM, R.K., MOLER, G.F., & KORFMACHER, W.A. (1980) Combined capillary gas chromatography/atmospheric pressure negative chemical ionization/mass spectrometry for the determination of 2,3,7,8-tetrachlorodibenzo-p-dioxin in tissue. Anal. Chem., 52: 2278-2282.

MITTLER, J.C., ERTEL, N.H., PENG, R.X., YANG, C.S., & KIERNAN, T. (1984) Changes in testosterone hydroxylase activity in rat testis following administration of 2,3,7,8-tetrachlorodibenzo-p-dioxin. Ann. N.Y. Acad. Sci., 438: 645-648.

MIVRA, H., OMORI, A., & SHIBUE, M. (1974) The effect of chlorophenols on the excretion of porphyrins in urine. Jpn. J. ind. Health, 16: 575-577.

MOLLER, M.E., GLOWINSKI, I.B., & THORGEIRSSON, S.S. (1984) The genotoxicity of aromatic amines in primary hepatocytes isolated from C57BL/6 and DBA/2 mice. Carcinogenesis, 5: 797-804.

MOORE, J.A., GUPTA, B.N., ZINKL, J.G., & VOS, J.G. (1973) Postnatal effects of maternal exposure to 2,3,7,8-tetrachlorodibenzo-p-dioxins (TCDD). Environ. Health Perspect., 5: 81-85.

MOORE, J.A., GUPTA, B.N., & VOS, J.G. (1976) Toxicity of 2,3,7,8-tetrachloro-dibenzofuran - preliminary results. In: Proceedings from the National Conference on Polychlorinated Biphenyls, Chicago, Illinois, 19-21 November, 1975, Research Triangle Park, North Carolina, Research Triangle Park Institute.

MOORE, J.A., MCCONNELL, E.E., DALGARD, D.W., & HARRIS, M.W. (1979) Comparative toxicity of three halogenated dibenzofurans in guinea pigs, mice and rhesus monkeys. Ann. N.Y. Acad. Sci., 320: 151-163.

MOORE, R.W. & PETERSON, R.E. (1985) Enhanced catabolism and elimination of androgens do not cause the androgenic deficiency in 2,3,7,8-tetrachlorodibenzo-p-dioxin-treated rats. Fed. Proc., 44: 518.

MOORE, R.W., POTTER, C.L., THEOBALD, H.M., ROBINSON, J.A., & PETERSON, R.E. (1985) Androgenic deficiency in male rats treated with 2,3,7,8-tetra- chlorodbenzo-p-dioxin. Toxicol. appl. Pharmacol., 79: 99-111.

MORITA, M. & OISHI, S. (1977) Clearance and tissue distribution of polychlorinated dibenzofurans in mice. Bull. environ. Contam. Toxicol., 18: 61-66.

MORITA, M., NAKAGAWA, J., & RAPPE, C. (1978) Polychlorinated dibenzofuran (PCDF) formation from PCB mixture by heat and oxygen. Bull. environ. Contam. Toxicol., 19: 665-670.

MORTELMANS, K., HAWORTH, S., SPECK, W., & ZEIGER, E. (1984) Mutagenicity testing of agent orange components and related chemicals. Toxicol. appl. Pharmarcol., 75: 137-146.

MOSES, M. & SELIKOFF, I.J. (1981) Soft tissue sarcomas, phenoxy herbicides, and chlorinated phenols. Lancet, 1: 1370.

MOSES, M., LILIS, R., CROW, K.D., THORNTON, J., FISCHBEIN, A., ANDERSON, H.A., & SELIKOFF, I.J. (1984) Health status of workers with past exposure to 2,3,7,8-tetrachloridibenzo-p-dioxin in manufacture of 2,4,5-trichlorophenoxyacetic acid: Comparison of findings with and without chloracne. Am. J. ind. Med., 5: 161-182

MOTTURA, A., ZEI, G., NUZZO, F., CRIMAUDO, C., GIORGI, R., VENERONI, P., PAGGINI, P., MACARELLI, P., FRACCARO, M., NICOLETTI, B., & DECARLI, L. (1981) Evaluation of results of chromosome analyses on lymphocytes of TCDD exposed subjects after the Seveso accident. Mutat. Res., 85: 238-239.

MUKITARI, H., BAARS, A.J., & BREIMER, D.D. (1981) Differences in inducibility of particulate and cytosolic rat liver glutathione S-transferase activities. Xenobiotica, 11: 367-371.

MULCAHY, M.T. (1980) Correspondence. Chromosome aberrations and "agent orange". Med. J. Aust., 2: 573-574.

MULLER, E. (1937) [Chloracne (caused by chlorinated benzenes). Inaugural Dissertation,] Speyer am Rhein, Pilger-Druckerei (Thesis, Friedrich-Wilhelm University, Breslau).

MURRAY, F.J., SMITH, F.A., NITSCHKE, K.D., HUMISTON, C.G., KOCIBA, R.J., & SCHWETZ, B.A. (1979) Three-generation reproduction study of rats given 2,3,7,8-tetrachlorodibenzo-p-dioxin (TCDD) in the diet. Toxicol. appl. Pharmacol., 50: 241-252.

NAGARKATTI, P.S., SWEENEY, G.D., GAULDIE, J., & CLARK, D.A. (1984) Sensitivity to suppression of cytotoxic T cells generation by 2,3,7,8-tetrachlorodibenzo-p-dioxin (TCDD) in dependent on the Ah genotype of the murine host. Toxicol. appl. Pharmacol., 72: 169-176.

NAGAYAMA, J., KURATSUNE, M., & MASUDA, Y. (1976) Determination of chlorinated dibenzofurans in kanechlors and "Yusho oil". Bull. environ. Contam. Toxicol., 15: 9-13.

NAGAYAMA, J., NISHIZUMI, M., & MASUDA, Y. (1979) [Subacute toxicity of polychlorinated dibenzofurans in mice.] Fukuoka Igakuzassh, 70: 109-113 (in Japanese).

NAGAYAMA, J., TOKUDOME, S., & KURATSUNE, M. (1980) Transfer of polychlorinated dibenzofurans to the foetuses and offspring of mice. Food Cosmet. Toxicol., 18: 153-157.

NAGAYAMA, J., KUROKI, H., MASUDA, Y., & KURATSUME, M. (1983) A comparative study of polychlorinated dibenzofurans, polychlorinated biphenyls and 2,3,7,8-tetrachlorodibenzo-p-dioxin on aryl hydrocarbon hydroxylase inducing potency in rats. Arch. Toxicol., 53: 177-184.

NAGAYAMA, J., KUROKI, H., MASUDA, Y., HANDA, S., & KURATSUNE, M. (1985a) Genetically mediated induction of aryl hydrocarbon hydroxylase activity in mice by polychlorinated dibenzofuran isomers and 2,3,7,8-tetrachlorodibenzo-p-dioxin. Arch. Toxicol., 56: 226-229.

NAGAYAMA, J., KIYOHARA, C., KURATSUNE, M., & MASUDA, Y. (1985b) Induction of aryl hydrocarbon hydroxylase activity in human lymphoblastoid cells by chlorinated dibenzofuran isomers and 2,3,7,8-tetrachlorodibenzo-p-dioxin. In: Keith, L.H., Rappe, C., & Choudhary, G., ed. Chlorinated dioxins and dibenzofurans in the total environment II, Stoneham, Maine, Butterworth Publishers, pp. 285-295.

NAU, H. & BASS, R. (1981) Transfer of 2,3,7,8-tetrachlorodibenzo-p-dioxin (TCDD) to the mouse embryo and fetus. Toxicology, 20: 299-308.

NAU, H., BASS, R., & NEUBERT, D. (1986) Transfer of 2,3,7,8-tetrachlorodibenzo-p-dioxin (TCDD) via placenta and milk, and postnatal toxicity in the mouse. Arch. Toxicol., 59: 36-40.

NCI (1977) Bioassay of dibenzo-p-dioxin for possible carcinogenicity, Washington, DC, National Cancer Institute, 104 pp (Technical Report No. 122).

NCI (1979) Bioassay of 2,7-dichlorodibenzo-p-dioxin (DCDD) for possible carcinogenicity, Washington, DC, National Cancer Institute, 103 pp (Technical Report No. 123).

NEAL, R.A., BEATTY, P.W., & GASIEWICZ, T.A. (1979) Studies of the mechanisms of toxicity of 2,3,7,8-tetrachlorodibenzo-p-dioxin (TCDD). Ann. N.Y. Acad. Sci., 320: 204-213.

NEBERT, D.W., ROBINSON, J.R., NIWA, A., KUMAKI, K., & POLAND, A.P. (1975) Genetic expression of aryl hydrocarbon hydroxylase activity in the mouse. J. cell. Physiol., 85: 393-414.

NEBERT, D.W., JENSEN, N.M., PERRY, J.W., & OKA, T. (1980) Association between ornithine decarboxylase induction and the Ah locus in mice treated with polycyclic aromatic compounds. J. biol. Chem., 255: 6836-6842.

NESTRICK, T.J., LAMPARSKI, L.L., & STEHL, R.H. (1979) Synthesis and identification of the 22 tetrachlorodienzo-p-dioxin isomers by high performance liquid chromatography and gas chromatography. Anal. Chem., 51: 2273-2281.

NESTRICK, T.J., LAMPARSKI, L.L., & TOWNSEND, D.I. (1980) Identification of tetrachlorodibenzo-p-dioxin isomers at the 1 ng level by photolytic degradation and patter recognition techniques. Anal. Chem., 52: 1865-1874.

NESTRICK, T.J., LAMPARSKI, L.L., FRAWLEY, N.N., HUMMEL, R.A., KOCHER, C.W., MAHLE, N.H., MCCOY, J.W., MILLER, D.L., PETERS, T.L., PILLEPICH, J.L., SMITH, W.E., & TOBEY, S.W. (1986) Perspectives of a large scale environmental survey for chlorinated dioxins: Overview and soil data. Chemosphere, 15: 1453-1460.

NEUBERT, D. & DILLMANN, I. (1972) Embryotoxic effects in mice treated with 2,4,5-trichlorophenoxyacetic acid and 2,3,7,8-tetrachlorodibenzo-p-dioxin. Naunyn-Schmiedeberg's Arch. Pharmacol., 272: 243-264.

NIEMANN, R.A., BRUMLEY, W.C., FIRESTONE, D., & SPHON, J.A. (1983) Analysis of fish for 2,3,7,8-tetrachlorodibenzo-p-dioxin by electron capture capillary gas chromatography. Anal. Chem., 55: 1497-1504.

NIH (1980a) Bioassay of 1,2,3,6,7,8- and 1,2,3,7,8,9-hexachlorodibenzo-p-dioxin for possible carcinogenicity (dermal study), Bethesda, Maryland, US Department of Health and Human Services, National Institutes of Health (DHSS Publication No. (NIH) 80-1758).

NIH (1980b) Bioassay of 1,2,3,6,7,8- and 1,2,3,7,8,9-hexachlorodibenzo-p-dioxin for possible carcinogenicity (gavage), Bethseda, Maryland, US Department of Health and Human Services, National Institutes of Health (DHHS Publication No. (NIH) 80-1754).

NIH (1982a) Carcinogenesis bioassay of 2,3,7,8-tetrachlorodibenzo-p-dioxin (CAS No 1746-01-6) in Osborne-Mendel rats and B6C3F1 mice (gavage study), Research Triangle Park, North Carolina, US National Institutes of Health, National Toxicology Program (NTP Technical Report Series No. 209).

NIH (1982b) Carcinogenesis bioassay of 2,3,7,8-tetrachlorodibenzo-p-dioxin (CAS No 1746-01-6) in Swiss-Webster mice (dermal study), Research Triangle Park, North Carolina, US National Institutes of Health, National Toxicology Program (NTP Technical Report Series No. 201).

NILSSON, C.A., ANDERSSON, K., RAPPE, C., & WESTERMARK, S.O. (1974) Chromatographic evidence for the formation of chlorodioxins from chloro-2-phenoxyphenols. J. Chromatogr., 96: 137-147.

NILSSON, C.A., NORSTROM, A., ANDERSSON, K., & RAPPE, C. (1978) Impurities in commercial products related to pentachlorophenol. In: Rao, K.R., ed. Pentachlorophenol: Chemistry, pharmacology and environmental toxicology, New York, London, Plenum Press, pp. 313-324.

NISBET, I.C.T. & PAXTON, M.B. (1982) Statistical aspects of three-generation studies of the reproductive toxicity of TCDD and 2,4,5,-T. Am. Stat., 36(3): 290-298.

NISHIZUMI, M. (1978) Acute toxicity of polychlorinated dibenzofurans in CF-1 mice. Toxicol. appl. Pharmacol., 45: 209-212.

NISHIZUMI, M., KURATSUNE, M., & MASSUDA, Y. (1975) [Comparison of hyperkeratosis induced by PCBs, PCDF and PCDD application. Polychlorinated biphenyls, polychlorinated dibenzofuran and polychlorinated dibenzodioxin.] Fukuoka Asa Med., 66: 600-604 (in Japanese).

NIWA, A., KUMAKI, K., & NEBERT, D.W. (1975) Induction of aryl hydrocarbon - hydroxylase activity in various cell cultures by 2,3,7,8-tetrachlorodibenzo-p-dioxin. Mol. Pharmacol., 11: 399-408.

NOLAN, R.J., SMITH, F.A., & HEFNER, J.G. (1979) Elimination and tissue distribution of 2,3,7,8-tetrachlorodibenzo-p-dioxin (TCDD) in female guinea pigs following a single oral dose. Tox. appl. Pharmacol., 48: 167 (abstract).

NORBACK, D.H. & ALLEN, J.R. (1973) Biological responses of the nonhuman primate, chicken, and rat to chlorinated dibenzo-p-dioxin ingestion. Environ. Health Perspect., 5: 233-240.

NORBACK, D.H., ENGBLOM, J.F., & ALLEN, J.R. (1975) Tissue distribution and excretion of octachlorodibenzo-p-dioxin in the rat. Toxicol. appl. Pharmacol., 32: 330-338.

NORMAN, L.R., JOHNSON, E.F., & MULLER-EBERHARD, U. (1978) Identification of the major cytochrome P-450 form transplacentally induced in neonatal rabbits by 2,3,7,8-tetrachlorodibenzo-p-dioxin. J. biol. Chem., 253: 8640-8647.

NORSTROM, R.J., HALLETT, D.J., SIMON, M., & MULVIHILL, M.J. (1982) Analysis of Great Lakes Herring Gull eggs for tetrachlorodibenzo-p-dioxins. In: Hutzinger, O., ed. Chlorinated dioxins and related compounds. Impact on the environment, Oxford, New York, Pergammon Press, pp. 173-182.

NORSTROM, R.J., SIMON, M., & WESELOH, D.V. (1986) Long-term trends of PCDD and PCDF contamination in the Great Lakes. Presented at Dioxin 86, 6th International Symposium on Chlorinated Dioxins and Related Compounds, Fukuoka, Japan, 16-19 September, 1986.

NORSTROM, R.J., SIMON, M., WHITEHEAD, P.E., KUSSAT, R., & GARRET, C. (1988) Level of polychlorinated dibenzo-p-dioxins (PCDDs) and polychlorinated dibenzofurans (PCDFs) in biota and sediments near potential sources of contamination in British Columbia, 1987, West Vancouver, British Columbia, Environment Canada (Analytical Report CRD-88-5).

NRC CANADA (1981) Polychlorinated dibenzo-p-dioxins. Limitation to the current analytical technique, Ottawa, National Research Council of Canada (Publication No. NRCC/NRC 18576).

NYGREN, M., RAPPE, C., LINDSTROM, G., HANSSON, M., BERGQVIST, P.-A., MARKLUND, S., DOMELLOF, L., HARDELL, L., & OLSSON, M. (1986) Identification of 2,3,7,8- substituted polychlorinated dioxins and dibenzofurans in environmental and human samples. In: Rappe, C., Choudhary, G., & Keith, L., ed. Chlorinated dioxins and dibenzofurans in perspective, Chelsea, Michigan, Lewis Publishers, pp. 17-34.

OBERG, T. & BERGSTROM, J. (1986) Combustion test data from a Swedish hazardous waste incinerator. Chemosphere, 15: 2045-2048.

OISHI, S. (1977) Influence of polychlorinated dibenzofurans (PCDFs) and polychlorinated biphenyls (PCBs) to serum protein components in rats. Bull. environ. Contam. Toxicol., 18: 773-777.

OISHI, S. & HIRAGA, K. (1980) Effect of polychlorinated biphenyl, dibenzofuran and dibenzo-p-dioxin on the susceptibility of male mice to endotoxin. J. environ. Sci. Health, B15: 77-85.

OISHI, S., MORITA, M., & FUKUDA, H. (1978) Comparative toxicity of polychlorinated biphenyls and dibenzofurans in rats. Toxicol. appl. Pharmacol., 43: 13-22.

O'KEEFE, P., MESELSON, M.S., & BAUGHMAN, R. (1977) Neutral clean-up procedure for 2,3,7,8-tetrachlorodibenzo-p-dioxin residues in bovine fat and milk. J. Assoc. Off. Anal. Chem., 61: 621-626.

O'KEEFE, P., MEYER, C., HILKER, D., ALDOVES, K., JELUS-TYROR, B., DILLON, K., DONNOLLY, R., HORN, E., & SLOAN, R. (1983) Analysis of 2,3,7,8-tetrachlorodibenzo-p-dioxin in Great Lakes fish. Chemosphere, 12: 325-332.

O'KEEFE, P., SILKWORTH, J.B., BIERTHY, J.F., SMITH, R.M., DECAPRIO, A.P., TURNER, J.N., EADON, G., HILKER, D.R., ALDOUS, K.M., KAMINSKY, L.S., & COLLINS, D.N. (1985) Chemical and biological investigations of a transformer accident at Binghamton, NY. Environ. Health Perspect., 60: 201-209.

OKEY, A.B. & VELLA, L.M. (1982) Binding of 3-methylchloanthrene and 2,3,7,8-tetrachlorodibenzo-p-dioxin to a common Ah receptor site in mouse and rat hepatic cytosols. Eur. J. Biochem., 127: 39-47.

OKEY, A.B., BONDY, G.P., MASON, M.E., KAHL, G.F., EISEN, H.J., GUENTHNER, T.M., & NEBERT, D.W. (1979) Regulatory gene product of the Ah locus. J. biol. Chem., 254: 11636-11648.

OKEY, A.B., BONDY, G.P., MASON, M.E., NEBERT, D.W., FORSTER-GIBSON, C.J., MUNCHAN, J., & DUFRESNE, M.J. (1980) Temperature-dependent cytosol-to-nucleus translocation of the Ah receptor for 2,3,7,8-tetrachlorodibenzo-p-dioxin in continuous cell culture lines. J. biol. Chem., 225: 11415-11422.

OKINO, S.T., QUATTROCHI, L.C., BARNES, H.J., OSANTO, S., GRIFFIN, K.J., JOHNSON, E.F., & TUKEY, R.H. (1985) Cloning and characterization of cDNAs encoding 2,3,7,8-tetrachlorodibenzo-p-dioxin-inducible rabbit mRNAs for cytochrome P-450 isozymes 4 and 6. Proc. Natl Acad. Sci. (USA), 82: 5310-5314.

OLIE, K., VERMEULEN, P.L., & HUTZINGER, O. (1977) Chlorodibenzo-p-dioxins and chlorodibenzofurans are trace components of fly ash and flue gas of some municipal incinerators in the Netherlands. Chemosphere, 8: 455-459.

OLIE, K., BERG, M.V.D., & HUTZINGER, O. (1983) Formation and fate of PCDD and PCDF from combustion processes. Chemosphere, 12: 627-636.

OLIVER, R.M. (1975) Toxic effects of 2,3,7,8-tetrachlorodibenzo-1,4-dioxin in laboratory workers. Br. J. ind. Med., 32: 49-53.

OLSON, J.A. & GUNNING, D. (1983) The storage form of vitamin A in rat liver cells. J. Nutr., 113: 2184-2191.

OLSON, J.R. (1986) Metabolism and disposition of 2,3,7,8-tetrachlorodibenzo-p-dioxin in guinea pigs. Toxicol. appl. Pharmacol., 85: 263-273.

OLSON, J.R., GASIEWICZ, T.A., & NEAL, R.A. (1980a) Tissue distribution, excretion, and metabolism of 2,3,7,8-tetrachlorodibenzo-p-dioxin (TCDD) in the golden Syrian hamster. Toxicol. appl. Pharmacol., 56: 78-85.

OLSON, J.R., HOLSCHER, M.A., & NEAL, R.A. (1980b) Toxicity of 2,3,7,8-tetrachlorodibenzo-p-dioxin in the golden syrian hamster. Toxicol. appl. Pharmacol., 55: 67-78.

ONO, M., WAKIMOTO, T., TATSUKAWA, R., & MASUDA, Y. (1986) Polychlorinated dibenzo-p-dioxins and dibenzofurans in human adipose tissues of Japan. Chemosphere, 15: 1629-1634.

ONTARIO (1985) Scientific criteria document for standard development. Polychlorinated dibenzo-p-dioxins (PCDDs) and polychlorinated dibenzofurans (PCDFs), Toronto, Ontario Ministry of the Environment (Report No. 4-84).

ONTARIO (1986) Drinking water survey St. Clair river - Detroit river area, Toronto, Ontario Ministry of the Environment.

ORR, J.B. & RICHARDS, M.B. (1934) Growth and vitamin A deficiency. Biochem. J., 28: 1259-1273.

OSBORNE, R. & GREENLEE, W.F. (1985) 2,3,7,8-Tetrachlorodibenzo-p-dioxin (TCDD) enhances terminal differentiation of cultured human epidermal cells. Toxicol. appl. Pharmacol., 77: 434-443.

OSBORNE, R., DOLD, K.M., & GREENLEE, W.F. (1984) Cell culture models to study mechanisms of toxicity of chlorinated aromatic compounds to skin and thymus. Chem. Ind. Inst. Toxicol., 4: 2-7.

OTT, M.G., HOLDER, B.B., & OLSON, R.D. (1980) A mortality analysis of employees engaged in the manufacture of 2,4,5-trichlorophenoxyacetic acid. J. occup. Med., 22: 47-50.

PAASIVIRTA, J., ENQVIST, J., RAISANEN, S., & PAASIVUO, P. (1977) On the limit of detection of TCDD in gas chromatography. Chemosphere, 6: 355.

PALAUSKY, J., HARWOOD, J.J., CLEVENGER, T.E., KAPILA, S., & YANDERS, A.F. (1986) Disposition of tetrachlorodibenzo-p-dioxin in soil. In: Rappe, C., Choudhary, G., & Keith, L., ed. Chlorinated dioxins and dibenzofurans in perspective, Chelsea, Michigan, Lewis Publishers, pp. 211-223.

PATTERSON, D.G., Jr, HOFFMAN, R.E., NEEDHAM, L.L., ROBERTS, D.W., BAGBY, J.R., PIRKLE, J.L., FALK, H., SAMPSON, E.J., & HOUK, V.N. (1986) 2,3,7,8-Tetrachlorodibenzo-p-dioxin levels in adipose tissue of exposed and control persons in Missouri. J. Am. Med. Assoc., 256: 2683-2686.

PATTERSON, J.M., MCHENRY, E.W., & CRANDALL, W.A. (1942) The physiological properties of vitamin A. 1. A specific effect upon body weight and body composition in the Albino rat. Biochem. J., 36: 792-794.

PAZDERNIK, T.L. & ROZMAN, K.K. (1985) Effect of thyroidectomy and thyroxine on 2,3,7,8-tetrachlorodibenzo-p-dioxin-induced immunotoxicity. Life Sci., 36: 695-703.

PAZDEROVA-VEJLUPKOVA, J., LUKAS, E., NEMCOVA, M., SPACILOVA, M., JIRASEK, L., KALENSKY, J., JOHN, J., JIRASEK, A., & PICKOVA, J. (1974) [Chronic intoxication by chlorinated hydrocarbons formed during the production of sodium 2,4,5-trichlorophenoxyacetate.] Pracov. Lek., 26: 332-339 (in Czech).

PAZDEROVA-VEJLUPKOVA, J., LUKAS, E., NEMCOVA, M., PICKOVA, J., & JIRASEK, L. (1980) [Chronic poisoning by 2,3,7,8-tetrachlorodibenzo-p-dioxin.] Pracov. Lek., 32: 204-209 (in Czech).

PAZDEROVA-VEJLUPKOVA, J., NEMCOVA, M., PICKOVA, J., JIRASEK, L., & LUKAS, E. (1981) The development and prognosis of chronic intoxication by tetrachlorodibenzo-p-dioxin in men. Arch. environ. Health, 36: 5-11.

PETERSON, R.E., MADHUKAR, B.V., YANG, K.H., & MATSUMURA, F. (1979a) Depression of adenosine triphosphatase activities in isolated liver surface membranes of 2,3,7,8-tetrahlorodibenzo-p-dioxin-treated rats: correlation with effects on ouabain biliary excretion and bile flow. J. Pharmacol. exp. Ther., 210: 275-210.

PETERSON, R.E., HAMADA, N., YANG, K.H., & MADHUKAR, B.V. (1979b) Reversal of 2,3,7,8-tetrachlorodibenzo-p-dioxin-induced depression of ouabain biliary excretion by pregnenolone-16-beta-carbonitrile and spironolactone in isolated perfused rat livers. Toxicol. appl. Pharmacol., 50: 407-416.

PHILIPPI, M., SCHMID, J., WIPF, H.K., & HUTTER, R. (1982) A microbial metabolite of TCDD. Experientia (Basel), 38: 659-661.

PIPER, W.N., ROSE, J.Q., & GEHRING, P.J. (1973) Excretion and tissue distribution of 2,3,7,8-tetrachlorodibenzo-p-dioxin in the rat. Adv. Chem. Ser., 120: 85-91.

PITOT, H.C. & SIRICA, A.E. (1980) The stages of initiation and promotion in hepatocarcinogenesis. Biochim. Biophys. Acta, 605: 191-215.

PITOT, H.C., GOLDSWORTHY, T., CAMPBELL, H.A., & POLAND, A. (1980) Quantitative evaluation of the promotion by 2,3,7,8-tetrachlorodibenzo-p-dioxin of hepatocarcinogenesis from diethylnitrosamine. Cancer Res., 40: 3616-3620.

POCCHIARI, F. (1978) 2,3,7,8-Tetrachlorodibenzo-para-dioxin decontamination. Ecol. Bull. (Stockholm), 27: 67-70.

POCCHIARI, F., DIDOMENICO, A., SILANO, V., & ZAPPONI, G. (1983) Environmental impact of the accidental release of tetrachlorodibenzo-p-dioxn (TCDD) at Seveso (Italy). In: Coulston, F. & Pocchiari, F., ed. Accidental exposure to dioxins. human health aspects, New York, London, Academic Press, pp. 5-35.

POELLINGER, L. & GULLBERG, D. (1985) Characterization of the hydrophobic properties of the receptor for 2,3,7,8-tetrachlorodibenzo-p-dioxin. Mol. Pharmacol., 27: 271-276.

POELLINGER, L., KURL, R.N., LUND, J., GILLNER, M., CARLSTEDT-DUKE, J., HOGBERG, B., & GUSTAFSSON. J.-A. (1982) High-affinity binding of 2,3,7,8-tetrachlorodibenzo-p-dioxin in cell nuclei from rat liver. Biochem. Biophys. Acta, 714: 516-523.

POELLINGER, L., LUND, J., HANSSON, L.-A., & GUSTAFSSON, J.-A. (1983) Physicochemical characterization of specific and non-specific polyaromatic hydrocarbon binders in rat and mouse liver cytosol. J. biol. Chem., 258: 13535-13542.

POHJANVIRTA, R. & TUOMISTO, J. (1986) Han/Wistar rats are exceptionally resistant to TCDD. II. Arch. Toxicol., 11 (Suppl.): 344-347.

POHLAND, A.E. & YANG, G.C. (1972) Preparation and characterization of chlorinated dibenzo-p-dioxins. J. agric. food Chem., 20(6): 1093-1099.

POIGER, H. & BUSER, H.R. (1983) Structure elucidation of mammalian TCDD-metabolites. In: Tucker, R.E., Young, A.L., & Gray, A.P., ed. Human and environmental risks of chlorinated dioxins and related compounds, New York, London, Plenum Press, pp. 483-492.

POIGER, H. & SCHLATTER, Ch. (1979) Biological degradation of TCDD in rats. Nature (London), 281: 706-707.

POIGER, H. & SCHLATTER, Ch. (1980) Influence of solvents and adsorbents on dermal and intestinal absorption of TCDD. Food Cosmet. Toxicol., 18: 477-481.

POIGER, H. & SCHLATTER, Ch. (1985) Influence of phenobarbital and TCDD on the hepatic metabolism of TCDD in the dog. Experientia (Basel), 41: 376-378.

POIGER, H. & SCHLATTER, Ch. (1986) Pharmacokinetics of 2,3,7,8-TCDD in man. Chemosphere, 15: 1489-1494.

POIGER, H., BUSER, H.R., WEBER, H., ZWEIFEL, U., & SCHLATTER, Ch. (1982) Structure elucidation of mammalian TCDD-metabolites. Experientia (Basel), 38: 484-486.

POIGER, H., BUSER, H.R., & SCHLATTER, Ch. (1984) The metabolism of 2,3,7,8-tetrachlorodibenzofuran in the rat. Chemosphere, 13: 351-357.

POLAND, A. & GLOVER, E. (1973a) Studies on the mechanism of toxicity of the chlorinated dibenzo-p-dioxins. Environ. Health Perspect., 5: 245-251.

POLAND, A. & GLOVER, E. (1973b) 2,3,7,8-Tetrachlorodibenzo-p-dioxin: A potent inducer of aminolevulinic acid synthetase. Science, 179: 476-477.

POLAND, A. & GLOVER, E. (1973c) Chlorinated dibenzo-p-dioxins: Potent inducers of aminolevulinic acid synthetase and aryl hydrocarbon hydroxylase. II. A study of the structure-activity relationship. Mol. Pharmacol., 9: 736-747.

POLAND, A. & GLOVER, E. (1974a) The induction of aryl hydrocarbon hydroxylase by 2,3,7,8-tetrachlorodibenzo-p-dioxin: Evidence for a receptor mutation in genetically non-responsive mice. Pharmacologist, 16: 240 (Abstract 282).

POLAND, A. & GLOVER, E. (1974b) Comparison of 2,3,7,8-tetrachlorodibenzo-p-dioxin, a potent inducer of aryl hydrocarbon hydroxylase, with 3-methylcholanthrene. Mol. Pharmacol., 10: 349-359.

POLAND, A. & GLOVER, E. (1974c) Genetic expression of aryl hydrocarbon hydroxylase activity. Induction of monooxygenase activities and cytochrome P1-450 formation by 2,3,7,8-tetrachlorodibenzo-p-dioxin in mice genetically "nonresponsive" to other aromatic hydrocarbons. J. biol. Chem., 249: 5599-5606.

POLAND, A. & GLOVER, E. (1975) Genetic expression of arylhydrocarbon hydroxylase by 2,3,7,8-tetrachlorodibenzo-p-dioxin: Evidence for a receptor mutation in genetically non-responsive mice. Mol. Pharmacol., 11: 389-398.

POLAND, A. & GLOVER, E. (1979) An estimate of the maximum in vivo covalent binding of 2,3,7,8-tetrachlorodibenzo-p-dioxin to rat liver protein, ribosomal RNA, and DNA. Cancer Res., 39: 3341-3344.

POLAND, A. & GLOVER, E. (1980) 2,3,7,8-Tetrachlorodibenzo-p-dioxin: Segregation of toxicity with the Ah-locus. Mol. Pharmacol., 17: 86-94.

POLAND, A. & KENDE, A. (1976) 2,3,7,8-Tetrachlorodibenzo-p-dioxin: Environmental contaminant and molecular probe. Fed. Proc., 35: 2404-2411.

POLAND, A. & KNUTSON, J.C. (1982) 2,3,7,8-Tetrachlorodibenzo-p-dioxin and related halogenated aromatic hydrocarbons: Examination of the mechanisms of toxicity. Annu. Rev. Pharmacol. Toxicol., 22: 517-554.

POLAND, A., SMITH, D., METTER, G., & POSSICK, P. (1971) A health survey of workers in a 2,4-D and 2,4,5-T plant. Arch. environ. Health, 22: 316-327.

POLAND, A., GLOVER, E., & KENDE, A.S. (1976) Stereospecific, high affinity binding of 2,3,7,8-tetrachlorodibenzo-p-dioxin by hepatic cytosol. Evidence that the binding species is receptor for induction of aryl hydrocarbon hydroxylase. J. biol. Chem., 251: 4936-4946.

POLAND, A., PALEN, D., & GLOVER, E. (1982) Tumor promotion by TCDD in HRS/J mice. Nature (Lond.), 300(5889): 271-273.

POLI, A., FRANCESCHINI, G., PUGLISI, L., & SIRTORI, C.R. (1980) Increased total and high density lipoprotein cholesterol with apoprotein changes resembling streptozotocin diabetes in tetrachlorodibenzodioxin (TCDD) treated rats. Biochem. Pharmacol., 29: 835-838.

POTTER, C.L., SIPES, I.G., & RUSSELL, D.H. (1982) Inhibition of ornithine decarboxylase activity by 2,3,7,8-tetrachlorodibenzo-p-dioxin. Biochem. Pharmacol., 31: 3367-3371.

POTTER, C.L., SIPES, I.G., & RUSSELL, D.H. (1983) Hypothyroxinemia and hypothermia in rats in response to 2,3,7,8-tetrachlorodibenzo-p-dioxin administration. Toxicol. appl. Pharmacol., 69: 89-95.

POTTER, C.L., MENAHAN, L.A., & PETERSON, R.E. (1986a) Relationship of alterations in energy metabolism to hypophagia in rats treated with 2,3,7,8-tetrachlorodibenzo-p-dioxin. Fundam. appl. Toxicol., 6: 89-97.

POTTER, C.L., MOORE, R.W., INHORN, S.L., HAGEN, T.C., & PETERSON, R.E. (1986b) Thyroid status and thermogenesis in rats treated with 2,3,7,8-tetrachlorodibenzo-p-dioxin. Toxicol. appl. Pharmacol., 84: 45-55.

PRATT, R.M., DENCKER, L., & DIEWERT, V.M. (1984) 2,3,7,8-Tetrachlorodibenzo-p-dioxin-induced cleft palate in the mouse: Evidence for alterations in palatal shelf fusion. Teratog. Carcinogen. Mutagen., 4: 427-436.

PRESTON, B.D., VAN MILLER, P.J., MOORE, R.W., & ALLEN, J.R. (1981) Promoting effects of polychlorinated biphenyls (Aroclor 1254) and polychlorinated dibenzofuran-free Aroclor 1254 on diethylnitrosamine-induced tumorigenesis in the rat. J. Natl Cancer Inst., 66: 509-515.

PUHVEL, S.M., SAKAMOTO, M., ERTL, D.C., & REISNER, R.M. (1982) Hairless mice as models for chloracne: A study of cutaneous changes induced by topical application of established chloracnegens. Toxicol. appl. Pharmacol., 64: 492-503.

PUHVEL, S.M., ERTL, D.C., & LYNBERG, C.A. (1984) Increased epidermal transglutaminase activity following 2,3,7,8-tetrachlorodibenzo-p-dioxin: In vivo and in vitro studies with mouse skin. Toxicol. appl. Pharmacol., 73: 42-47.

PUHVEL, S.M., SAKAMOTO, M., & REISNER, R.M. (1986) Localization of TCDD in hairless mouse skin. Chemosphere, 15: 2065-2067.

QUILLEY, C.P. & RIFKIND, A.B. (1986) Prostaglandin release by the chick embryo heart is increased by 2,3,7,8-tetrachlorodibenzo-p-dioxin and by other cytochrome P-448 inducers. Biochem. biophys. Res. Commun., 136(2): 582-589.

RAMSEY, J.C., HEFNER, J.G., KARBOWSKI, R.J., BRAUN, W.H., & GEHRING, P.J. (1982) The in vivo biotransformation of 2,3,7,8-tetrachlorodibenzo-p-dioxin (TCDD) in the rat. Toxicol. appl. Pharmacol., 65: 180-184.

RAPPE, C. (1978a) Chemical background of the phenoxy acids and dioxins. Ecol. Bull. (Stockholm), 27: 28-30.

RAPPE, C. (1978b) Decontamination of products formed during the industrial preparation of 2,4,5-trichlorophenol. In: Cattabeni, F., Cavallero, A., & Galli, G., ed. Dioxin: toxicological and chemical aspects, New York, SP Medical and Scientific Books, pp. 179-183.

RAPPE, C. (1984) Analysis of polychlorinated dioxins and furans. Environ. Sci. Technol., 18: 78A-90A.

RAPPE C. (1985) Problems in analysis of PCDDs and PCDFs and presence of these compounds in human milk, Copenhagen, WHO Regional Office for Europe (ICP/CEH/501/05/7).

RAPPE, C. (1987) Global distribution of polychlorinated dioxins (PCDDs) and dibenzofurans (PCDFs). In: Solving hazardous waste problems: Learning from dioxins, New York, American Chemical Society, pp. 20-23 (ACS Symposium Series No. 338).

RAPPE, C. & BUSER, H.R. (1980) Chemical properties and analytical methods. In: Kimbrough, R.D., ed. Halogenated biphenyls, terphenyls, naphthalenes, dibenzodioxins and related products, Amsterdam, Oxford, New York, Elsevier Science Publishers, pp. 41-80.

RAPPE, C. & KJELLER, L.-O. (1987) PCDDs and PCDFs in environmental samples air, particulates, sediments and soil. Chemosphere, 16: 1775-1780.

RAPPE, C. & NYGREN, M. (1984) Chemical analysis of human samples. Identification and quantification of polychlorinated dioxins and dibenzofurans. In: de Serres, F.J. & Pero, R.W., ed. Individual susceptibility to genotoxic agents in the human population, New York, London, Plenum Press, pp. 305-314.

RAPPE, C., BUSER, H.R., & BOSHARDT, H.P. (1978) Identification and quantification of polychlorinated dibenzo-p-dioxins (PCDDs) and dibenzofurans (PCDFs) in 2,4,5-T-ester formulations and herbicide orange. Chemosphere, 7: 431-438.

RAPPE, C., BUSER, H.R., KUROKI, H., & MASUDA, Y. (1979) Identification of polychlorinated dibenzofurans (PCDFs) retained in patients with Yusho. Chemosphere, 4: 259-266.

RAPPE, C., BUSER, H.R., STALLING, D.L., SMITH, L.M., & DOUGHERTY, R.C. (1981) Identification of polychlorinated dibenzofurans in environmental samples. Nature (Lond.), 292: 524-526.

RAPPE, C., MARKLUND, S., BERGQVIST, P.-A., & HANSSON, M. (1983a) Polychlorinated dibenzo-p-dioxins, dibenzofurans and other polynuclear aromatics formed during incineration and polychlorinated biphenyl fires. In: Choudhary, G., Keith, L.H., & Rappe, C., ed. Chlorinated dioxins and dibenzofurans in the total environment, Boston, Butterworth Publishers, pp. 99-124.

RAPPE, C., MARKLUND, S., NYGREN, M., & GARA, A. (1983b) Parameters for identification and confirmation in trace analyses of polychlorinated dibenzo-p-dioxins and dibenzofurans. In: Choudhary, G., Keith, L.H., & Rappe, C., ed., Chlorinated dioxins and dibenzofurans in the total environment, Boston, Butterworth Publishers, pp. 240-259.

RAPPE, C., NYGREN, M., BUSER, H.R., MASUDA, Y., KUROKI, H., & CHEN, P.H. (1983c) Identification of polychlorinated dioxins (PCDDs) and dibenzofurans (PCDFs) in human samples, occupational exposure and Yusho patients. In: Tucker, R.E., Young, A.L., & Gray, A.P., eds. Human and environmental risks of chlorinated dioxins and related compounds, New York, London, Plenum Press, pp. 241-254.

RAPPE, C., BERGQVIST, P.-A., & MARKLUND, S. (1985a) Analysis of polychlorinated dibenzofurans and dioxins in ecological samples. In: Keith, L.H., Rappe, C., & Choudhary, G., ed. Chlorinated dioxins and dibenzofurans in the total environment II, Boston, Butterworth Publishers, pp. 135-138.

RAPPE, C., MARKLUND, S., KJELLER, L-O., BERGQVIST, P.-A., & HANSSON, M. (1985b) Composition of polychlorinated dibenzofurans (PCDF) formed in PCB fires. In: Keith, L.H., Rappe, C., & Choudhary, G., ed. Chlorinated dioxins and dibenzofurans in the total environment II, Boston, Butterworth Publishers, p. 401-424.

RAPPE, C., NYGREN, M., MARKLUND, S., KJELLER, L.-O., BERGQVIST, P.A., & HANSON, M. (1985c) Assessment of human exposure to polychlorinated dibenzofurans and dioxins. Environ. Health Perspect., 60: 303-304.

RAPPE, C., KJELLER, L.-O., & MARKLUND, S. (1985d) PCDF isomers and isomer levels found in PCBs. In: Komai, R.Y. & Addis, G., ed. Proceedings of a Workshop on PCB By-Product Formation, Palo Alto, California, 4-6 December, 1984, Palo Alto, California, Electric Power Research Institute, pp. 20-23.

RAPPE, C., KJELLER, L.-O., MARKLUND, S., & NYGREN, M. (1986a) Electrical PCB accident, an update. Chemosphere, 15: 1291-1295.

RAPPE, C., NYGREN, M., HANSSON, M., & KAHN, P.C. (1986b) Analysis of adipose tissue and blood samples from Vietnam veterans. Clean-up, analysis and quality control, P 41, In: Dioxin 86, 6th International Symposium on Chlorinated Dioxins and Related Compounds, Fukuoka, Japan, 16-19 September, 1986.

RAPPE, C., ANDERSSON, R., BERGQVIST, P.-A., BROHEDE, C., HANSSON, M., KJELLER, L.-O., LINDSTROM, G., MARKLUND, S., NYGREN, M., SWANSON, S.E., TYSKLIND, M., & WIBERG, K. (1987) Overview on environmental fate of chlorinated dioxins and dibenzofurans, sources, levels and isomeric pattern in various matrices. Chemosphere, 16: 1603-1618.

RAPPE, C., NYGREN, M., LINDSTROM, G., BUSER, H.R., BLASER, O., & WUTHRICH, C. (1987) Polychlorinated dibenzofurans and dibenzo-p-dioxins and other chlorinated contaminants in cow milk from various locations in Switzerland. Environ. Sci, Technol., 21: 964-970.

REGGIANI, G. (1978) Medical problems raised by the TCDD contamination in Seveso, Italy. Arch. Toxicol., 40: 161-188.

REGGIANI, G. (1980a) Acute human exposure to TCDD in Seveso, Italy. J. Toxicol. environ. Health, 6: 27-43.

REGGIANI, G. (1980b) Toxicology of TCDD and related compounds: observation in man. In: Hutzinger, O., Frei, R.W., Merian, E., & Pocchiari, F., ed. Chlorinated dioxins and related compounds. Impact on the environment, Oxford, New York, Pergamon Press, pp. 463-493.

REGGIANI, G. (1983a) Anatomy of TCDD spill: The Seveso accident. Curr. Dev., 2: 269-341.

REGGIANI, G. (1983b) An overview on the health effects of halogenated dioxins and related compounds - the Yusho and Taiwan episodes. In: Coulston, F. & Pocchiari, F., ed. Accidental exposure to dioxins. Human health aspects, New York, London, Academic Press, pp. 39-67.

REGIONE LOMBARDIA (1984) Final report and recommendations of the 6th International Steering Committee Meeting, Milan, 19-21 February, 1984, Milan, Regione Lombardia, pp. 1-17.

RICE, R.H. & CLINE, P.R. (1984) Opposing effects of 2,3,7,8-tetrachlorodibenzo-p-dioxin and hydrocortisone on growth and differentiation of cultured malignant human keratinocytes. Carcinogenesis, 5(3): 367-371.

RICE, R.H., CLINE, P.R., & COE, E.L. (1983) Mutually antagonistic effects of hydrocortisone and retinylacetate on envelope competence in cultured malignant human keratinocytes. J. invest. Dermatol., 81: 176s-178s.

RICHERT, J., VON (1962) [On neurological complications in a case of chlorinated hydrocarbon poisoning accompanied by chloracne.] Nervenarzt, 33(4): 180-184 (in German).

RIKANS, L.E., GIBSON, D.D., & MCCAY, P.B. (1979) Evidence for the presence of cytochrome P-450 in rat mammary gland. Biochem. Pharmacol., 28: 3039-3042.

RISSE-SUNDERMAN, A. (1959) [Intoxication by chloro-aromatics,] Cologne-Lindenburg, University of Cologne, Department of Dermatology (Thesis) (in German).

RIZZARDINI, M., ROMANO, M., TURSI, F., SALMONA, F., VECCHI, A., SIRONI, M., GIZZI, F., BENFENATI, E., GARATTINI, S., & FANELLI, R. (1983) Toxicological evaluation of urban waste incinerator emissions. Chemosphere, 12: 559-564.

ROBERTSON, L.W., REGEL, U., FILSER, J.G., & OESCH, F. (1985) Absence of lipid peroxidation as determined by ethane exhalation in rats treated with 2,3,7,8-tetrachlorodibenzo-p-dioxin (TCDD). Arch. Toxicol., 57: 13-16.

ROGERS, A.M., ANDERSEN, M.E., & BACK, K.C. (1982) Mutagenicity of 2,3,7,8-tetrachlorodibenzo-p-dioxin and perfluoro-n-decanoic acid in L5178Y mouse-lymphoma cells. Mutat. Res., 105: 445-449.

ROMKES, K., PISKORSKA-PLISZCZYNSKA, J., & SAFE, S. (1987) Effects of 2,3,7,8-tetrachlorodibenzo-p-dioxin on hepatic and uterine estrogen receptor levels in rats. Toxicol. appl. Pharmacol., 87: 306-314.

ROSE, J.Q., RAMSEY, J.C., WENTZLER, T.H., HUMMEL, R.A., & GEHRING, P.J. (1976) The fate of 2,3,7,8-tetrachlorodibenzo-p-dioxin following single and repeated oral doses to the rat. Toxicol. appl. Pharmacol., 36: 209-226.

ROZMAN, K. (1984) Hexadecane increases the toxicity of 2,3,7,8-tetrachlorodibenzo-p-dioxin (TCDD): Is brown adipose tissue the primary target in TCDD-induced wasting syndrome? Biochem. biophys. Res. Commun., 125(3): 996-1004.

ROZMAN, K., ROZMAN, T., & GREIM, H. (1984) Effect of thyroidectomy and thyroxine on 2,3,7,8-tetrachlorodibenzo-p-dioxin (TCDD) induced toxicity. Toxicol. appl. Pharmacol., 72: 372-376.

ROZMAN, K., ROZMAN, T., SCHEUFLER, E., PAZDERNIK, T., & GREIM, H. (1985a) Thyroid hormones modulate the toxicity of 2,3,7,8-tetrachlorodibenzo-p-dioxin (TCDD). J. Toxicol. environ. Health, 16: 481-491.

ROZMAN, K., HAZELTON, G.A., KLAASSEN, C.D., ARLOTTO, M.P., & PARKINSON, A. (1985b) Effect of thyroid hormones on liver microsomal enzyme induction in rats exposed to 2,3,7,8-tetrachlorodibenzo-p-dioxin. Toxicology, 37: 51-63.

ROZMAN, K., PEREIRA, D., & IATROPOULOS, M.J. (1986) Histopathology of interscapular brown adipose tissue, thyroid, and pancreas in 2,3,7,8-tetra-chlorodibenzo-p-dioxin (TCDD)-treated rats. Toxicol. appl. Pharmacol., 82: 551-559.

RYAN, J.J., LAU, P.-Y., PILON, J.C., & LEWIS, D. (1983a) 2,3,7,8-Tetrachlorodibenzo-p-dioxin and 2,3,7,8-tetrachlorodibenzofuran residues in great lakes commercial and sport fish. In: Choudhary, G., Keith, L.H., & Rappe, C., ed. Chlorinated dioxins and dibenzofurans in the total environment, Boston, Buttersworth Publishers, pp. 87-97.

RYAN, J.J., PILON, J.C., CONACHER, H.B.S., & FIRESTONE, D. (1983b) Inter-laboratory study on determination of 2,3,7,8-tetrachlorodibenzo-p-dioxin in fish. J. Assoc. Off. Anal. Chem., 66: 700-707.

RYAN, J.J., LIZOTTE, R., SAKUMA, T., & MORI, B. (1985) Chlorinated dibenzo-p-dioxins, chlorinated dibenzofurans and pentachlorophenol in Canadian chicken and pork samples. J. agric. food Chem., 33: 1021-1026.

RYAN, J.J., SCHECTER, A., SUN, W.-F., & LIZOTTE, R. (1986) Distribution of chlorinated dibenzo-p-dioxins and chlorinated dibenzofurans in human tissues from the general population. In: Rappe, C., Choudhary, G., & Keith, L., ed. Chlorinated dioxins and dibenzofurans in perspective, Chelsea, Michigan, Lewis Publishers, pp. 3-16.

RYHAGE, R. (1964) Use of mass spectrometer as a detector and analyzer for effluents emerging from high temperature gas liquid chromatography columns. Anal. Chem., 36: 759-764.

SACCHI, G.A., VIGANO, P., FORTUNATI, G., & COCUCCI, S.M. (1986) Accumulation of 2,3,7,8-tetrachlorodibenzo-p-dioxin from soil and nutriculture solution by bean and maize plants. Experientia (Basel), 42: 586-588.

SAFE, S.H. & SAFE, L.M (1984) Synthesis and characterization of twenty-two purified polychlorinated dibenzofuran congeners. J. agric. food Chem., 32: 68-71.

SAFE, S.H., MASON, G., KEYS, B., FARRELL, K., ZMUDZKA, B., SAWYER, T., PISKORSKA-PLISZEZYNSKA, J., SAFE, L.M., ROMKES, M., & BANDIERA, S. (1986) Polychlorinated dibenzo-p-dioxins and dibenzofurans: correlation between in vitro and in vivo structure-activity relationships (SARs). Chemosphere, 15: 1725-1731.

SAFE, S.H., MASON, G., FARRELL, K., KEYS, B., PISKORSKA-PLISZCZYNSKA, J., MADGE, J.A., & CHITTIM, B. (1987) Validation of in vitro bioassays for 2,3,7,8-TCDD equivalents. Chemosphere, 16: 1723-1728.

SAI (SYSTEMS APPLICATIONS, INC.) (1980) Human exposure to atmospheric concentration of selected chemicals, Springfield, Virginia, National Technical Information Service, Vol. 1 (Report prepared for US Environmental Protection Agency, Research Triangle Park, North Carolina) (PB 81-193252).

SANDERMANN, W. (1984a) [Dioxin. The history of the discovery of 2,3,7,8-tetrachlorodibenzo-p-dioxin (TCDD, dioxin, Seveso poison.] Naturwiss. Rundsch., 37(5): 173-178 (in German).

SANDERMANN, W. (1984b) [Breakdown of dioxin by beta-radiation. The history of the discovery of 2,3,7,8-tetrachlorodibenzo-p-dioxin (Second communication).] Naturwiss. Rundsch., 37(11): 445-446 (in German).

SANDERMANN, W., STOCKMANN, H., & GASTEN, R. (1957) [On the pyrolysis of pentachlorphenol.] Chem. Ber., 90: 690-692 (in German).

SANGER, V.L., SCOTT, L., HAMDY, A., GALE, C., & POUNDEN, W.D. (1958) Alimentary toxemia in chickens. J. Am. Vet. Med. Assoc., 133: 172-176.

SARNA, L.P., HODGE, P.E., & WEBSTER, G.R.B. (1984) Octanol-water partition coefficients of chlorinated dioxins and dibenzofurans by reversed-phase HPLC using several C18 columns. Chemosphere, 13: 975-983.

SAWAHATA, T., OLSON, J.R., & NEAL, R.A. (1982) Identification of metabolites of 2,3,7,8-tetrachlorodibenzo-p-dioxin (TCDD) formed on incubation with isolated rat hepatocytes. Biochem. biophys. Res. Commun., 105: 341-346.

SAWYER, T.W. & SAFE, S. (1985) In vitro AHH induction by polychlorinated biphenyl and dibenzofuran mixtures: Additive effects. Chemosphere, 14: 79-84.

SAWYER, T.W., JONES, D., ROSANOFF, K., MASON, G., PISKORSKA-PLISZCZYNSKA, J., & SAFE, S. (1986) The biologic and toxic effects of 2,3,7,8-tetrachlorodibenzo-p-dioxin in chickens. Toxicology, 39: 197-206.

SCHANTZ, S.L., BARSOTTI, D.A., & ALLEN, J.R. (1978) Toxicological effects produced in nonhuman primates chronically exposed to fifty parts per trillion 2,3,7,8-tetrachlorodibenzo-p-dioxin (TCDD). Toxicol. appl. Pharmacol., 48(1): A180.

SCHECTER, A., WEERASINGHE, W.C.A., GROSS, M., & DEKIN, A. (1986a) Human tissue levels of PCDDs and PCDFs in over one hundred year old frozen Eskimo tissue, meat, and California redwood charcoal and their relation to the trace chemistry theory of dioxin origin. In: Dioxin 86. 6th International Symposium on Chlorinated Dioxins and Related Compounds, Fukuoka, Japan, 16-19 September, 1986, p.135.

SCHECTER, A.J., RYAN, J.J., & CONSTABLE, J.D. (1986b) Chlorinated dibenzo-p-dioxin and dibenzofuran levels in human adipose tissue and milk samples from the north and south of Vietnam. Chemosphere, 15: 1613-1620.

SCHILLER, C.M., WALDEN, R., & SHOAF, C.R. (1982) Studies on the mechanism of 2,3,7,8-tetrachlorodibenzo-p-dioxin toxicity: Nutrient assimilation. Fed. Proc., 41: 1426 (Abstract).

SCHILLER, C.M., ADCOCK, C.M., MOORE, R.A., & WALDEN, R. (1985) Effect of 2,3,7,8-tetrachlorodibenzo-p-dioxin (TCDD) and fasting on body weight and lipid parameters in rats. Toxicol. appl. Pharmacol., 81: 356-361.

SCHILLER, C.M., ADCOCK, C.M., SGIAF, C.R., & WALDEN, R. (1986) Effects of adenine and its isomer 4-aminopyrazolo-(3,4-d)-pyrimidine on 2,3,7,8-tetrachlorodibenzo-p-dioxin-induced mortality in rats. Toxicol. appl. Pharmacol., 84: 369-378.

SCHOENY, R. (1982) Mutagenicity testing of chlorinated biphenyls and chlorinated dibenzofurans. Mutat. Res., 101: 45-56.

SCHULZ, K.H. (1968) [On the symptoms and etiology of chloracne.] Arbeitsmed. Sozialmed. Arbeitshyg., 3: 25-29 (in German).

SCHWETZ, B.A., NORRIS, J.M., SPARSCHU, G.L., ROWE, V.K., GEHRING, P.J., EMERSON, J.L., & GEHRING, C.G. (1973) Toxicology of chlorinated dibenzo-p-dioxins. Environ. Health Perspect., 5: 87-99.

SEEFELD, M.D. & PETERSON, R.E. (1983) 2,3,7,8-Tetrachlorodibenzo-p-dioxin-induced weight loss: A proposed mechanism. In: Tucker, R.E., Young, A.L., & Gray, A.P., ed. Human and environmental risks of chlorinated dioxins and related compounds, New York, London, Plenum Press, pp. 405-412 (Environmental Science Research Series).

SEEFELD, M.D. & PETERSON, R.E. (1984) Digestible energy and efficiency of feed utilization in rats treated with 2,3,7,8-tetrachlorodibenzo-p-dioxin. Toxicol. appl. Pharmacol., 74: 214-222.

SEEFELD, M.D., CORBETT, S.W., KEESEY, R.E., & PETERSON, R.E. (1984a) Characterization of the wasting syndrome in rats treated with 2,3,7,8-tetrachlorodibenzo-p-dioxin. Toxicol. appl. Pharmacol., 73: 311-322.

SEEFELD, M.D., KEESEY, R.E., & PETERSON, R.E. (1984b) Body weight regulation in rats treated with 2,3,7,8-tetrachlorodibenzo-p-dioxin. Toxicol. appl. Pharmacol., 76: 526-536.

SEILER, J.P. (1973) A survey on the mutagenicity of various pesticides. Experientia (Basel), 29: 622-623.

SHADOFF, L.A., HUMMEL, R.A., & LAMPARSKI, L. (1977) A research for 2,3,7,8-tetrachlorodibenzo-p-dioxin (TCDD) in an environment exposed annually to 2,4,5-trichlorophenoxyacetic acid ester (2,3,5-T) herbicides. Bull. environ. Contam. Toxicol., 18: 478-485.

SHARMA, R.P. & GEHRING, P.J. (1979) Effects of 2,3,7,8-tetrachlorodibenzo-p-dioxin (TCDD) on splenic lymphocyte transformation in mice after single and repeated exposures. Ann. N.Y. Acad. Sci., 320: 487-497.

SHARMA, R.P., KOCIBA, R.J., & GEHRING, P.J. (1984) Immunotoxicologic effects of 2,3,7,8-tetrachlorodibenzo-p-dioxin (TCDD) in rabbits. J. environ. Pathol. Toxicol. Oncogen., 5(4/5): 321-328.

SHEFFIELD, A. (1985) Sources and releases of PCDDs and PCDFs to the Canadian environment. Chemosphere, 14: 811-814.

SHIGEMATSU, N., ISHIMARU, S., SAITO, R., IDEDA, T., MATSUBA, K., SUGIYAMA, K., & MASUDA, Y. (1978) Respiratory involvement in polychlorinated biphenyls poisoning. Environ. Res., 16: 92-100.

SHIREMAN, R.B. & WEI, CHENG-I. (1986) Uptake of 2,3,7,8-tetrachlorodibenzo-p-dioxin from plasma lipoproteins by cultured human fibroblasts. Chem.-biol. Interact., 58: 1-12.

SHIVERICK, K.T. & MUTHER, T.F. (1983) 2,3,7,8-Tetrachlorodibenzo-p-dioxin (TCDD) effects on hepatic microsomal steroid metabolism and serum estradiol of pregnant rats. Biochem. Pharmacol., 32: 991-995.

SHOAF, C.R. & SCHILLER, C.M. (1981) Studies on the mechanism of 2,3,7,8-tetrachlorodibenzo-p-dioxin (TCDD) toxicity-lipid assimilation. II. Pharmacologist, 23: 176 (Abstract).

SILKWORTH, J., MCMARTIN, D., DECAPRIO, A., REJ, R., O'KEEFE, P., & KAMINSKY, L. (1982) Acute toxicity in guinea pigs and rabbits of soot from a polychlorinated biphenyl-containing transformer fire. Toxicol. appl. Pharmacol., 65: 425-439.

SIMPSON, C.F., PRITCHARD, W.R., & HARMS, R.H. (1959) An endotheliosis in chickens and turkeys caused by an unidentified dietary factor. J. Am. Vet. Med. Assoc., 134: 410-416.

SLONECKER, P.J., PYLE, J.R., & CANTRELL, J.S. (1983) Identification of polychlorinated dibenzo-p-dioxin isomers by powder X-ray diffraction with electron capture gas chromatography. Anal. Chem., 55: 1543-1547.

SMITH, A.G., FRANCIS, J.E., KAY, S.J.E., & GREIG, J.B. (1981) Hepatic toxicity and uroporphyrinogen decarboxylase activity following a single dose of 2,3,7,8-tetrachlorodibenzo-p-dioxin to mice. Biochem. Pharmacol., 30: 2825-2830.

SMITH, A.G., FRANCIS, J.E., & GREIG, J.B. (1985) Continued depression of hepatic uroporphyrinogen decarboxylase activity caused by hexachlorobenzene 2,3,7,8-tetrachlorodibenzo-p-dioxin despite regeneration after partial hepatectomy. Biochem. Pharmacol., 34: 1817-1820.

SMITH, A.H., FISHER, D.O., GILES, H.J., & PEARCE, N. (1983) The New Zealand soft tissue sarcoma case-control study: Interview findings concerning phenoxyacetic acid exposure. Chemosphere, 12: 565-571.

SMITH, F.A., SCHWETZ, B.A., & NITSCHKE, K.D. (1976) Teratogenicity of 2,3,7,8-tetrachlorodibenzo-p-dioxin in CF-1 mice. Toxicol. appl. Pharmacol., 38: 517-523.

SMITH, R.M., O'KEEFE, P.W., ALDOUS, K.M., HILKER, D.R., & O'BRIEN, J.E. (1983) 2,3,7,8-Tetrachlorodibenzo-p-dioxin in sediment samples from love canal storm sewers and creeks. Environ. Sci. Technol., 17: 6-10.

SODERKVIST, P., POELLINGER, L., & GUSTAFSSON, J.-A. (1986) Carcinogen-binding proteins in the rat ventral prostate: Specific and nonspecific high-affinity binging sites for benso(a)pyrene, 3-methylcholanthrene, and 2,3,7,8-tetrachlorodibenzo-p-dioxin. Cancer Res., 46: 651-657.

SOUTHERLAND, J.H., KUYKENDAL, W.B., LAMASON, W.H. II, & OBERACKER, D.A. (1987) Assessment of combustion sources as emitters of chlorinated dioxin compounds: A report on the result of tier 4 of the national dioxin strategy. Chemosphere, 16: 2161-2168.

SPARSCHU, G.L., DUNN, F.L., & ROWE, V.K. (1971) Study of the teratogenicity of 2,3,7,8-tetrachlorodibenzo-p-dioxin in the rat. Food Cosmet. Toxicol., 9: 405-412.

SPITSBERGEN, J.M., SCHAT, K.A., KLEEMAN, J.M., & PETERSON, R.E. (1986) Interactions of 2,3,7,8-tetrachlorodibenzo-p-dioxin (TCDD) with immune responses of rainbow trout. Vet. Immunol. Immunopathol., 12: 263-280.

STALLING, D.L., SMITH, L.M., PETTY, J.D., HOGAN, J.W., JOHNSON, J.L., RAPPE, C., & BUSER, H.R. (1983) Residues of polychlorinated dibenzo-p-dioxins and dibenzofurans in laurentian great lakes fish. In: Tucker, R.E., Young, A.L., & Gray, A.P., ed. Human and environmental riks of chlorinated dioxins and related compounds, New York, London, Plenum Press, pp. 221-240.

STEHL, R.H. & LAMPARSKI, L.L. (1977) Combustion of several 2,4,5-trichloro-phenoxy compounds: formation of 2,3,7,8-tetrachlorodibenzo-p-dioxin. Science, 197: 1008-1009.

STEHL, R.H., PAPENFUSS, R.R., BREDEWEG, R.A., & ROBERTS, R.W. (1973) The stability of pentachlorophenol and chlorinated dioxins to sunlight, heat, and combustion. Adv. Chem. Ser., 120: 119-125.

STEHR, P.A., STEIN, G., FALK, H., SAMPSON, E., SMITH, S.M., STEINBERG, K., WEBB, K., AYRES, S., SCHRAMM, W., DONNELL, H.D., & GEDNEY, W.B. (1986) A pilot epidemiologic study of possible health effects associated with 2,3,7,8-tetrachloro-dibenzo-p-dioxin contaminations in Missouri. Arch. environ. Health, 41: 16-21.

STEINBERG, K.K., MACNEIL, M.L., KARON, J.M., STEHR, P.A., NEESE, J.W., & NEEDHAM, L.L. (1985) Assessment of 2,3,7,8-tetrachlorodibenzo-p-dioxin exposure using a modified d-glucaric acid assay. J. Toxicol. environ. Health, 16: 743-752.

STEINER, M., BORGES, H., FREEDMAN, L., & GRAY, S.J. (1968) Effects of starvation on the tissue composition of the small intestine in the rat. Am. J. Physiol., 215: 75-77.

STEWARD, A.R. & BYARD, J.L. (1981) Induction of benzo(a)pyrene metabolism by 2,3,7,8-tetrachlorodibenzo-p-dioxin in primary cultures of adult rat hepatocytes. Toxicol. appl. Pharmacol., 59: 603-616.

STOHS, S.J., HASSAN, M.Q., & MURRAY, W.J. (1983) Lipid peroxidation as a possible cause of TCDD toxicity. Biochem. biophys. Res. Commun., 111: 854-859.

SUN, T.-T., SHIH, C., & GREEN, H. (1979) Keratin cytoskeletons in epithelial cells of internal organs. Proc. Natl Acad. Sci. (USA), 76: 2813-2817.

SUN, T.-T., EICHNER, R., NELSON, W.G., TSENG, S.C.G., WEISS, R.A., JARVINEN, M., & WOODCOCK-MITCHELL, J. (1983a) Keratin classes: Molecular markers for different types of epithelial differentiation. J. invest. Dermatol., 81: 109-115.

SUN, T.-T., EICHNER, R., NELSON, W.G., VIDRICH, A., & WOODCOCK-MITCHELL, J. (1983b) Keratin expression during normal epidermal differentiation. In: Seji, M. & Bernstein, I.A., ed. Current problems in dermatology. Normal and abnormal epidermal differentiation, New York, Karger, pp. 277-291.

SUNDSTROM, G., JENSEN, S., JANSSON, B., & ERNE, K. (1979) Chlorinated phenoxyacetic acid derivatives and tetrachlorodibenzo-p-dioxin in foliage after application of 2,4,5-trichlorophenoxyacetic acid esters. Arch. environ. Contam. Toxicol., 8: 441-448.

SUSKIND, R.R. & HERTZBERG, V.S. (1984) Human health effects of 2,4,5-T and its toxic contaminants. J. Am. Med. Assoc., 251: 2372-2380.

SUSKIND, R.R., CLEVELAND, F., KEENAN, C., AKIN, R., DAVIS, A., & KEHOE, R.A. (1953) Report on a clinical and environmental survey, Nitro, West Virginia, Monsanto Chemical Co..

SUTER-HOFMANN, M. & SCHLATTER, Ch. (1985) Toxicity of particulate emissions from a municipal incinerator: critique of the concept of TCDD-equivalents. Chemosphere, 15: 1733-1743.

SWEENEY, G.D. & JONES, K.G. (1983) Studies of the mechanism of action of hepatotoxicity of 2,3,7,8-tetrachlorodibenzo-p-dioxin (TCDD) and related compounds. In: Tucker, R.E., Young, A.L., & Gray, A.P., ed. Human and environmental risks of chlorinated dioxins and related compounds, New York, London, Plenum Press, pp. 415-422.

SWEENEY, G.D., JONES, K.G., COLE, F.M., BASFORD, D., & KRESTYNSKI, F. (1979) Iron deficiency prevents liver toxicity of 2,3,7,8-tetrachlorodibenzo-p-dioxin. Science, 204: 332-335.

SWIFT, L.L., GASIEWICZ, T.A., DUNN, G.D., SOULE, P.D., & NEAL, R.A. (1981) Characterization of the hyperlipidemia in guinea pigs induced by 2,3,7,8-tetrachlorodibenzo-p-dioxin. Toxicol. appl. Pharmacol., 59: 489-499.

SWITZERLAND (1982) Environmental pollution due to dioxins and furans from chemical rubbish incineration plants, Bern, Ministry of Environment, Federal Swiss Government.

TAYLOR, M.L., TIERNAN, T.O., RAMALINGAM, B., WAGEL, D.J., GARRETT, J.H., SOLCH, J.G., & FERGUSON, G.L. (1985) Synthesis, isolation, and characterization of the tetrachlorinated dibenzo-p-dioxins and other related compound. In: Keith, L., Rappe, C., & Choudhary, G., ed. Chlorinated dioxins and dibenzofurans in the total environment. II, Boston, Butterworth Publishers, pp. 17-35.

TELEGINA, K.A. & BIKBULATOVA, L.I. (1970) [Affection of the follicular apparatus of the skin in workers occupied in production of butyl ether of 2,3,4-trichlorphenoxyacetic acid.] Vestn. Dermat. Venerol (Moscow), 44: 35-39 (in Russian).

TELEKY, L. (1913) [Chlorine and hydrochloric acid. German Empire.] Wiener Arb. Geb. Soz. Med., 4: 55-56 (in German).

TENCHINI, M.L., CRIMAUDO, C., PACCHETTI, G., MOTTURA, A., AGOSTI, S., & DE CARLI, L. (1983) A comparative cytogenetic study on cases of induced abortions in TCDD-exposed and non-exposed women. Environ. Mutagen., 5: 73-85.

THIBODEAUX, L.J. (1983) Offsite transport of 2,3,7,8-tetra-chlorodibenzo-p-dioxin from a production disposal facility. In: Choudhary, G., Keith, L.H., & Rappe, C., ed. Chlorinated dioxins and dibenzofurans in the total environment, Boston, Butterworth Publishers, pp. 75-85.

THIESS, A.M., FRENTZEL-BEYME, R., & LINK, R. (1982) Mortality study of persons exposed to dioxin in a trichlorophenol-process accident that occurred in the BASF AG on November 17, 1953. Am. J. ind. Med., 3: 179-189.

THIGPEN, J.E., FAITH, R.E., MCCONNELL, E.E., & MOORE, J.A. (1975) Increases susceptibility to bacterial infection as a sequela of exposure to an environmental contaminant 2,3,7,8-tetrachlorodibenzo-p-dioxin (TCDD). Infect. Immun., 12: 1319-1324.

THOMAS, P.T., & HINSDILL, R.D. (1979) The effect of perinatal exposure to tetrachlorodibenzo-p-dioxin on the immune response of young mice. Drug chem. Toxicol., 2: 77-98

THUNBERG, T. & HAKANSSON, H. (1983) Vitamin A (retinol) status in the Gunn rat: the effect of 2,3,7,8-tetrachlorodibenzo-p-dioxin. Arch. Toxicol., 53: 225-233.

THUNBERG, T., AHLBORG, U.G., & JOHNSSON, H. (1979) Vitamin A (retinol) status in the rat after a single oral dose of 2,3,7,8-tetrachlorodibenzo-p-dioxin. Arch. Toxicol., 42: 265-274.

THUNBERG, T., AHLBORG, U.G., HAKANSSON, H., KRANTZ, C., & MONIER, M. (1980) Effect of 2,3,7,8-tetrachlorodibenzo-p-dioxin on the hepatic storage of retinol in rats with different dietary supplies of vitamin A (retinol). Arch. Toxicol., 45: 273-285.

THUNBERG, T., AHLBORG, U.G., & WAHLSTROM, B. (1984) Comparison between the effects of 2,3,7,8-tetrachlorodibenzo-p-dioxin and six other compounds on the vitamin A storage, the UDP-glucuronosyltransferase and the aryl hydrocarbon hydroxylase activity in the rat liver. Arch. Toxicol., 55: 16-19.

TIERNAN, T.O. (1983) Analytical chemistry of polychlorinated dibenzo-p-dioxins and dibenzofurans: A review of the current status. In: Choudhary, G., Keith, L., & Rappe, C., ed. Chlorinated dioxins and dibenzofurans in the total environment, Boston, Butterworth Publishers, pp. 211-237.

TOFILON, P.J. (1980) Depressed guinea pig testicular microsomal cytochrome P-450 content by 2,3,7,8-tetrachlorodibenzo-p-dioxin. Life Sci., 27: 871-876.

TOFILON, P.J. & PIPER, W.N. (1982) 2,3,7,8-Tetrachlorodibenzo-p-dioxin-mediated depression of rat testicular heme synthesis and microsomal cytochrome P-450. Biochem. Pharmacol., 31: 3663-3666.

TOGNONI, G. & BONACCORSI, A. (1982) Epidemiological problems with TCDD. Drug Metab. Rev., 13: 447-469.

TOSINE, H., SMILLIE, D., & REES, G.A.V. (1983) Comparative monitoring and analytical methodology for 2,3,7,8-TCDD in fish. In: Tucker, R.E., Young, A.L., & Gray, A.P., ed. Human and environmental risks of chlorinated dioxins and related compounds, New York, London, Plenum Press, pp. 127-142.

TOTH, K., SOMFAI-RELLE, S., SUGAR, J., & BENCE, J. (1979) Carcinogenicity testing of herbicide 2,4,5-trichlorophenoxyethanol containing dioxin and of pure dioxin in Swiss mice. Nature (Lond.), 278: 548-549.

TSUKAMOTO, H., MAKISUMI, S., HIROSE, H., KOJIMA, T., FUKUMOTO, H., FUKOMOTO, K., KURATSUNE, M., NISHIZUMI, M., SHIBATA, M., NAGAI, J., YAE, Y., SAWADA, K., FURUKAWA, M., YOSHIMURA, H., TATSUMI, K., OGURI, K., SHIMENO, H., KENO, K., KOBAYASHI, H., YANO, T., ITO, A., OKADA, T., INAGAMI, K., KOGA, T., TOMITA, Y., KOGA, T., YAMADA, Y., MIYAGUCHI, M., SUGANO, M., HORI, K., TAKESHITA, K., MANAKO, K., NAKAMURA, Y., & SHIGEMORI, N. (1969) [The chemical studies on detecton of toxic compounds in rice bran oils used by the patients of Yusho.] Fukuoka Acta med., 6: 496-512 (in Japanese).

TSYRLOV, I.B., CHASOVNIKOVA, O.B., GRISHANOVA, A.YU., & LYAKHOVICH, V.V. (1986) Reappraisal of the liver benzpyrene hydroxylase synthesized de novo after treatment of rats with 2,3,7,8-tetrachlorodibenzo-p-dioxin and 3-methylcholanthrene. FEBS Lett., 198: 225-228.

TUCKER, A.N., VORE, S.J., & LUSTER, M.I. (1986) Supppression of B cell differentiation by 2,3,7,8-tetrachlorodibenzo-p-dioxin. Mol. Pharmacol., 29: 372-377.

TUKEY, R.H., HANNAH, R.R., NEGISHI, M., NEBERT, D.W., & EISEN, H.J. (1982a) The Ah locus: Correlation of intranuclear appearance of inducer-receptor complex with induction of cytochrome P1-450 mRNA. Cell, 31: 275-284.

TUKEY, R.H., NEGISHI, M., & NEBERT, D.W. (1982b) Quantitation of hepatic cytochrome P1-450 mRNA with the use of a cloned DNA probe. Effects of various P-450 inducers in C57BL/6N and DBA/2N mice. Mol. Pharmacol., 22: 779-786.

TULP, M. & HUTZINGER, O. (1978) Rat metabolism of polychlorinated dibenzo-p-dioxins. Chemosphere, 9: 761-768.

TUNG, T.T. (1973) Le cancer primaire du foie au Vietnam. Chirurgie, 99: 427-436.

TURNER, J.N. & COLLINS, D.N. (1983) Liver morphology in guinea pigs administered either pyrolysis products of a polychlorinated biphenyl trans former fluid or 2,3,7,8-tetrachlorodibenzo-p-dioxin. Toxicol. appl. Pharmacol., 67: 417-429.

TUTEJA, N., GONZALEZ, F.J., & NEBERT, D.W. (1985) Developmental and tissue-specific differential regulation of the mouse dioxin-inducible P1-450 and P3-450 genes. Dev. Biol., 112: 177-184.

UMBREIT, T.H., PATEL, D., & GALLO, M.A. (1985) Acute toxicity of TCDD contaminated soil from an industrial site. Chemosphere, 14(6/7): 945-947.

UMBREIT, T.H., HESSE, E.J., & GALLO, M.A. (1986a) Bioavailability of dioxin in soil from a 2,4,5-T manufacturing site. Science, 232: 497-499.

UMBREIT, T.H., HESSE, E.J., & GALLO, M.A. (1986b) Comparative toxicity of TCDD contaminated soil from Times Beach, Missouri, and Newark, New Jersey. Chemosphere, 15: 2121-2124.

UOTILA, P., PARKKI, M.G., & AITO, A. (1978) Quantitative and qualitative changes in the metabolism of benzo(a)pyrene in rat tissues after intragastric administration of TCDD. Toxicol. appl. Pharmacol., 46: 671-683.

US EPA (1982) Environmental monitoring at Love Canal, Washington, DC, US Environmental Protection Agency, Office of Research and Development, Vol. I (EPA/600/4-82-030a).

US EPA (1985) Health assessment document for polychlorinated dibenzo-p-dioxins, Washington, DC, US Environmental Protection Agency, Office of Health and Environmental Assessment (EPA/600/8-84/0146).

US EPA (1987) Interim procedures for estimating risk associated with exposures to mixtures of chlorinated dibenzo-p-dioxins and -dibenzofurans (CDDs and CDFs). Risk assessment forum, Washington, DC, US Environmental Protection Agency, 48 pp (EPA/625/3-87/012).

VAHRENHOLT, F. (1977) [Seveso - An unparalleled catastrophe.] Umwelt, 1: 59, 60, 62, 64 (in German).

VAN, D.D. (1984) Herbicides as a possible cause of liver cancer. In: Westing, A.H., ed. Herbicides in war, the long-term ecological and human consequences, London, Taylor and Francis, pp. 119-121.

VAN DEN BERG, M., OLIE, K., & HUTZINGER, O. (1983) Uptake and selective retention in rats of orally administered chlorinated dioxins and dibenzofurans from fly-ash and fly-ash extract. Chemosphere, 12(4/5): 537-544.

VAN DEN BERG, M., VAN GREEVENBROEK, M., & OLIE, K. (1986a) Bioavailability of PCDDs and PCDFs on fly ash after semi-chronic oral ingestion by the rat. Chemosphere, 15(4): 509-518.

VAN DEN BERG, M., DE VROOM, E., & OLIE, K. (1986b) Bioavailability of PCDDs and PCDFs on fly ash after semi-chronic oral ingestion by guinea pig and syrian golden hamster. Chemosphere, 15(4): 519-533.

VAN DEN BERG, M., VAN DER WIELEN, F.W.M., & OLIE, K. (1986) The presence of PCDDs and PCDFs in human breast milk from the Netherlands. Chemosphere, 15: 693-706.

VAN LOGTEN, M.J., GUPTA, B.N., MCCONNELL, E.E., & MOORE, J.A. (1980) Role of the endocrine system in the action of 2,3,7,8-tetrachlorodibenzo-p-dioxin (TCDD) on the thymus. Toxicology, 15: 135-144.

VAN MILLER, J.P., MARLAR, R.J., & ALLEN, J.R. (1976) Tissue distribution and excretion of tritiated tetrachlorodibenzo-p-dioxin in non-human primates and rates. Food Cosmet. Toxicol., 14: 31-34.

VAN MILLER, J.P., LALICH, J.J., & ALLEN, J.R. (1977) Increased incidence of neoplasms in rats exposed to low levels of 2,3,7,8-tetrachlorodibenzo-p-dioxin. Chemosphere, 61: 625-632.

VECCHI, A., MANTOVANI, A., SIRONI, M., LUINI, W., CAIRO, M., & GARATTINI, S. (1980) Effect of acute exposure to 2,3,7,8-tetrachlorodibenzo-p-dioxin on humoral antibody production in mice. Chem.-biol. Interact., 30: 337-342.

VECCHI, A., SIRONI, M., CANEGRATI, M.A., RECCHIA, M., & GARATTINI, S. (1983) Immunosuppressive effect of 2,3,7,8-tetrachlorodibenzo-p-dioxin in strains of mice with different susceptibility to induction of aryl hydrocarbon hydroxylase. Toxicol. appl. Pharmacol., 68: 434-441.

VEERKAMP, W., WEVER, J., & HUTZINGER, O. (1981) The metabolism of some chlorinated dibenzofurans by rats. Chemosphere, 10: 397-403.

VILLENUEVE, E.C., JENNINGS, R.W., BURSE, V.M., & KIMBROUGH, R.D. (1974) Evidence of chlorodibenzo-p-dioxin and chlorodibenzofuran in hexachlorobenzene. J. agric. food Chem., 22: 916-917.

VINOPAL, J.H. & CASIDA, J.E. (1973) Metabolic stability of 2,3,7,8-tetra-chlorodibenzo-p-dioxin in mammalian liver microsomal systems and in living mice. Arch. environ. Contam. Toxicol., 1: 122-132.

VISWANATHAN, T.S. & KLEOPFER, R.D. (1986) The presence of hexachloroxanthene at Missouri dioxin sites, In: Rappe, C., Choudhary, G., & Keith, L., ed. Chlorinated dioxins and dibenzofurans in perspective, Chelsea, Michigan, Lewis Publishers, pp. 201-210.

VOS, J.G. & BEEMS, R.B. (1971) Dermal toxicity studies of technical polychlorinated biphenyls and fractions thereof in rabbits. Toxicol. appl. Pharmacol., 19: 617-633.

VOS, J.G. & KOEMAN, J.H. (1970) Comparative toxicologic study with polychlorinated biphenyls in chickens with special reference to porphyria, edema formation, liver necrosis, and tissue residues. Toxicol. appl. Pharmacol., 17: 656-668.

VOS, J.G. & MOORE, J.A. (1974) Suppression of cellular immunity in rats and mice by maternal treatment with 2,3,7,8-tetrachlorodibenzo-p-dioxin. Int. Arch. Allergy, 47: 777-794.

VOS, J.G., KOEMAN, J.H., VAN DER MAAS, H.L., TEN NOEVER DE BRAUW, M.C., & DE VOS, R.H. (1970) Identification and toxicological evaluation of chlorinated dibenzofuran and chlorinated napthalene in two commercial polychlorinated biphenyls. Food Cosmet. Toxicol., 8: 625-633.

VOS, J.G., MOORE, J.A., & ZINKL, J.G. (1973) Effect of 2,3,7,8-tetrachlorodibenzo-p-dioxin on the immune system of laboratory animals. Environ. Health Perspect., 5: 149-162.

VOS, J.G., MOORE, J.A., & ZINKL, J.G. (1974) Toxicity of 2,3,7,8-tetrachlorodibenzo-p-dioxin (TCDD) in C57 Bl/6 mice. Toxicol. appl. Pharmacol., 29: 229-241.

VOS, J.G., KREEFTENBERG, J.G., ENGEL, H.W.B., MINDERHOUD, A., & VAN NOORLE JANSEN, L.M. (1978a) Studies on 2,3,7,8-tetrachlorodibenzo-p-dioxin-induced immune suppression and decreased resistance to infection: Endotoxin hypersensitivity, serum zinc concentrations and effect of thymosin treatment. Toxicology, 9: 75-86.

VOS, J.G., KREEFTENBERG, J.G., & KATER, L. (1978b) Immune suppression by TCDD. In: Cattabeni, F., Cavallaro, A., & Galli, ed. Dioxin (TCDD), New York, John Wiley & Sons, Halsted Press Division, pp. 163-175.

WAHLE, P. (1914) [On two cases of chloracne.] Inaugural dissertation for the Doctorate in Medicine, Surgery and Obstetrics of the Medical Faculty, University of Leipzig (in German).

WALDEN, R. & SCHILLER, C.M. (1985) Short communications. Comparative toxicity of 2,3,7,8-tetrachlorodibenzo-p-dioxin (TCDD) in four (sub)strains of adult male rats. Toxicol. appl. Pharmacol., 77: 490-495.

WARD, C.T. & MATSUMURA, F. (1978) Fate of 2,3,7,8-tetrachlorodibenzo-p-dioxin (TCDD) in a model aquatic environment. Arch. environ. Contam. Toxicol., 7: 349-357.

WAUER, (1918) [Occupational illness caused by chlorinated hydrocarbons (perna disease).] Zentralbl. Gewerbehyg., 6: 100-101 (in German).

WEBER, H., & BIRNBAUM, L. S. (1985) 2,3,7,8-Tetrachlorodibenzo-p-dioxin (TCDD) and 2,3,7,8-tetrachlorodibenzofuran (TCDF) in pregnant C57Bl/6N mice: Distribution to the embryo and excretion. Arch. Toxicol., 57: 159-162.

WEBER, H., POIGER, H., & SCHLATTER, Ch. (1982a) Acute oral toxicity of TCDD-metabolites in male guinea pigs. Toxicol. Lett., 14: 117-122.

WEBER, H., POIGER, H., & SCHLATTER, Ch. (1982b) Fate of 2,3,7,8-tetrachlorodibenzo-p-dioxin metabolites from dogs in rats. Xenobiotica, 12: 353-357.

WEBER, H., LUZI, P., RESI, L., TANGANELLI, P., LOVATI, M.R., & POLI, A. (1983) Natural history of TCDD-induced liver lesions in rats as observed by transmission electron microscopy during a 32-week period after a single intraperitoneal injection. J. Toxicol. environ. Health, 12: 533-540.

WEBER, H., LAMB, J.C., HARRIS, M.W., & MOORE, J.A. (1984) Teratogenicity of 2,3,7,8-tetrachlorodibenzofuran (TCDF) in mice. Toxicol. Lett., 20: 183-188.

WEBER, H., HARRIS, M.W., HASEMAN, J.K., & BIRNBAUM, L.S. (1985) Teratogenic potency of TCDD, TCDF and TCDD-TCDF combinations in C57Bl/6N mice. Toxicol. Lett., 26: 159-167.

WEBSTER, G.R.B., FRIESEN, K.J., SARNA, L.P., & MUIR, D.C.G. (1985) Environmental fate modelling of chlorodioxins: Determination of physical constants. Chemosphere, 14: 609-622.

WEDEL, J., VON, HOLLA, W.A., & DENTON, J. (1943) Observations on the toxic effects resulting from exposure to chlorinated naphtalene and chlorinated phenyls with suggestions for prevention. Rubber Age, 53: 419-426.

WEISSBERG, J.B. & ZINKL, J.G. (1973) Effects of 2,3,7,8-tetrachlorodibenzo-p-dioxin upon hemostasis and hematologic function in the rat. Environ. Health Perspect., 5: 119-123.

WESTING, A.H., (1984) Herbicides in war: past and present. In: Westing, A.H., ed. Herbicides in war, the long-term ecological and human consquences, London, Taylor and Francis.

WHITE, K.L., Jr, LYSY, H.H., MCCAY, J.A., & ANDERSON, A.C. (1986) Modulation of serum complement levels following exposure to polychlorinated dibenzo-p-dioxins. Toxicol. appl. Pharmacol., 84: 209-219.

WHITLOCK, J.P. & GALEAZZI, D.R. (1984) 2,3,7,8-Tetrachlorodibenzo-p-dioxin receptors in wild type and variant mouse hepatoma cells. J. biol. Chem., 259:. 980-985.

WHO/EURO (1987) Dioxins and furans from municipal incinerators, Copenhagen, WHO Regional Office for Europe (Environmental Health Series 17).

WIKLUND, K. & HOLM, L.-E. (1986) Soft tissue sarcoma risk in Swedish agricultural and forestry workers. J. Natl Cancer Inst., 76: 229-234.

WILLEY, J.C., SALADINO, A.J., OZANNE, C., LECHNER, J.F., & HARRIS, C.C. (1984) Acute effects of 12-O-tetradecanoylphorbol-13-acetate, teleocidin B, or 2,3,7,8-tetrachlorodibenzo-p-dioxin on cultured normal human bronchial epithelial cells. Carcinogenesis, 5: 209-215.

WILLIAMS, D.T., CUNNINGHAM, H.M., & BLANCHFIELD, B.J. (1972) Distribution and excretion studies of octachlorodibenzo-p-dioxin in the rat. Bull. Environ. Contam. Toxicol., 7: 57-62.

WIPF, H.K. & SCHMID, J. (1983) Seveso - An environmental assessment. In: Tucker, R.E., Young, A.L., & Gray, R., ed. Human and environmental risks of chlorinated dioxins and related compounds, New York, London, Plenum Press, pp. 255-276.

WIPF, H.K., HOMBERGER, E., NEUNER, N., RANALDER, U.B., VETTER, W., & VUILLEUMIER, J.P. (1982) TCDD-levels in soil and plant samples from the Seveso area. In: Hutzinger, O., Frei, R.W., Merian, E., & Pocchiari, F., ed. Chlorinated dioxins and related compounds. Impact on the environment, Oxford, New York, Pergamon Press, pp. 115-127.

WOLF, G. (1980) Vitamin A. In: Alfin-Slater, R.B. & Kritchevsky, D., ed. Human nutrition, a comprehensive treatise. Part B. Nutrition and the adult, New York, London, Plenum Press, Vol. 3, pp. 97-203.

WOODS, J.S. (1973) Studies of the effects of 2,3,7,8-tetrachlorodibenzo-p-dioxin on mammalian hepatic delta-aminolevulinic acid synthetase. Environ. Health Perspect., 5: 221-225.

WROBLEWSKI, V.J. & OLSON, J.R. (1985) Hepatic metabolism of 2,3,7,8-tetrachlorodibenzo-p-dioxin (TCDD) in the rat and guinea pig. Toxicol. appl. Pharmacol., 81: 231-240.

WU, Y.C., LO, Y.C., KAO, H.Y., PAN, C.C., & LIN, R.Y. (1984) Cell-mediated immunity in patients with polychlorinated biphenyl poisoning. J. Formoson Med. Assoc., 83: 419-429.

YAMAGISHI, T., MIYAZAKI, T., AKIYAMA, K., MORITA, M., NAKAGAWA, J., HORII, S., & KANEKO, S. (1981) Polychlorinated dibenzo-p-dioxins and dibenzofurans in commercial diphenyl ether herbicides, and in fresh water fish collected from the application area. Chemosphere, 10: 1137-1144.

YANG, K.H., CROFT, W.A., & PETERSON, R.E. (1977) Effects of 2,3,7,8-tetrachlorodibenzo-p-dioxin on plasma disappearance and biliary excretion of foreign compounds in rats. Toxicol. appl. Pharmacol., 40: 485-496.

YANG, K.H., CHOI, E.J., & CHOE, S.Y. (1983a) Cytotoxicity of 2,3,7,8-tetrachlorodibenzo-p-dioxin on primary cultures of adult rat hepatocytes. Arch. environ. Contam. Toxicol., 12: 183-188.

YANG, K.H., YOO, B.S., & CHOE, S.Y. (1983b) Effects of halogenated dibenzo-p-dioxins on plasma disappearance and biliary excretion of ouabain in rats. Toxicol. Lett., 15: 259-264.

YOCKIM, R.S., ISENSEE, A.R., & JONES, G.E. (1978) Distribution and toxicity of TCDD and 2,4,5-T in an aquatic model ecosystem. Chemosphere, 7: 215-220.

YOSHIHARA, S., NAGATA, K., YOSHIMURA, H., KUROKI, H., & MASUDA, Y. (1981) Inductive effect on hepatic enzymes and acute toxicity of individual polychlorinated dibenzofuran congeners in rats. Toxicol. appl. Pharmacol., 59: 580-588.

YOSHIMURA, H., KAMIMURA, H., OGURI, K., HONDA, Y., & NAKANO, M. (1986) Stimulating effect of activated charcoal beads on fecal excretion. Chemosphere, 15(3): 219-227.

YOUNG, A.L. (1983) Long-term studies on the persistence and movement of TCDD in a natural ecosystem. In: Tucker, R.E., Young, A.L., & Gray, P., ed. Human and environmental risks of chlorinated dioxins and related compounds, New York, London, Plenum Press, pp. 173-190.

YOUNG, A.L., KANG, H.K., & SHEPARD, B.M. (1983) Clorinated dioxins as herbicide contaminants. Environ. Sci. Technol., 17: 530A-532A.

YOUNG, A.L., THALKEN, C.E., & WARD, W.E. (1975) Studies of the ecological impact of repetitive aerial applications of herbicides on the ecosystem of test area C-52A, Eglin Air Force Base, Florida, Washington, DC, US Department of Defence, 127 pp. (Final Report October 1975).

YOUNG, A.L., THALKEN, C.E., ARNOLD, E.L., CUPELLO, J.M., & COCKERHAM, L.G. (1976) Fate of 2,3,7,8-tetrachlorodibenzo-p-dioxin (TCDD) in the environment: Summary and decontamination recommendations, US Air Force Academy, Colorado, Washington, DC, US Department of Defence (Document 19 USAFA TR-76-8).

ZACK, J.A. & GAFFEY, W.R. (1983) A mortality study of workers employed at the Monsanto Company Plant in Nitro, West Virginia. Environ. Sci. Res., 26: 575-591.

ZACK, J.A. & SUSKIND, R.R. (1980) The mortality experience of workers exposed to tetrachlorodibenzodioxin in a trichlorophenol process accident. J. occup. Med., 22: 11-14.

ZEDDA, S., CIRLA, A.M., & SALA, C. (1976) [Accidental tetrachlorodibenzoparadioxin contamination. Considerations on the I.C.M.E.S.A. episode.] Med. Lav., 67: 371-378 (in Italian).

ZELIKOV, A.K. & DANILOV, L.N. (1974) Occupational dermatoses (acnes) in workers engaged in production of 2,4,5-trichlorophenol. Sov. Med., 7: 145-146.

ZINKL, J.G., VOS, J.G., MOORE, J.A., & GUPTA, B.N. (1973) Hematologic and clinical chemistry effects of 2,3,7,8-tetrachlorodibenzo-p-dioxin in laboratory animals. Environ. Health Perspect., 5: 111-118.

RESUME ET RECOMMANDATIONS

1. Résumé

1.1 Sources

Les dibenzo-para-dioxines polychlorées (PCDD) et les dibenzofurannes polychlorés (PCDF) constituent deux séries d'hydrocarbures aromatiques tricycliques halogénés de propriétés physico-chimiques très voisines, présentes un peu partout dans l'environnement. Leur origine n'est pas naturelle et ils ne sont pas produits intentionnellement. On connait 75 isomères (isomérie de position) pour les PCDD et 135 pour les PCDF.

Les sources les plus importantes de contamination par ces deux séries de composés sont les suivantes:

- contamination de produits chimiques du commerce, par exemple chlorophénols et dérivés, PCB;
- incinération de déchets municipaux, de déchets dangereux et de déchets d'hôpitaux, ainsi que de boues provenant du traitement des effluents;
- fonctionnement des véhicules automobiles;
- utilisation de combustibles fossiles;
- surchauffe et émissions de foyers faisant intervenir des béniphyles polychlorés (PCB);
- élimination de déchets industriels provenant, par exemple, de la production de chlorophénols et de leurs dérivés, du traitement du bois par le chlorophénol, de l'emploi de PCB liquides dans l'appareillage électrique et du traitement du papier et de la pâte à papier.

1.2 Concentrations dans l'environnement et voies d'exposition

D'après les quelques données dont on dispose, la concentration de ces composés serait très faible dans l'air, le sol et les sédiments, de l'ordre du femtogramme (fg) par mètre cube dans l'air et du nanogramme (ng) par kilogramme dans le sol et les sédiments. On a observé des concentrations allant jusqu'à 50 mg/kg, aussi bien pour les PCDD que pour les PCDF, dans certains organismes aquatiques à l'état naturel. On dispose de très peu de données sur la contamination de l'eau de boisson et des denrées alimentaires vendues dans le commerce.

Pour ce qui est de la population en général, l'exposition à ces composés semble principalement associée à la chaîne alimentaire.

Certains travailleurs peuvent être très exposés lorsqu'ils sont affectés à la production, la mise en oeuvre ou à la destruction de matériaux contenant des PCDD ou des PCDF, ainsi que leurs précurseurs. Pour ce personnel, l'inhalation et les contacts cutanés constituent les principales voies d'exposition à prendre en compte.

1.3 Toxicocinétique, biotransformation et surveillance biologique

La biodisponibilité des PCDD et des PCDF dépend de la matrice au sein de laquelle ils sont incorporés et de la voie d'exposition. On ne dispose pour aucune des espèces en cause de données sur la biodisponibilité par inhalation.

On ignore la quantité absorbée par l'homme en cas d'exposition, par quelque voie que ce soit.

Les études sur des rongeurs à qui l'on a administré une ou plusieurs doses de 2,3,7,8-TCDD par voie orale montrent qu'environ la moitié de la dose administrée est absorbée dans les voies digestives. La demi-vie d'élimination se situe, d'après la littérature, entre 12 et 94 jours chez les rongeurs. Chez le singe rhésus, la demi-vie de la 2,3,7,8-TCDD est d'environ 1 an dans le tissu adipeux.

Les observations concernant la toxicocinétique des PCDD chez les animaux sont limitées, en dehors du cas de la 2,3,7,8-TCDD. Pour ce dérivé, on a observé une demi-vie de l'ordre de 2 à 8 jours chez le rat, la souris et le singe et de plus de 20 jours chez le cobaye. Chez le rat, on a constaté que la pentachlore-2,3,4,7,8 dibenzofuranne s'élimine moins rapidement que la 2,3,7,8-TCDD.

Les études sur la rétention tissulaire des PCDD et des PCDF chez diverses espèces exposées à des mélanges synthétiques ou à des échantillons prélevés dans l'environnement et contenant des PCDD ou des PCDF montrent que la durée de rétention des divers analogues est très variable selon qu'ils sont ou non substitués en 2, 3, 7, ou 8 par un atome de chlore.

D'après quelques observations effectuées sur l'homme, la demi-vie serait de 2 à 6 ans pour certains PCDD et PCDF substitués en 2, 3, 7 et 8.

Les PCDD et les PCDF s'accumulent principalement dans les graisses; ils sont également excrétés dans le lait et traversent la barrière placentaire. On en trouve également à faible concentration, dans le sang et les organes vitaux.

La distribution tissulaire chez l'homme est encore mal élucidée, encore qu'il semble que le rapport des concentrations dans les tissus adipeux et dans le foie soit plus élevé que chez les rongeurs.

Dans l'ensemble de la population, on observe une concentration résiduelle de PCDD dans le tissu adipeux qui atteint 20 mg/kg, en l'absence de toute exposition particulière connue; mais des chiffres plus élevés ont été signalés quelquefois, sans aucun signe de maladie. Dans les deux cas, les groupes de population étudiés n'avaient pas été constitués par sondage aléatoire. Dans ces échantillons, on a observé les PCDD et les PCDF les plus substitués par du chlore, en particulier des octachlorodibenzo-p-dioxines. La concentration tissulaire des TCDD avait tendance à augmenter avec l'âge.

1.4 Effets sur la santé

1.4.1 Animaux

Les effets toxiques et biologiques découlant de l'exposition aux 2,3,7,8-TCDD dépendent de divers facteurs, dont l'espèce, la souche, l'âge et le sexe des animaux d'expérience. Entre autres signes de toxicité observés chez plusieurs espèces animales, on note une perte de poids, une hépatoxicité, une porphyrie, une atteinte cutanée, des lésions gastriques, une atrophie du thymus, une atteinte du système immunitaire, des effets tératogènes, des effets sur la reproduction et des effets cancérogènes. Les TCDD exercent des effets biologiques extrêmement divers, notamment l'induction de certaines enzymes et une carence en vitamine A. Ces effets ne sont pas tous observés chez la même espèce animale. Les effets toxiques les plus caractéristiques qu'on retrouve chez tous les animaux de laboratoire sont la perte de poids, l'atrophie du thymus et l'immunotoxicité. Chez l'homme, une chloracné et des lésions cutanées de ce type constituent les signes les plus fréquents d'une intoxication par les 2,3,7,8-TCDD; on observe également des lésions cutanées chez le rhésus, la souris glabre et le lapin. En revanche, l'exposition au 2,3,7,8-TCDD ne provoque ni chloracné ni lésions cutanées de ce type chez la plupart des rongeurs. De nombreuses lésions toxiques s'observent principalement au niveau des tissus épithéliaux.

Des effets ont été observés sur la reproduction chez le rhésus et chez le rat. La plus faible dose exerçant un effet serait de l'ordre de 1-2 ng/kg de poids corporel par jour. Dans deux études de cancérogénicité chez le rat, on a obtenu un épithélioma hépatocellulaire avec des doses respectives d'environ 0,1 et 0,01 µg/kg de poids corporel par jour. Une dose réduite à 0,001 µg/kg de poids corporel se traduit par une modification des hépatocytes au niveau de certains foyers ou territoires. L'incidence de certaines tumeurs à déterminisme hormonal était plus faible que chez les animaux témoins.

Apparemment, les TCDD n'ont pas de propriétés mutagènes et ne devraient donc pas être génotoxiques. Il faut donc admettre que les effets cancérogènes s'expliquent par un mécanisme indirect.

Plusieurs autres PCDD et PCDF déterminent des manifestations analogues à celles que provoquent les 2,3,7,8-TCDD, mais leur activité est très inégale. On connaît 12 isomères qui présentent une toxicité plus élevée, à savoir les tétra-, penta-, hexa- et heptaCDD ou CDF qui possèdent quatre atomes de chlore symétriques deux à deux, en poisition 2,3,7 et 8. Des études prolongées sur l'animal ont révélé l'action cancérogène d'un mélange de deux hexachlorodibenzo-p-dioxines (1,2,3,7,8,9- et 1,2,3,6,7,8-hexaCDD), mais en présence de doses plus élevées que celles qu'on avait utilisées dans l'étude des TCDD. La dibenzo-p-dioxine et la dichloro-2,7 dibenzo-p-dioxine ne se sont pas révélées cancérogènes. Les activités relatives, toxiques et biologiques, des PCDD et des PCDF ont été estimées au moyen d'études de courte durée chez le rat et en culture de cellules mammaliennes.

Selon les espèces, les animaux présentent une sensibilité très inégale aux effets biologiques et toxiques des PCDD et PCDF substitués en 2,3,7,8. Par exemple, la DL_{50} par voie orale varie, pour les 2,3,7,8-TCDD, de 0,6 µg/kg de poids corporel chez le cobaye à 5051 µg/kg chez le hamster doré syrien. Les différences considérables de sensibilité vis-à-vis des 2,3,7,8-TCDD et des composés apparentés qu'on observe ainsi chez les diverses espèces et souches est impossible à expliquer par les différences qu'on constate dans la toxicocinétique. La toxicité et la toxicocinétique des TCDD chez les singes sont à peu près les mêmes que chez l'homme. Chez des souris de lignée pure, on a des raisons de penser que la concentration cellulaire du récepteur aux Ah est partiellement corrélée avec la sensibilité à l'action biologique et toxique de ces composés. Le récepteur a été retrouvé chez d'autres espèces, notamment chez l'homme. Cependant, l'abondance relative du récepteur aux Ah selon les espèces n'explique pas entièrement les différences de sensibilité.

1.4.2 Homme

Malgré de nombreuses études cliniques et études de suivi post-thérapeutiques, aucun effet général persistant bien net n'a été mis en évidence, si ce n'est une chloracné, à la suite d'expositions professionnelles ou accidentelles aux PCDD et aux PCDF. D'autres effets ont été notés mais aucun n'est persistant, en dehors de la chloracné et, peut-être, de troubles fonctionnels minimes.

Dans quelques études épidémiologiques consacrées à des cas d'exposition à un mélange de dioxines, de furannes et d'autres produits chimiques, on a fait état d'une augmentation de l'incidence des cancers de localisations diverses, mais plusieurs facteurs ne permettent pas de faire entièrement foi à ces observations.

Lors de l'accident de Seveso, le seul effet nocif indiscutable a été la chloracné. Cette affection (193 cas) s'est déclarée en 1976 et 1977 et elle était encore active en 1984 chez 20 des victimes. De nombreuses études ont été consacrées à la recherche de liens possibles entre l'exposition à l'Agent orange et des effets nocifs chez les civils ou les militaires, au Viet Nam. Cependant, les données dont on dispose à l'heure actuelle ne permettent pas de conclure catégoriquement à l'existence d'effets sur la reproduction ou d'autres effets biologiques notables.

Lors de l'incident survenu au Missouri, les enfants chez qui l'on avait observé des signes aigus d'intoxication lors de la contamination, en 1971, sont, semble-t-il, aujourd'hui en bonne santé. En outre, des études épidémiologiques poursuivies dans ce même Etat au sein de populations plus longuement exposées à des concentrations plus faibles de dioxine n'ont jusqu'ici révélé aucun effet appréciable sur la santé. Mais si aucun symptôme clinique n'a été observé, on a constaté un effet sur l'immunité à médiation cellulaire.

Les seuls cas d'intoxication humaine par les PCDF pour lesquels on dispose d'observations circonstanciées concernent la contamination d'huile de riz par des PCDF, des PCB et des PCQ, observée à Yusho au Japon, en 1968, et Yu-cheng à Taiwan, en 1979. Au total, plusieurs milliers de personnes ont été gravement intoxiquées. Il semble très probable que les PCDF sont à incriminer dans ces intoxications. La symptomatologie générale était analogue à celle qui accompagne les intoxications par les TCDD, compte tenu des différences traduisant l'intensité de l'exposition et la structure d'âge et de sexe des groupes exposés.

A Yusho, l'apport quotidien moyen de PCDF substitués en 2,3,7,8 a été estimé à 0,1-0,2 µg/kg de poids corporel sur plusieurs mois, alors que la dose pathogène minimale a été estimée à 0,05-0,1 µg/kg de poids corporel par jour, sur 30 jours.

1.5 Conclusion

Les PCDD et les PCDF se rencontrent dans tout l'environnement et il est probable que chacun en est porteur. Ces composés déterminent parfois des effets toxiques complexes en cas d'exposition professionnelle ou accidentelle.

D'après les observations faites à Yusho, les expériences conduites chez des espèces sensibles de singes, et compte tenu de certaines hypothèses concernant l'activité relative des PCDD et des PCDF, il se peut que l'homme et certains singes présentent une sensibilité comparable à l'égard de ces composés. Cependant, les incertitudes concernant la dose effectivement reçue et les difficultés de l'évaluation des effets toxiques autres que la chloracné interdisent, dans le cas de l'homme, une conclusion catégorique quant à la résistance relative de l'homme aux effets toxiques de ces composés. Il convient de limiter l'exposition aux plus faibles niveaux compatibles avec les impératifs pratiques.

2. Recommandations

1. Des études interlaboratoires de validation, selon une sorte de "poule" avec protocoles normalisés de contrôle et d'assurance de qualité, sont indispensables pour améliorer les méthodes d'analyse.

   La méthodologie de l'échantillonnage, les méthodes d'analyse et l'interprétation des données doivent être optimalisées et normalisées avant le démarrage des enquêtes.

2. Des données complémentaires sont nécessaires sur l'origine des PCDD et des PCDF, sur leur répartition dans l'environnement et sur leur destinée.

   D'autres observations sont indispensables au sujet de la présence des PCDD ou des PCDF dans l'environnement, notamment sur l'évolution des concentrations dans le temps et sur la détermination des profils isomériques, notamment dans les produits alimentaires, dans l'air ambiant et dans les sédiments.

3. Il serait bon de faire des observations sur les effets qu'exercent les PCDD et les PCDF sur la biocénose.

4. Des données plus complètes sont nécessaires en ce qui concerne la biodisponibilité des PCDD et des PCDF provenant de diverses matrices, dans l'environnement et dans la ration alimentaire. L'exposition à ces sources devrait être mise en corrélation avec les pratiques agricoles et industrielles.

5. Il convient de mettre au point et de valider des méthodes chimiques et biologiques plus simples et moins coûteuses pour rechercher la présence de PCDD et de PCDF.

6. Des études sur les mécanismes toxiques des PCDD et des PCDF sont nécessaires pour élucider les différences observées dans les effets produits chez les diverses espèces et permettre une extrapolation à l'homme.

7. Il importe de poursuivre l'étude de l'immunotoxicité, notamment en ce qui concerne la fonction des lymphocytes T cytotoxiques. En particulier, il est capital d'étudier la nature et la durée des effets sur le système immunitaire d'une exposition pendant la période périnatale.

8. Des études de toxicité à long terme devraient être effectuées, notamment des études de reproduction sur plusieurs générations chez diverses espèces, au moyen de trois des PCDD et des PCDF les plus répandus, à savoir le 2,3,4,7,8-pentaCDF, le 1,2,3,7,8-pentaCDD et l'octaCDD.

9. Etant donné que l'homme est exposé à des mélanges complexes de PCDD et de PCDF, il faut poursuivre la mise au point et la validation de divers systèmes d'épreuve, notamment des cultures de cellules humaines en vue d'apprécier l'activité toxique de ces composés et de leurs mélanges. Ces systèmes permettront d'étudier les mécanismes d'action, les relations structure/activité et les effets interactifs.

10. Il serait bon d'étudier la charge de l'organisme en PCDD et PCDF et d'établir une corrélation entre cette charge, les effets cliniques constatés et les résultats des examens de laboratoire. Le suivi de groupes exposés antérieurement est important à cet égard.

EVALUATION DES DANGERS POUR LA SANTE DE L'HOMME DE L'EXPOSITION AUX DIBENZO-P-DIOXINES POLYCHLORES (PCDD) ET AUX DIBENZOFURANNES POLYCHLORES (PCDF)

1. Introduction

Pour évaluer les dangers que représentent les PCDD et les PCDF pour la santé humaine, il faut connaître à la fois l'intensité de l'exposition et les effets biologiques correspondants.

Il est fort difficile d'évaluer l'exposition humaine. Plusieurs méthodes sont possibles, par exemple:

a) Utilisation de modèles physiologiques classiques de l'inhalation, de l'ingestion et de l'absorption cutanée. Il faut connaître de façon précise la concentration des produits en cause dans les différents milieux et dans les denrées alimentaires, ainsi que leur biodisponibilité.

b) Estimations de l'apport sur la base de modèles pharmacocinétiques simples et des teneurs observées dans les divers tissus humains en vue d'une évaluation précise de l'exposition. Il faut en outre connaître en détail l'apport, la distribution, le métabolisme et l'élimination des PCDD et des PCDF chez l'homme.

2. Evaluation de l'exposition

2.1 Sources de contamination

Les principales sources de PCDD et de PCDF identifiées jusqu'ici sont les contaminants contenus dans les produits chimiques vendus dans le commerce (voir section 3.3), les émissions par suite de combustion (voir section 3.5) et l'élimination de déchets industriels contenant des PCDD ou des PCDF (sections 3.4, 3.5.9 et 3.5.10).

Dans certains cas, on peut estimer au niveau local la contribution relative de ces diverses sources. Mais, les méthodes et les données dont on dispose aujourd'hui ne permettent pas de conclusions définitives quant à leur importance relative au niveau d'un pays ou du monde entier.

2.2 Concentrations dans le milieu ambiant

Les données restreintes dont on dispose montrent que la concentration atmosphérique résiduelle est très faible (fg/m^3) pour les 2,3,7,8-tétrachloro-PCDD ou PCDF ainsi que pour les dérivés pentachlorés ou hexachlorés. (Si l'on tient compte des analogues heptachlorés ou octachlorés, on observe des concentrations de l'ordre du picogramme par mètre cube).

D'après les rares données disponibles, il est peu probable qu'on trouve des tétrachloro-2,3,7,8-PCDD ou PCDF ni des dérivés pentachlorés ou hexachlorés dans une eau de boisson traitée, même à la concentration de 1 pg/litre (voir section 5.2). Dans tous les échantillons de sols et de sédiments analysés (provenant de régions industrialisées ou non), la concentration de PCDD et de PCDF allait de quelques nanogrammes à plusieurs centaines de nanogrammes par kilogramme (la concentration la plus élevée concernant les sédiments et le sol en zone urbaine).

On ne connaît pas la concentration résiduelle des PCDD et des PCDF dans les végétaux en général.

Des concentrations atteignant 50 ng/kg ont été observées chez des poissons capturés dans la nature pour les mêmes dérivés (principalement les dérivés tétrachlorés et pentachlorés). Le plus souvent, ces composés ont été observés dans des poissons gras ou des poissons qui se nourrissent sur le fond (voir section 4.4.2).

Les observations concernant les organismes terrestres ne permettent pas d'estimer les concentrations résiduelles (voir section 4.4.3). Dans trois échantillons d'un mélange de différents laits de vache, on a trouvé, pour le lait entier, une concentration maximale de 100 pg/kg (voir section 5.4). La contamination des autres denrées alimentaires vendues dans le commerce est également très mal connue. L'analyse de plusieurs échantillons de poulet et de porc montre que ces produits contiennent environ 5-30 ng/kg d'analogues fortement chlorés. Le profil de ces analogues n'est pas le même que chez les organismes aquatiques (voir section 5.4).

Les données disponibles ne permettent pas d'évaluer l'exposition globale de la population dans son ensemble. Elles suffisent pour une évaluation limitée de l'exposition dans le cas des populations locales. Compte tenu des concentrations environnementales examinées ci-dessus et des hypothèses habituelles sur l'apport d'aliments, d'air et d'eau, les denrées alimentaires risquent davantage de contribuer notablement à l'exposition aux PCDD/PCDF que l'air, tandis que l'eau de boisson est sans doute beaucoup moins en cause.

2.3 Modalités d'exposition

Chez l'homme, le tissu adipeux contient des tétrachloro-2,3,7,8 PCDD/PCDF ainsi que des dérivés pentachlorés et hexachlorés. Cette contamination s'explique sans doute par une exposition aux produits présents dans l'environnement, aux concentrations indiquées plus haut.

En outre, les nourrissons peuvent être exposés par l'intermédiaire du lait maternel et les jeunes enfants par l'ingestion de terre contaminée. Mais, dans la plupart des cas, ce dernier mode d'exposition ne devrait être pris en compte que dans les régions fortement polluées.

Certaines populations sont particulièrement exposées à l'occasion d'accidents survenus dans l'industrie (et des opérations de nettoyage ultérieures) lors de la production et de l'utilisation normales de chlorophénols, d'herbicides phénoxylés et de PCB. En pareil cas, ce sont l'inhalation et le contact cutané qui constituent les modes d'exposition les plus importants. Cependant, on ne dispose pas de données quantitatives sur la nature et la concentration des contaminants.

Sur la base des valeurs indiquées plus haut pour les concentrations dans le milieu ambiant et des hypothèses habituelles sur les paramètres physiologiques et les valeurs de l'apport, il est probable que l'ingestion constitue le mode d'exposition essentiel. L'inhalation de l'air ambiant ne devrait pas poser de problème encore qu'un air fortement contaminé puisse contribuer sensiblement à l'exposition. En général, il n'est pas possible actuellement d'estimer l'importance relative de l'exposition par voie cutanée.

2.4 Biodisponibilité

On ne dispose d'aucune donnée sur la biodisponibilité provenant d'études sur l'homme. L'expérimentation animale montre que la biodisponibilité des PCDD ou des PCDF après ingestion dépend de la matrice du produit ingéré. Les données disponibles au sujet de l'apport par voie orale sont résumées au tableau 46.

Des études sur des rats glabres montrent que l'exposition cutanée par contact de la peau intacte avec un sol contaminé représente environ 1-2%. On ne dispose d'aucune donnée pour l'exposition par inhalation.

3. Résultats de l'exposition animale

3.1 Toxicocinétique des 2,3,7,8-TCDD

Des études sur des rongeurs à qui l'on administrait du 2,3,7,8-TCDD par voie orale, en une ou plusieurs prises, ont montré que l'absorption dans les voies digestives était d'au moins 50% chez le rat, le cobaye et le hamster, mais de moins de 30% chez la souris (tableau 40). Les valeurs indiquées pour la demi-vie d'élimination étaient de l'ordre de 12-31 jours pour le rat, la souris et le hamster et de 22-94 jours pour le cobaye (tableau 41). Cependant, la plupart de ces études ont été effectuées en utilisant des doses toxiques. La demi-vie des 2,3,7,8-TCDD chez les primates est mal connue mais il semble, d'après les données disponibles pour le rhésus, que la demi-vie apparente soit de l'ordre de 1 an dans les tissus adipeux.

Les 2,3,7,8-TCDD ne s'accumulent pas dans les tissus animaux. Chez les rongeurs, l'accumulation intervient principalement au niveau du foie et du tissu adipeux (tableaux 42 à 44). Chez des rhésus (tableau 45), on a observé une concentration élevée de ces mêmes produits dans le tissu adipeux, le foie, la peau et les muscles.

Chez des rats ayant reçu quotidiennement pendant 2 ans des 2,3,7,8-TCDD à raison de 1 ng/kg de poids corporel, on a observé une accumulation de 540 ng/kg de poids corporel dans le foie où l'on a également noté certaines altérations morphologiques. Des quantités du même ordre ont été notées chez le péromysque après exposition à un sol contenant des 2,3,7,8-TCDD à la concentration de 10-710 ng/kg (Cockherham et al., 1980). L'exposition des animaux, au niveau de l'ensemble de leur corps, à un sol présentant de telles teneurs peut donc se traduire par une concentration tissulaire qui a des effets observables chez les animaux d'expérience.

Les TCDD sont en grande partie éliminés dans les déjections, encore qu'il existe une certaine excrétion urinaire. Elle est plus importante chez le hamster que chez les autres espèces étudiées.

La transformation des 2,3,7,8-TCDD en métabolites à caractère polaire plus prononcé s'observe chez toutes les espèces animales étudiées (voir section 6.2 et tableau 62). L'élimination fécale et urinaire des métabolites est rapide chez toutes ces espèces, sauf chez le cobaye. Les métabolites connus sont beaucoup moins toxiques que les composés dont ils dérivent.

3.2 Toxicocinétique des PCDD et des PCDF autres que les TCDD

En dehors du cas des dérivés tétrachlorés, les observations sur la toxicocinétique des PCDD chez les animaux sont limitées. De ce point de vue, les PCDF ont été davantage étudiés. La demi-vie des 2,3,7,8-TCDF serait de l'ordre de 2 à 8 jours chez le rat, la souris et le rhésus et de plus de 20 jours chez le cobaye (tableau 65). Les études sur le rat montrent que les 2,3,7,8-pentaCDF se fixent davantage dans les tissus que les 2,3,7,8-TCDF (65% et 3,8% respectivement, au bout de 5 jours).

La rétention tissulaire des PCDD et des PCDF chez diverses espèces exposées à des mélanges de synthèse ou à des échantillons prélevés dans l'environnement et contenant des PCDD et des PCDF se révèle très inégale selon que les produits sont ou non substitués par des atomes de chlore dans toutes les positions 2,3,7 et 8.

3.3 Effets toxiques des 2,3,7,8-TCDD

Les effets toxiques et biologiques découlant de l'exposition aux 2,3,7,8-TCDD dépendent de divers facteurs, dont l'espèce, la souche, l'âge et le sexe des animaux d'expérience. Entre autres signes de toxicité observés chez plusieurs espèces animales, on note une perte de poids, une hépatoxicité, une porphyrie, une atteinte cutanée, des lésions gastriques, une atrophie du thymus, une atteinte du système immunitaire, des effets tératogènes, des effets sur la reproduction et des effets cancérogènes. Les TCDD exercent des effets biologiques extrêmement divers, notamment l'induction de certaines enzymes et une carence en vitamine A. Ces effets ne sont pas tous observés chez la même espèce animale. Les effets toxiques les plus caractéristiques qu'on retrouve chez tous les animaux de laboratoire sont la perte de poids, l'atrophie du thymus et l'immunotoxicité. Chez l'homme, une chloracné et des lésions cutanées apparentées constituent les signes les plus fréquents d'une intoxication par les 2,3,7,8-TCDD; on observe également des lésions cutanées chez le rhésus, la souris glabre et le lapin. En revanche, l'exposition au 2,3,7,8-TCDD ne provoque ni chloracné ni lésions cutanées de ce type chez le rat, la plupart des souris, le cobaye et le hamster. Les lésions toxiques observées sont fréquemment soit des lésions hyperplasiques/métaplasiques, soit des lésions hypoplasiques et elles intéressent principalement les tissus épithéliaux.

Des effets toxiques sur la reproduction ont été observés chez les singes rhésus: la plus faible dose sans effets observables serait, d'après les calculs, de 1 à 2 ng/kg de poids corporel par jour. Il se peut qu'il existe une dose sans effets observables de 1 ng/kg de poids corporel par jour chez le rat, s'agissant des effets sur la reproduction (Murray et al., 1979; Nisbet & Paxton, 1982).

Lorsqu'on compare les études consacrées à la production de cancers chez le rat par Kociba et al. (1978) et par le NTP (1982a, b), il apparaît clairement que les tumeurs hépatiques, notamment les épithéliomas hépatocellulaires, s'obtiennent à des doses similaires. Bien que le NTP ainsi que Kociba et al. (1978) aient observé une augmentation de l'incidence des tumeurs au niveau d'autres organes, les résultats ne sont pas analogues dans les deux études. Cela tient peut-être, en partie, à des différences dans les doses administrées (gavage ou exposition par incorporation à des aliments broyés) et dans les souches. Dans l'étude de Kociba, l'administration d'une dose de 10 ng/kg de poids corporel a provoqué une augmentation de l'incidence des nodules néoplasiques (hyperplasiques) chez les femelles, tandis qu'une dose de 1 ng/kg de poids corporel se traduisait par un gonflement des hépatocytes en foyers ou par places. A ces doses, l'incidence de certaines tumeurs à déterminisme hormonal était plus faible chez les animaux d'expérience que chez les témoins, ce qui donne à penser que les 2,3,7,8-TCDD déterminent des altérations au niveau des glandes endocrines. Compte tenu de ces résultats de l'expérimentation animale et des données dont on dispose au sujet de l'homme, le CIRC (1982, suppl. 4) est arrivé à la conclusion que les preuves de cancérogénicité des TCDD étaient suffisantes chez les animaux, mais insuffisantes chez l'homme.

Apparemment, les TCDD n'ont pas de propriétés mutagènes et ne devraient donc pas être génotoxiques. Leur action cancérogène est donc attribuée à un mécanisme indirect (épigénétique).

3.4 Effets toxiques des PCDD et des PCDF autres que les TCDD

Plusieurs autres PCDD et PCDF provoquent les mêmes symptômes que les 2,3,7,8-TCDD, mais leur activité est très inégale (tableaux 56, 62). Pour résumer, il existe 12 isomères qui présentent une toxicité élevée, à savoir les tétra-, penta-, hexa- et heptaCDD et CDF contenant quatre atomes de chlore symétriques deux à deux en position 2,3,7 et 8. On a montré, lors d'études prolongées sur l'animal, qu'un mélange de deux hexaCDD (1,2,3,7,8-9 et 1,2,3,6,7,8-haxaCDD) était cancérogène, mais à des doses plus élevées que celles utilisées dans l'étude des TCDD. La dioxine non substituée et la dichloro-2,7 dioxine n'ont manifesté aucun pouvoir cancérogène.

L'activité relative, toxique et biologique, des PCDD et des PCDF a été estimée au moyen d'études de courte durée chez le rat et d'études en culture de cellules mammaliennes. Comme critères, on a retenu l'inhibition de la prise de poids, l'atrophie du thymus, l'induction d'enzymes, la tératogénicité, la production d'acné et la kératinisation. En l'absence d'observations sur la toxicité à long terme, les résultats fournis par ces épreuves de durée limitée constituent actuellement la seule source qui permette un classement par toxicité en vue de l'évaluation des dangers pour la santé de l'homme.

Les études consacrées à des mélanges de ces composés ont mis en évidence une synergie additive tout au plus.

3.5 Etude des différences interspécifiques

La sensibilité aux effets biologiques et toxiques des 2,3,7,8-TCDD est très inégale selon les espèces. Par exemple, la DL_{50} par voie orale varie de 0,6 µg/kg de poids corporel chez le cobaye à 5051 µg/kg de poids corporel chez le hamster doré syrien (tableau 47); en outre, on a signalé des différences prononcées de DL_{50} chez différentes souches de la même espèce (par exemple le rat et la souris). La toxicité et la toxicocinétique des TCDD sont très analogues chez les singes et chez l'homme. Cependant, il est impossible d'expliquer les différences considérables de sensibilité, selon le sexe et la souche, aux 2,3,7,8-TCDD et aux composés analogues par les différences qu'on observe sur le plan toxicocinétique. Les observations montrent que, chez des souris de lignée pure, l'abondance cellulaire du récepteur Ah est partiellement corrélée avec la sensibilité aux effets biologiques et toxiques de ces composés. On a également repéré ce récepteur chez d'autres espèces, notamment chez l'homme. Cependant, l'abondance relative de ce récepteur selon les espèces n'explique pas les différences de sensibilité aux 2,3,7,8-TCDD; cette constatation n'a rien d'étonnant quand on sait qu'il existe des mécanismes de toxicité complexes et encore inconnus qui font intervenir de multiples facteurs en plus du récepteur aux Ah.

4. Effets sur la santé de l'homme

4.1 PCDD

La population générale est exposée à de faibles quantités de PCDD et de PCDF présentes dans des mélanges complexes qui ne provoquent aucun cas de maladie. Lors de quelques incidents, par exemple à Seveso et à Yusho, des ouvriers et d'autres personnes sont tombés malades à la suite d'une exposition à des quantités plus élevées d'un nombre restreint de ces composés.

Dans le cas de l'exposition professionnelle ou accidentelle, l'effet clinique le plus net réside dans une chloracné. D'autres effets (tableau 64) ont été observés mais, à part la chloracné et peut-être des troubles fonctionnels mineurs, aucun n'a été durable.

Dans certaines des études de mortalité réalisées, on a fait état d'une augmentation de l'incidence des cancers de diverses localisations, mais le trop petit nombre de cas incite à la prudence.

L'impression générale qui se dégage des études de suivi est que les effets généraux aigus des TCDD, même lorsqu'ils sont graves, sont habituellement réversibles, à l'exception de la chloracné, ou s'améliorent peu à peu après l'arrêt de l'exposition. A Seveso, le seul effet nocif sur la santé qui soit indiscutable a été la chloracné: sur les 193 cas qui se sont déclarés en 1976 et 1977, 20 présentaient encore des symptômes actifs en 1984. De nombreuses études ont été consacrées à la recherche de liens possibles entre l'exposition à l'Agent orange, au Viet Nam, et divers effets sur la santé, tant chez les civils que chez les militaires. Cependant, les données dont on dispose à ce jour ne permettent pas de conclure catégoriquement à l'existence d'effets biologiques notables, en particulier sur la reproduction (voir section 9.2).

Dans un certain nombre d'études, on a comparé les populations exposées à divers groupes témoins sur la base du dosage des lipides sériques, d'épreuves de la fonction hépatique et de divers autres paramètres. Bien que dans ces études ainsi que dans des études de cas isolés, on ait signalé des différences statistiquement significatives, il est impossible de formuler des conclusions définitives par suite du manque d'uniformité, de diverses insuffisances sur le plan technique et de l'impossibilité d'exclure les facteurs de confusion.

Lors de la contamination accidentelle survenue en 1971 au Missouri (Etats-Unis d'Amérique), des enfants ont manifesté des signes d'intoxication aiguë mais ils sont aujourd'hui en bonne santé, semble-t-il. Les études épidémiologiques conduites dans le même Etat sur des populations durablement exposées à des concentrations plus faibles n'ont jusqu'ici révélé aucun effet biologique notable. Cependant, malgré l'absence de manifestations cliniques, certains signes témoignent d'une action sur le système immunitaire à médiation cellulaire.

La gamme des effets des TCDD sur la santé humaine reste à préciser. On peut conclure que, dans l'ensemble, les observations concernant l'exposition et les effets sur la santé ne permettent pas d'établir pour l'homme des relations dose/effet ou dose/réponse.

En dépit de nombreuses études cliniques et études de suivi, aucun effet général persistant bien net n'a été observé, à l'exception de la chloracné. Compte tenu de ce qu'on sait actuellement, il semble peu probable que l'exposition aux TCDD ait des séquelles toxicologiques permanentes, graves et invalidantes.

4.2 PCDF

Les seuls cas d'intoxication humaine par les PCDF pour lesquels on dispose d'informations circonstanciées concernent les incidents survenus à Yusho, au Japon (1968) et à Yu-cheng, à Taiwan (1979), à la suite d'une contamination d'huile de riz par des PCDF, des PCD et des PCQ (voir section 11.1). Au total, plusieurs milliers de personnes ont été gravement intoxiquées. La récapitulation des données montre que, selon toute vraisemblance, il faut incriminer les PCDF. La symptomatologie générale était sensiblement la même que lors d'une intoxication par les PCDD. Les différences reflètent peut-être l'intensité de l'exposition et la structure, par âge et sexe, de la population exposée. Dans le cas des malades de Yusho, les estimations de l'apport quotidien moyen de PCDF pendant plusieurs mois ont abouti à une dose de 0,9 µg/kg de poids corporel pour les PCDF totaux, de 0,1-0,2 µg/kg pour les tétrachloro-2,3,7,8 dibenzofurannes ainsi que les penta- et hexaPCDF, à quoi il faut ajouter 150 µg pour les PCB et 148 µg pour les PCQ par kg de poids corporel (Hayabuchi et al., 1979). La dose pathogène minimale a été estimée à 0,6 mg de PCDF totaux par personne sur 30 jours, ce qui correspond à une dose quotidienne de 0,05-0,1 µg/kg de poids corporel pour les PCDF substitués en 2,3,7 et 8. Quoi qu'il en soit, les données disponibles sont insuffisantes pour qu'on puisse se prononcer sur la valeur de la dose qui serait sans danger pour l'homme.

4.3 Charge de l'organisme humain et cinétique

Chez l'homme, la concentration résiduelle des TCDD dans le tissu adipeux s'élève jusqu'à 20 mg/kg dans la population générale, en dehors de toute exposition précise connue, mais elle peut atteindre une valeur plus élevée dans certains cas sans entraîner de manifestations pathologiques. Aucune des populations ainsi étudiées n'avait été constituée par sondage aléatoire. Les autres PCDD et PCDF contenant un plus grand nombre d'atomes de chlore, en particulier les octaDD, se rencontrent également dans ces échantillons (voir tableaux 29, 30). Les concentrations moyennes semblent augmenter avec l'âge.

Dans certaines situations, on a observé des concentrations plus élevées (de l'ordre de quelques microgrammes par kilogramme) qui ne s'accompagnaient d'aucune manifestation pathologique.

Lors des accidents de Yusho et de Yu-cheng, les symptômes observés étaient associés à des concentrations de PCDF plus élevées; par exemple, on a trouvé, un an après exposition à de l'huile de riz contaminée, une concentration de 6,9 µg/kg de tissu adipeux pour les pentachloro-2,3,4,7,8 dibenzofurannes.

D'après les données très limitées dont on dispose, la concentration dans la population générale du 2,3,4,7,8-pentaCDF, par exemple, semble cent fois plus faible que la concentration observée chez les victimes de l'accident de Yusho.

Aucune comparaison de ce type n'est possible pour les PCDD.

Des données limitées montrent que, à l'exception des TCDF, les isomères chlorés en position 2,3,7 et 8 font l'objet d'une rétention sélective.

D'après une étude expérimentale unique, la demi-vie des TCDD serait de 5 ans chez l'homme. Une autre étude a permis d'évaluer cette demi-vie à 2-6 ans pour les 1,2,3,6,7,8-hexaCDD, les 1,2,3,4,6,7,8-heptaCDD, les octaCDD, les 1,2,3,4,6,7,8-heptaCDF et les octaCDF. Ces observations devront être complétées car elles proviennent d'études qui portaient sur deux sujets seulement, sans compter que la toxicinétique de ces types de composés ne se ramène peut-être pas simplement à une cinétique du premier ordre. Cependant, même si les données actuelles ont des limites, il est clair que la demi-vie de ces composés est de l'ordre d'une ou plusieurs années.

Les valeurs indiquées pour la demi-vie sont très différentes chez l'homme et chez les rongeurs. Mais, les expériences conduites sur les animaux ont généralement été exécutées au moyen de doses toxiques. En outre, les animaux qui ont une moindre longévité ont un métabolisme plus important de sorte qu'il est normal que la demi-vie soit plus courte.

Les PCDD et les PCDF sont essentiellement retenus dans les graisses, mais ces produits sont aussi excrétés dans le lait (tableau 39) et traversent la barrière placentaire. On les trouve aussi, à plus faibles concentrations, dans le sang et les organes vitaux. La distribution entre les différents tissus humains est mal connue mais selon certains, le rapport des concentrations dans le tissu adipeux et dans le foie est plus élevé chez l'homme que chez les rongeurs. Cependant, cette conclusion repose sur des données fort restreintes fondées sur des pièces d'autopsie. Il reste donc à voir si elle vaut pour la population dans son ensemble.

Les voies de pénétration dans l'organisme humain sont encore mal connues mais on admet que l'apport alimentaire représente l'essentiel. Cependant, le nourrisson représente un cas particulier puisque, par suite du passage transplacentaire, il peut y avoir une exposition in utero. D'après les dosages effectués jusqu'ici dans le lait maternel, ce dernier pourrait être une source importante de contamination.

Il n'existe aucune donnée concernant la dose des PCDD qui est toxique pour l'homme. Toutefois, lors des accidents de Yusho et de Yu-cheng, les victimes avaient absorbé une dose totale de l'ordre de 3,3-3,8 mg pour les PCDF totaux et de 400-500 µg pour les PCDF substitués en 2,3,7 et 8. Il n'existe aucune donnée fiable sur les doses sans effet nocif.

5. Conclusions générales

Les PCDD et les PCDF se rencontrent dans tout l'environnement et il est probable que chacun en est porteur. Parfois, ces produits déterminent des effets toxiques complexes à la suite d'une activité professionnelle ou accidentelle.

D'après les observations faites à Yusho, les expériences conduites chez des espèces sensibles de singes et compte tenu de certaines hypothèses concernant l'activité relative des PCDD et des PCDF, il se peut que l'homme et certains singes présentent une sensibilité comparable à l'égard de ces composés. Cependant, les incertitudes concernant la dose effectivement reçue et les difficultés de l'évaluation des effets toxiques autres que la chloracné interdisent, dans le cas de l'homme, une conclusion catégorique quant à la résistance relative de l'homme aux effets toxiques de ces composés. Il convient de limiter l'exposition aux plus faibles niveaux compatibles avec les impératifs pratiques.

RECOMMENDATIONS

1. Des études interlaboratoires de validation, selon une sorte de "poule" et l'utilisation de protocoles normalisés de contrôle et d'assurance de qualité, sont indispensables pour améliorer les méthodes d'analyse. La méthodologie de l'échantillonnage, les méthodes d'analyse et l'interprétation des données doivent être optimalisées et normalisées avant le démarrage des enquêtes.

2. Des données complémentaires sont nécessaires sur l'origine des PCDD et des PCDF, sur leur répartition dans l'environnement et sur leur destinée. D'autres observations sont indispensables au sujet de la présence des PCDD ou des PCDF dans l'environnement, notamment sur l'évolution des concentrations dans le temps et sur la détermination des profils isomériques, notamment dans les produits alimentaires, dans l'air ambiant et dans les sédiments.

3. Il serait bon de faire des observations sur les effets qu'exercent les PCDD et les PCDF sur la biocénose.

4. Des données plus complètes sont nécessaires en ce qui concerne la biodisponibilité des PCDD et des PCDF provenant de diverses matrices, dans l'environnement et dans la ration alimentaire. L'exposition à ces sources devrait être mise en corrélation avec les pratiques agricoles et industrielles.

5. Il convient de mettre au point et de valider des méthodes chimiques et biologiques plus simples et moins coûteuses pour rechercher la présence de PCDD et de PCDF.

6. Des études sur les mécanismes toxiques des PCDD et des PCDF sont nécessaires pour élucider les différences observées dans les effets produits chez les diverses espèces et permettre une extrapolation à l'homme.

7. Il importe de poursuivre l'étude de l'immunotoxicité, notamment en ce qui concerne la fonction des lymphocytes T cytotoxiques. En particulier, il est capital d'étudier les effets sur le système immunitaire d'une exposition à la période périnatale et de la durée de cette action.

8. Des études de toxicité à long terme devraient être effectuées, notamment des études de reproduction sur

plusieurs générations chez diverses espèces, au moyen de trois des PCDD et des PCDF les plus répandus, à savoir le 2,3,4,7,8-pentaCDF, le 1,2,3,7,8-pentaCDD et l'octaCDD.

9. Etant donné que l'homme est exposé à des mélanges complexes de PCDD et de PCDF, il faut poursuivre la mise au point et la validation de systèmes d'épreuve, permmettant notamment l'étude des réactions des tissus humains en vue d'apprécier l'activité toxique de ces composés et de leurs mélanges. Ces systèmes permettront d'étudier les mécanismes d'action, les relations structure/activité et les effets interactifs.

10. Il serait bon d'étudier la charge de l'organisme en PCDD et PCDF et d'établir une corrélation entre cette charge, les effets cliniques constatés et les résultats des examens de laboratoire. Le suivi des groupes exposés antérieurement est important à cet égard.